Human Sleep

Research and Clinical Care

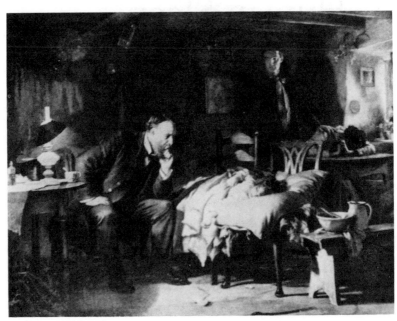

The Doctor, by Luke Fildes, 1891, is a vivid portrayal of a physician studying his sleeping patient.

Human Sleep
Research and Clinical Care

Wallace B. Mendelson, M.D.
Director of Sleep–Wake Study Program
State University of New York at Stony Brook
Stony Brook, New York

PLENUM MEDICAL BOOK COMPANY
NEW YORK AND LONDON

Library of Congress Cataloging in Publication Data

Mendelson, Wallace B.
  Human sleep.

  Includes bibliographies and index.
  1. Sleep disorders. 2. Sleep—Physiological aspects. 3. Hypnotics. I. Title. [DNLM: 1.
Sleep—drug effects. 2. Sleep—physiology. 3. Sleep Disorders. WL 108 M537h]
  RC547.M47   1987   616.8'49   87-7372
  ISBN 0-306-42627-7

First Printing—December 1987
Second Printing—June 1989

The author has written this book as a private individual. The views expressed here
do not necessarily reflect those of the State University of New York.

© 1987 Plenum Publishing Corporation
233 Spring Street, New York, N.Y. 10013

Plenum Medical Book Company is an imprint of Plenum Publishing Corporation

For Nina

Preface

Sleep plays an important role in the history of the neurosciences. On Easter Monday in 1920, Otto Loewi was awakened in the night by a dream in which he conceived of neurotransmitters communicating across the synapse. He quickly made notes, but in the morning he could not understand his scribbles. The following night, the dream came again. He wrote down his thoughts more carefully and, the next day, conducted the crucial experiment that launched modern neurophysiology (Koelle, 1986).

Since the beginning of the modern era of sleep research in the 1950s, we have used the principles of neurotransmission to explore the regulation of sleep. Without resorting excessively to comments on blind men and elephants, however, it is fair to say that the phenomena of sleep and waking can be approached from many perspectives. Among other things, sleep is a process that can be described electrically, an experience that so far defies physiological measurements, and a social behavior. In this book, I have tried to describe the physiology and pharmacology of sleep (Part I) and to relate them to clinical sleep disorders (Part II). Having neither the skill nor the grandiosity of Rousseau, I have made no attempt to write an encyclopedia of all that is known on the subject. Rather, I think of this book as more of a snapshot, giving a picture of where we are, and it is hoped, a history of how we got here.

Renoir, who knew a few things about making pictures, also made a comment that seems relevant to this endeavor. It was his belief that before painting a bowl of flowers, one should arrange them carefully; the next step was to turn them around and paint them from the other side. He meant that sometimes the effort to impose a certain order on observations can cause one to miss the inherent meaning. After some years of observing the processes of sleep, I can understand this. It is a common experience for most of us to think that we have finally found a pleasing pattern in the data; then a new observation is made and we find ourselves looking at it all from a new, unexplained perspective. A number of times in this book we will see how, despite our best efforts, the flowers have managed to rearrange themselves.

One of the special qualities of sleep research is that it covers such a wide range of human experience. Consequently, there is a tremendous amount of anecdotal material available, and one of the hardest parts of writing a textbook is resisting the temptation to include the colorful stories that might appear in my lectures. I have found, for instance, that I never really understood the power of circadian rhythms until a trip to Florida. There I saw fishermen wading in a lake among sedentary alligators, who spend their daytime digesting and resting. In the folk culture of the area, it was known that one may walk among the alligators during the day—but never at night. So, if in the midst of a discussion of sleep apnea I reveal yet another story about a Western gunslinger who was chased by Wild Bill Hickock because he shot a man for snoring too loudly, I hope I will be forgiven.

I am indebted to Miodrag Radulovacki, Laurence S. Jacobs, Dennis L. Murphy, Gary Miller, Phil Skolnick, Judith L. Rapoport, Joseph V. Martin, and Steven P. James for their helpful suggestions on various chapters. I have certainly learned from discussions with Richard R. Bootzin. My wife, Nina Crimm Mendelson, photographed the illustrations of "Flaming June," "The Sentinel," and "The Doctor."

Wallace B. Mendelson

Stony Brook, New York

Contents

II   Pathology of Sleep

Commonly Used Abbreviations

ACTH	Adrenocorticotropic hormone
AMPT	Alpha-methyl-paratyrosine
AOAA	Aminooxyacetic acid
ASDC	Association of Sleep Disorder Centers
AVT	Arginine vasotocin
BZ	Benzodiazepine
cps	Cycles per second (also Hertz or Hz)
DBE	Disordered breathing event
DIMS	Disorder of initiating and maintaining sleep
DOES	Disorder of excessive sleepiness
DSIP	Delta sleep-inducing peptide
DST	Dexamethasone suppression test
EEG	Electroencephalogram
EMG	Electromyogram
EOG	Electrooculogram
FSH	Follicle-stimulating hormone
GABA	Gamma-aminobutryic acid
GH	Growth hormone
5-HTP	5-Hydroxytryptophan
L-DOPA	L-Dihydroxyphenylalanine
LH	Luteinizing hormone
MAO	Monoamine oxidase
MDP	Muramyl dipeptide
MMPI	Minnesota Multiphasic Personality Inventory

MSLT	Multiple sleep latency test
MWT	Maintenance of wakefulness test
NE	Norepinephrine
PB	Pentobarbital
PCPA	Parachlorophenylalanine
PGO	Pontine-geniculate-occipital
PLM	Periodic leg movement
PRC	Phase response curve
PRL	Prolactin
REM	Rapid eye movement
ROE	Range of entrainment
RTSW	Repeated test of sustained wakefulness
SCN	Suprachiasmatic nucleus
TRH	Thyrotropin-stimulating hormone
TSH	Thyroid-stimulating hormone

PART I

Physiology and Pharmacology of Sleep

CHAPTER 1

An Introduction to
Sleep Studies

Although spontaneous electrical discharges in the brains of animals were reported as early as 1875, the first recordings from humans were performed by Hans Berger in 1929. Over the next decade, Berger wrote a remarkable series of papers confirming previous animal studies and showing that the electrical activity was derived from neuronal tissue, that it responded to sensory stimulation, and that abnormal discharges occurred during epileptic seizures (Berger, 1929, 1938). He used the term electroencephalogram (EEG) to refer to his recordings of this electrical activity.

In 1937, Loomis, Harvey, and Hobart described the results of 30 all-night EEG recordings from humans. They discovered that, in terms of EEG observations, sleep is made up of a series of discontinuous stages. Changes between these stages occurred spontaneously, apparently as a result of "internal stimuli." Although the classification has evolved, the principle that sleep is made up of discrete, recurring stages, regulated by neural mechanisms, is basic to much of modern sleep research. These concepts led the way to the discovery some years later of rapid eye movement (REM) sleep.

The formal description of REM sleep was anticipated by clinical observations before the advent of the electroencephalogram. Griesinger in 1868 (and others later) suggested that dreaming is associated with periods of eye movements. Freud (1895) mentioned that the major muscles of the body become very relaxed during dreaming. He speculated that this was a mechanism that prevented one from acting out one's dreams. MacWilliam (1923) distinguished between "undisturbed" and "disturbed" sleep. The latter was associated with increased blood pressure and pulse rate and changes in respiratory rate. In 1953, Aserinsky and Kleitman described periods of sleep characterized by conjugate rapid eye movements. During these periods, the EEG showed an activated pattern consisting of low amplitude waves generally of 15–20 and 5–8 cycles per second (cps). Associated with this sleep stage were increased heartbeat and respiration rates. Aserinsky and Kleitman awakened subjects during this REM sleep and found that about three-fourths of them reported experiencing dreams involving visual imagery. Another small percent reported "the feeling of having dreamed" but could not recall details. When subjects were awakened during sleep that did not contain rapid eye movements (non-REM sleep), only about 9% described dreams and another 9% reported the feeling of having been dreaming.

In the next few years after the description of REM sleep, two findings, in particular, led to a more complete understanding of its physiology. Jouvet and Michel (1959) reported that there was a marked decrease in muscle tone during REM sleep in animals; this was confirmed in humans by Ralph Berger in 1961. The second finding was a report by Dement and Kleitman in 1957 that REM sleep recurred in a cyclic fashion throughout the night, with interspersed periods of non-REM sleep. Each REM–non-REM cycle was thought to last 90–100 min. Dement and Kleitman then proposed a classification system in which REM was differentiated from non-REM sleep, which in turn was divided into four stages. This was the basis of an approach to classification that, with some revisions (Rechtschaffen and Kales, 1968), is still in use. Authors such as Oswald (1962) and Jouvet (1962) began to emphasize the concept that sleep is not a unitary process but rather is composed of REM sleep and non-REM sleep, which differ fundamentally in most physiological parameters. Thus, REM sleep, non-REM sleep, and waking have come to be thought of as the three *states of consciousness*.

An improved understanding of sleep stages comes from studies of various physiological differences between species, changes with age, and effects of sleep deprivation. The results of some of these approaches will be described briefly in this chapter. For further information on the development of sleep research, the reader may wish to see historical reviews written by some of the men who helped create that history (Dement and Mitler, 1974; Bremer, 1974; Jouvet, 1969).

TECHNIQUES OF HUMAN SLEEP STUDIES

Sleep studies on humans are usually performed by using a polygraph to record three types of data: the electroencephalogram (EEG), the electrooculogram (EOG), and the electromyogram (EMG). These measures, described by Rechtschaffen and Kales (1968), may be summarized as follows:

1. EEG. Electrodes (generally concave metallic disks) placed on the scalp are affixed by small gauze patches that have been covered with collodion, a sticky proteinaceous substance. The surface of the electrode that touches the skin has been coated with a jelly that facilitates transmission of electric potentials. The electrode is usually attached to the scalp above the ear, 2 inches below the top of the skull (technically referred to as C_3 or C_4). A second electrode is often placed in the occipital area (O_1 or O_2), where alpha waves are more prominent. This is particularly useful in defining the transition from wakefulness to sleep. Recordings may be made from either the left or right sides, since for these purposes the signals from each of the two homologous areas are generally the same. The polygraph amplifies and traces on paper an electrical signal that represents the difference in voltage between these electrodes and a relatively electrically neutral area (the *reference lead*). The latter lead is usually placed on the earlobe or on the mastoid bone behind the ear (A_1 or A_2). This arrangement is referred to as *unipolar recording*.

2. EOG. Electrodes are attached with plastic tape to the skin beside the outer corners (canthi) of the eyes. The signal that represents the difference between each eye lead and the reference electrode is amplified and traced on paper. When the eyes move conjugately, as if following a moving object, the tracings of the two eye channels appear as mirror images of each other.

3. EMG. Two electrodes are attached beneath the chin and the difference between the potentials of these two electrically active electrodes is amplified and traced on paper (*bipolar recording*). The amplitude (vertical height) of the signal is considered to be proportional to the degree of muscle tone.

POLYSOMNOGRAPHY

In addition to sleep staging, which is derived from the EEG, EOG, and EMG, a substantially more elaborate recording procedure (polysomnography) is generally performed in diagnosing a variety of sleep disorders. Other measures used in polysomnography include:

1. Anterior tibialis EMG. Two electrodes are placed on the leg to detect periodic leg movements, which are characteristic of nocturnal myoclonus (Chapter 11).

2. Nasal and oral air flow. Temperature-sensitive electrodes (thermistors) are placed next to the mouth and nose. Working on the principle that exhaled air is warmer than ambient air, they give a representation of air flow during respiration in sleep. Alternatively, devices measuring expiratory CO_2 may be used. Episodes of decreased air flow (disordered breathing events) are characteristic of sleep apnea syndrome (Chapter 6).

3. Blood oxygen saturation. The oxygen-carrying capacity of the blood is recorded, often from an oximeter that passes a beam of light across the earlobe or fingertip, and senses the light absorption of oxygenated and reduced hemoglobin. The data are recorded in terms of percentage oxygen saturation. Sensors on the skin which measure partial pressures of oxygen are also available.

4. Chest and abdominal movement. Respiratory effort can be measured several different ways. One common technique uses mercury-filled strain gauges in which electrical resistance changes with stretching due to movement of the chest and abdomen. Alternatively, pneumatic and electrical inductance devices may be employed.

5. Electrocardiogram (EKG). An EKG channel is employed to determine heart rate and the possible presence of cardiac arrhythmias. This is particularly important in the study of apneic patients.

STAGES OF SLEEP

Determination of sleep stage is based on the combined information from the EEG, EOG, and EMG. Records are read in *epochs* (usually 20 or 30 sec long); that is, the dominant sleep stage is determined for each sequential 20- or 30-sec period. The most widely accepted criteria for defining the stages are those of Rechtschaffen and Kales (1968), which should be carefully studied by any serious student of the subject. In summary, sleep stages may be defined as follows.

Waking

During relaxed wakefulness (Fig. 1-2), with the eyes closed, the EEG predominantly shows sinusoidal alpha waves (8–14 cps) intermixed with lower amplitude irregular beta waves (15–35 cps). Muscle tone is generally high, and irregular eye movements may be present. As the subject becomes drowsier, alpha activity decreases, and the eyes may roll slowly.

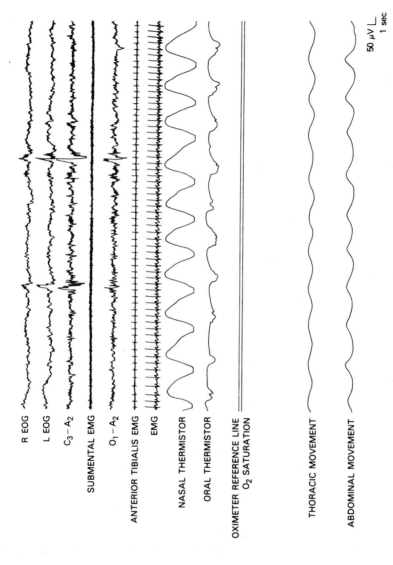

FIGURE 1-1. A normal polysomnogram. EOG, electrooculogram; EMG, electromyogram.

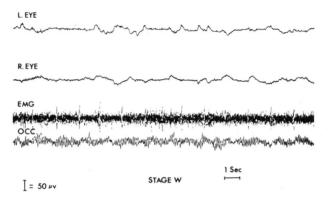

L. EYE

R. EYE

EMG

OCC.

I = 50 μv   STAGE W   1 Sec

FIGURE 1-2. Relaxed wakefulness in a normal young adult male whose eyes are closed. In Fig. 1-2 through 1-6, the following abbreviations are used: L.EYE, electrooculogram (left eye); R.EYE, electrooculogram (right eye); EMG, submental electromyogram; OCC, unipolar electroencephalogram (occipital area).

Non-REM Sleep

Stage 1

Alpha activity in stage 1 (Fig. 1-3) is greatly decreased to less than 50% of the subject's normal recording. A low-amplitude, mixed-frequency signal is primarily made up of beta and the slower theta (4–7 cps) activity. As the subject progresses toward stage 2, the slower activity predominates.

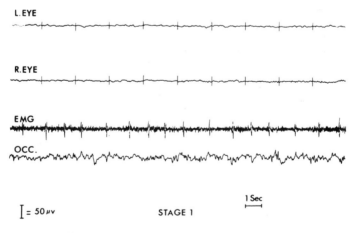

L. EYE

R. EYE

EMG

OCC.

I = 50 μv   STAGE 1   1 Sec

FIGURE 1-3. Polygraphic recording of stage 1 sleep.

Stage 2

This is composed of a largely theta background, and is character-ized by the appearance of two types of intermittent events, spindles and K complexes (Fig. 1-4). A *spindle* is a brief burst of rhythmic 12–14 cps waves, lasting at least 0.5 sec. A *K complex* is a high-amplitude negative wave followed by a positive wave. Sometimes brief bursts of low-amplitude 12–14 cps activity may be superimposed on the K com-plex. It should be noted that, in addition to its spontaneous appearance during stage 2 sleep, the K complex can occur at other times during sleep, as in a response to auditory stimuli.

Stages 3 and 4

These stages are characterized by the appearance of high amplitude (at least 75 μV) and slow (0.5–3 cps) delta waves. Collectively, these stages are often referred to as *slow-wave sleep* or *delta sleep*. When delta activity is between 20 to 50% of the record, stage 3 is scored (Fig. 1-5). In stage 4 (Fig. 1-6), delta activity makes up more than 50% of the ep-och. As we will see in Chapter 9, the amount of power in delta waves is sometimes measured electronically for research purposes. Sleep indles may or may not be present during stages 3 and 4.

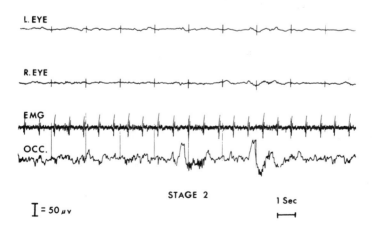

FIGURE 1-4. Polygraphic recording of stage 2 sleep.

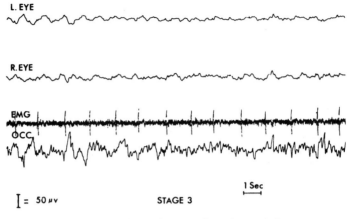

FIGURE 1-5. Polygraphic recording of stage 3 sleep.

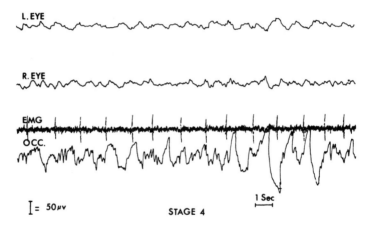

FIGURE 1-6. Polygraphic recording of stage 4 sleep.

REM Sleep

During REM sleep, the EEG returns to a mixed frequency pattern similar to that seen in stage 1. In contrast to stage 2, there are no sleep spindles or K complexes. The EMG drops to very low amplitude, indicating the decrease in tone of the submental muscles. Conjugate rapid eye movements appear. The frequency of eye movements in each epoch of REM sleep (*REM density*) is often calculated. Discontinuous events such as eye movements that occur in REM sleep are known as

phasic events; ongoing processes, such as muscle hypotonia and activated EEG, are *tonic* components.

THE REM–NON-REM CYCLE

Sleep stages do not occur at random but rather appear in cyclic
fashion (Fig. 1-7). In general, a normal young adult goes from waking
into a period of non-REM sleep (stages 1–4) lasting 70 to 90 min before
the first REM period. (The duration of this portion of sleep is referred
to as the *REM latency*, an important measure that may be altered in various conditions including narcolepsy and depression.) In an idealized
situation, the sequence of stages during this period before the first
REM sleep is: waking, stage 1, stage 2, stage 3, stage 4, stage 3, stage
2. At this point, the first REM period occurs, followed by a repetition of
non-REM sleep stages (stage 2, stage 3, stage 4, stage 3, stage 2) and
then another REM sleep period. This interval—from the beginning of
one REM period to the beginning of the next—is the definition of a
sleep cycle employed in this book. It should be noted, however, that it
can also be defined in other ways, such as from the beginning of one
non-REM sleep episode to the next (Feinberg, 1974). The latter method,
though less widely followed, is useful in that it includes an evaluation
of the first episode of slow-wave sleep in calculations involving cyclic
phenomena.

The duration of the REM-to-REM cycle is generally thought to be
about 90 min but may vary from 70 to 120 min. Feinberg (1976) has em-

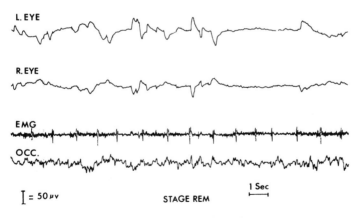

L. EYE

R. EYE

EMG

OCC.

I = 50 μv   STAGE REM   1 Sec

FIGURE 1-7. Polygraphic recording of REM sleep.

phasized that the mean duration of sleep cycles may change during the night curvilinearly, with different patterns of change in different age groups. The content of the sleep cycle changes as the night progresses (Feinberg, 1974). Excluding the first cycle, subsequent cycles show progressively less slow-wave sleep. The amount in the first cycle is age dependent, decreasing as one becomes older. With the exception of the elderly, the REM episode in the first cycle is shorter than those in subsequent cycles, in which it gets progressively longer. As we will see in Chapter 9, this natural progression may also be altered in depression, in which the first REM period may be fairly long. In general, though, slow-wave sleep is greatest early at night and decreases as the night advances; REM sleep is relatively brief early in sleep, and increases later in the night.

SLEEP STAGES AND AGE

As can be seen in Fig. 1-8, total sleep time and total nightly amount of individual sleep stages are age dependent (Feinberg and Carlson, 1968; Roffwarg, Muzio, and Dement, 1966; Kupfer and Reynolds, 1983). In general, total sleep time is greatest in infancy and decreases in childhood. It remains relatively stable starting in the young adult years until old age, when it declines. The amount of waking time after sleep onset also increases across the lifetime. Thomas Jefferson vividly described some of these qualities of the sleep of the elderly in this letter written when he was 76:

> I am not so regular in my sleep as the doctor (referring to Dr. Benjamin Rush), devoting to it from five to eight hours, according to my company or

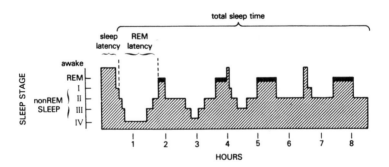

FIGURE 1-8. Graph of an idealized sequence of sleep stages in a normal young adult.

the book I am reading interests me; and I never go to bed without an hour, or half hour's previous reading of something moral, wherein to ruminate in the intervals of sleep. But whether I retire to bed early or late, I rise with the sun.

Letter to Dr. Vine Utley, 1819

The proportion of the various sleep stages also changes across one's lifetime. Percentage REM sleep is highest in infancy and childhood, drops and then levels off in adulthood, and declines in old age. Stage 4 sleep is highest in infancy and may be thought of as following a hyperbolic curve that decreases with age. Typical values for the whole night in a young adult might be as follows: 50% stage 2, 25% REM, 10% stage 3, 10% stage 4, and 5% stage 1.

Other changes in the sleep EEG occur across the lifetime. The amplitude of delta waves declines in old age (Feinberg, 1974; Blois *et al.*, 1983), and the relation of amplitude and frequency of EEG waves changes. In general, the two are inversely related; that is, waves of lower frequency have higher amplitudes. There is some evidence that in the non-REM sleep EEG of the elderly this relationship is diminished (Feinberg *et al.*, 1984). In terms of the two-process model of sleep regulation (to be discussed later in this chapter), the elderly may also display a reduced decay rate of process S (see p. 282) (Borbely, 1987).

EFFECTS OF TEMPORAL VARIABLES ON SLEEP

The duration of wakefulness before sleep is inversely related to the time it takes to fall alseep (*sleep latency*). Although it makes sense that the longer a person has been awake, the more quickly he falls alseep, it is perhaps surprising that sleep latency is strongly influenced by the time of day sleep occurs (Webb and Agnew, 1975). It is easier to fall asleep at midnight than at 4:00 PM, even when the length of prior wakefulness is held constant. Influences of the time of the 24-hr day on sleep are the topic of Chapter 10.

The length of wakefulness before sleep is directly related to the total amount of delta sleep (Webb and Agnew, 1971). There is some evidence that during prolonged periods of sleep in normal conditions (Gagnon and de Koninck, 1984), or temporal isolation (Weitzman *et al.*, 1980), delta sleep may reappear after 12 hr or so. Although other explanations are available, this raises the possibility that it, like many aspects of sleep, is also influenced by rhythmic processes.

REM sleep, in contrast to delta sleep, is much more clearly influenced by time of day than by the length of the prior wakefulness. It occurs more frequently during the morning hours than the afternoon

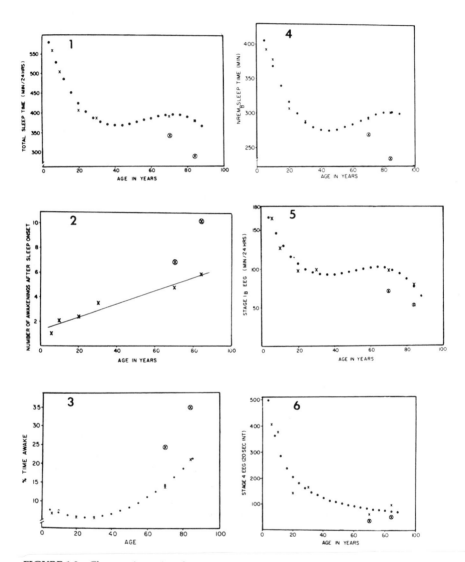

FIGURE 1-9. Changes in major sleep parameters with age. (From Feinberg *et al.*, 1968. Reprinted by permission.)

and evening, and this effect is relatively independent of the length of wakefulness before sleep and the amount of prior sleep (Weitzman *et al.*, 1970, 1974; Carskadon and Dement, 1975; Taub and Berger, 1973; Hume and Mills, 1975). Thus, naps in the afternoon have more delta sleep than naps in the morning because of the increased period of wakefulness since arising in the morning. Furthermore, following an afternoon nap, delta sleep is reduced during nocturnal sleep for similar reasons.

In summary, temporal variables—age, length of time asleep, length of wakefulness before the sleep period, and time of the 24-hr day at which sleep occurs—are important determinants of sleep characteristics. The underlying physiological and biochemical mechanisms for some of these temporal effects are discussed in Chapter 10.

PHYSIOLOGICAL VARIABLES IN SLEEP STAGES

In addition to the physiological changes that largely define REM sleep, such as decreased muscle tone, a variety of metabolic and autonomic nervous system changes occur (Berger, 1969). During REM sleep there is increased cerebral blood flow (Reivich *et al.*, 1968), brain temperature (Kawamura and Sawyer, 1965), and oxygen consumption (Brebbia and Altshuler, 1965). Erections may occur in the male during REM sleep, an observation used clinically in studying nocturnal penile tumesence (NPT) to evaluate impotence (Wasserman *et al.*, 1980). It will be recalled from the earlier historical review that periodic increases in blood pressure and pulse and respiration rate during sleep were noted even before the use of the EEG (MacWilliam, 1923). Subsequent polygraphic studies found increased variability of these measures during REM sleep (Snyder *et al.*, 1964). Indeed, later studies of REM sleep have shown loss of temperature regulation (Parmeggiani, 1980) and complex changes in cardiovascular (Mancia and Zanchetti, 1980) and respiratory (Sullivan, 1980) activity. This apparent autonomic dysregulation is the reason that in sleep apnea syndromes the apneas of REM sleep are often the most severe (Chapter 6).

SLEEP DEPRIVATION

A classic technique for determining the function of a physiological process has been to remove it, or to prevent it from occurring, and see what happens. Sleep deprivation studies, however, have been less revealing of the functions of sleep. Investigators have performed three different types of sleep deprivation studies: total sleep deprivation, selective sleep stage deprivation, and partial sleep deprivation.

Total Sleep Deprivation

Animal studies indicate that sleep deprivation for up to 33 days results in severe pathology or death (Rechtschaffen *et al.*, 1983). In humans, total sleep deprivation of 150–200 hr has been associated with the occurrence of brief psychotic episodes in some subjects but apparently does not result in long-term psychological effects (Pasnau, Naitoh, and Kollar, 1968; Gulevich, Dement, and Johnson, 1966). Lindbergh had such an experience during his Atlantic crossing. He described "the only occasion in my life when I saw and conversed with ghosts. . . . I can still see those phantoms clearly in memory, but after I landed at Paris I could not remember a single word they said" (Gill, 1977). Such observations have led some authors to speculate that sleep deprivation psychosis might be an aid in understanding schizophrenia (Luby and Gottlieb, 1966). It has become apparent, however, that florid psychotic states following sleep deprivation occur in only a very small number of cases. Tyler (1955), for instance, found such changes in only 7 of 350 subjects kept awake for 112 hr. They are very infrequent in persons who have been sleep deprived for less than 100 hr (Johnson, 1969).

Changes in mood and performance, in contrast to obvious psychotic states, do occur fairly consistently in persons undergoing prolonged sleep deprivation. Fatigue, irritability, feelings of persecution, and episodes of misinterpretation of stimuli have been reported (Johnson, 1969). Morris and Singer (1961), using projective tests on subjects kept awake for 72–98 hr, emphasized that various disturbances in perception, orientation, and attentiveness were functions of the previous personality of the subject. Williams, Lubin, and Goodnow (1959) concluded that the unevenness of test results in sleep-deprived subjects was primarily the result of a defect in attentiveness.

EEG studies of sleep-deprived subjects show lower amounts of alpha activity, which has been interpreted by various authors as demonstrating increased or decreased activation (Johnson, Slye, and Dement, 1965). During periods of decreased alpha activity, tracking performance may be poorer and subjective ratings of feeling and effort may deteriorate (Naitoh *et al.*, 1969). In the recovery sleep after extremely long periods of sleep deprivation, stage 4 and REM sleep increase above baseline values (Kales *et al.*, 1970).

In contrast to the extremely long deprivation periods described above, most persons have experienced the uncomfortable feelings that occur after one or two nights of sleep loss. Although complaints of irritability, fatigue, poor concentration, and feelings of depersonalization are commonly made, objective psychological testing has been less consistent in showing changes in mood. Roth *et al.* (1974) deprived 11 normal males of one night's sleep and found that tests showed higher scores on "sleepiness," "friendliness," and "aggression." After 24 hr of deprivation, there may be decreased "vigor" and increased "fatigue" and "confusion" (Hartmann, Orzack, and Branconnier, 1974b). Performance on a variety of psychological tests may be impaired; it has been suggested that this is the result of periodic lapses, in which the encoding of data into short-term memory is decreased (Polzella, 1975). Whether a person remains inactive or exercises periodically during two nights of sleep deprivation seems to make little difference on performance scores (Webb and Agnew, 1973).

Sleep deprivation may lead to transient neurological symptoms. Sassin (1970) found that subjects deprived of sleep for 6 hr developed weakness of neck flexion, hand tremors, horizontal nystagmus, and other signs. Gunderson, Dunne, and Feyer (1973) described seizures in nonepileptic soldiers who had been continuously awake for at least 24 hr while traveling. In patients with a known seizure disorder, EEG recordings obtained during sleep may accentuate epileptic discharges that are otherwise poorly seen. This effect may be enhanced even more by obtaining sleep recordings following a full day and night of wakefulness (Scollo-Lavizzari, Pralle, and de la Cruz, 1975).

Total sleep deprivation may also potentially benefit patients with depression. A review of the literature found that 852 patients have been treated with sleep deprivation, with improvement in 57.9% (Gillin, 1983). These studies will be discussed in detail in Chapter 9.

Selective Sleep Stage Deprivation

If subjects are deprived of a sleep stage, an excessive amount of that stage will occur during recovery sleep. This is referred to as the *rebound phenomenon* and may be seen following either REM (Clemes and Dement, 1967; Dement, Greenberg, and Klein, 1966a) or stage 4 (Agnew, Webb, and Williams, 1964) deprivation. Decreased REM or stage 4 sleep can be produced by mechanically arousing a subject whenever the polygraph indicates that the subject is entering that stage. When subjects are deprived of REM sleep in this manner of several nights, it is found that they must be aroused progressively more and more often. This is considered to be a manifestation of an increase in hypothetical *REM pressure*. Another method of producing decreased REM sleep is to administer a variety of drugs including alcohol, many hypnotics, stimulants, and antidepressants (Chapter 2). When such drugs are discontinued, a REM sleep rebound usually occurs. This was originally thought to be the cause of subjectively disturbed sleep during withdrawal; subsequent studies have shown disturbed sleep during withdrawal without REM rebound in some situations, suggesting the presence of a more complex mechanism (Chapter 8). Decreased REM sleep may also be produced by causing a subject to sleep for a fewer number of hours (partial sleep deprivation), since most REM sleep occurs in the later hours of sleep.

REM sleep deprivation studies have been reviewed by Ellman *et al.* (1978). Animal studies indicate that REM deprivation increases cortical excitability (Owen and Bliss, 1970; Cohen, Thomas, and Dement, 1970), alters food consumption (Elomaa and Johansson, 1980), and may increase stimulus-evoked aggressive (Morden *et al.*, 1968) and sexual (Dement, 1965) behavior. REM sleep deprivation has been reported to impair memory of past events and acquisition of new data (Stern, 1970; Harris, Overstreet, and Orbach, 1982; Dushenko and Sterman, 1984) and to alter monoamine metabolism (Semba, 1983) and behavioral responses to catecholaminergic and serotonergic agonists (Mogilnicka, 1981; Tufik, 1981).

In 1963, Dement and Fisher described psychological difficulties in 21 subjects who were REM sleep deprived for two to seven nights. Later, Dement (1964) reported even more dramatic disturbances in two subjects who were REM sleep deprived for 15 and 16 nights by a combination of awakenings and amphetamine administration. Different studies have failed to confirm these findings (Kales *et al.*, 1964; Snyder, 1963; Foulkes *et al.*, 1968), and it now seems unlikely that REM sleep deprivation has serious psychological consequences. On the contrary, some studies suggest that REM deprivation may, in fact, be beneficial in certain situations, such as treating depression (Chapter 9).

NATURAL LONG, SHORT, AND VARIABLE SLEEPERS

Sleep deprivation studies demonstrate the great difficulty encountered by most people who are denied more than a few hours of sleep in a 24-hr period. Some people, however, normally sleep very little without difficulty. Napoleon, Thomas Edison, and Chou En-lai were all said to have required little sleep. Meddis *et al.* (1973) studied a 70-year-old woman who claimed to have slept for only 1 hr a night for many years. She seemed puzzled why other people slept for long periods and "wasted so much time." During a 5-day study period in the laboratory, she averaged 67 min of sleep within a 24-hr period without any indication that she felt fatigued. Her sleep consisted of 16.5% REM sleep, 9.3% stage 4, 23.3% stage 3, and 50.9% stage 2. Similarly, Jones and Oswald (1968) studied two unusually short sleepers, men who had slept about 2¾ hr a day for many years. When studied in the laboratory, both men showed high proportions of delta sleep and REM sleep, as well as short REM latencies. Such natural short sleepers should be distinguished from chronic insomniacs, who often have relatively little deficit in total sleep time, but who feel substantial daytime distress at having poor quality sleep (Chapter 12).

There are also natural long sleepers. Albert Einstein was said to have slept a great deal. Little is known about why one person sleeps a long time, whereas another sleeps a little. Laboratory studies indicate that natural long and short sleepers have equal amounts of delta sleep, but that long sleepers have much more REM sleep than short sleepers (Webb and Agnew, 1970; Webb and Friel, 1971; Hartmann, Chung, and Chien, 1971). Using a variety of scholastic, personality, and medical measures, Webb and his associates found no revealing differences between their natural long sleepers (greater than 9½ hr sleep a day) and their short sleepers (less than 5½ hr sleep a day). Hartmann, Baekeland, and Zwilling (1972), however, described their short sleepers (defined by less than 6 hr of sleep a day) to be more efficient, hardworking, conformist, and less creative than long sleepers (defined by more than 9 hr). Hartmann's subjects were older and more set in their sleep habits than Webb's subjects; also, they were obtained by newspaper advertisements rather than by population surveys. Hartmann (1973) also described a group of people he called variable sleepers, who needed more sleep at times of stress, worry, depression, and increased mental activity and who needed less sleep at times when everything was going well.

In summary, people differ in their subjective sleep requirements, but it is not known why. Questions such as "How much sleep should I get?" cannot be answered by referring to tables, as in looking up an ideal body weight for a given height. Each person seems to have his or her own requirement for sleep. In terms of factors known to determine human sleep characristics, age, sex, and temporal variables are important, as are individual differences. Theories on the function and regulation of sleep must ultimately account for these known variables.

REGULATION OF SLEEP

Passive versus Active Regulation

As early as the last quarter of the nineteenth century, there began to be interest in the possibility that areas of the brain stem are concerned with the regulation of sleep and wakefulness. After the worldwide epidemic of viral encephalitis in the 1920s, von Economo (1929) described two syndromes—one of excessive sleep and the other of sleeplessness—and attributed them to lesions of the mesencephalic tegmentum and posterior hypothalamus, and of the basal forebrain and striate structures, respectively. In 1935, Bremer reported that if the midbrain of a cat is severed at the intercollicular level below the nucleus of the third cranial nerve, the animal appears to be sleeping, has the high-amplitude slow EEG waves characteristic of sleep, and cannot be aroused by ordinary sensory stimulation (Bremer, 1974; Brazier, 1973). This type of preparation (*cerveau isolé*) in effect, separates the cerebrum from the rest of the brain. A lower section at the first cervical segment of the spinal cord (*encephale isolé*) allows the animal to retain behavioral and EEG signs of wakefulness. Bremer and others writing in this period believed that the sleep of the *cerveau isolé* cat resulted from a lack of adequate sensory stimulation, which they felt was necessary to maintain wakefulness. Sleep was thus considered to be a passive phenomenon. Although sleep might be regulated by specific neuroanatomical loci, it was thought to be primarily a resting state entered by the brain when there was inadequate stimulation from a number of specific sensory modalities.

One of the major advances in understanding sleep came with the discovery by Moruzzi and Magoun (1949) of the reticular activating system, an anatomically diffuse network running throughout the brain stem. Histologically, this system is characterized by cellular polymorphism, dendrites lacking regional characteristics, and other features (Morgane and Stern, 1974). Electrical stimulation of the reticular activating system by a current with a frequency of 100–300 cps was found to arouse sleeping animals. It was thought that stimulation of this diffuse system (rather than of specific sensory tracts) led to arousal; when the reticular activating system was not actively stimulating the cerebrum, mechanisms in the thalamus and lower pons tended to synchronize the firing of cortical neurons, resulting in the slow waves seen in sleep. This, too, is basically a passive concept of sleep.

Several types of studies, outlined by Jouvet (1969), brought this passive view of sleep into question. First, it was shown that electrical stimulation of various areas of the brain could produce sleep (Hess, 1929, 1944; see also Parmeggiani, 1964). These studies argued against sleep being a passive process; rather, it appeared that some types of stimulation result in sleep. There were many difficulties, however. Only certain low frequencies were effective, and formal analyses demonstrating that the appearance of sleep was statistically significant (rather than having occurred randomly) were often lacking. A second support for an active view of sleep came from studies demonstrating that lesions in the midpons greatly decreased sleep (Batini *et al.*, 1958, 1959). Although this region was poorly localized, it seemed likely that brain loci that could actively inhibit the reticular activating system existed. Perhaps the final, strongest support for an active view of sleep was the discovery of REM sleep, which was discussed earlier (Aserinsky and Kleitman, 1953). It became clear that sleep was not a unitary phenomenon but rather that it was composed of at least two distinct states: REM and non-REM sleep. Thus, there appeared to be mechanisms not only for changing from sleep to wakefulness, but also between different types of sleep.

As Jouvet (1969) pointed out, while sleep was viewed as a passive phenomenon, its regulation could be thought of in terms of "dry" neurophysiology, a concept of F.O. Schmidt (1962) (dry referred to those aspects of neurophysiology that are essentially electrical). Hence, in the passive concept of sleep, decreased activity of the reticular activating system was considered to be the result of such phenomena as decreased afferent input and neuronal fatigue. With the active concept of sleep, many phenomena were observed that were difficult to explain in terms of this dry neurophysiology. First, the circadian and ultradian rhythms of the sleep stages, and the REM rebound phenomenon that may occur over many days, run very different time courses than electrical potentials of the brain, which are measured in milliseconds. It seemed more likely that issues of regulation of these phenomena could be resolved in the realm of "wet" neurophysiology (the study of neurohumors). As it turned out, this approach was very fruitful.

Neurotransmitters

Pharmacological and Anatomical Approaches

Two types of studies yielded valuable information on the possible role of neurotransmitters in the regulation of sleep. The first involved infusions into animals of acetylcholine, the catecholamines norepinephrine and dopamine, and the indoleamine serotonin. Such studies were often done in young birds because their blood–brain barrier is permeable to these substances (e.g., see Spooner and Winters, 1965). Alternatively, precursors of these substances, which can enter the mammalian brain, have been used in a variety of animals and humans. Such studies showed that these compounds, which presumably transmit impulses between neurons, are profoundly involved in the regulation of sleep. This pharmacological approach is the basis of much of the work to be described here.

The second type of study employing a biochemical approach to neurochemical control mechanisms resulted from the discovery that certain monoamines, when exposed to formaldehyde vapor, produced compounds that fluoresce (Falck *et al.*, 1962). Before the development of a technique based on this observation, the diffuse, polymorphous nature of the reticular formation had made identification of neuroanatomical pathways difficult. By using histofluorescence, it became possible to identify cellular pathways on the basis of their neurotransmitters. It was found that serotonin-containing neurons are located largely in the *raphe nuclei* in the lower midbrain and upper pons. Noradrenergic neurons are found throughout the brain stem reticular formation, with highest concentration in the *locus ceruleus* in the pons (Ungerstedt, 1971).

Studies of the cholinergic system have not had the benefit of histological techniques as effective as those for monoamines (Morgane and Stern, 1974; Morgane, 1982). At present, the relatively diffuse cholinergic tracts are identified indirectly by testing for the presence of the enzyme acetylcholinesterase. Shute and Lewis (1967) suggest that these tracts fall into two general pathways. The *dorsal tegmental pathway* is centered in the nucleus cuneiformis of the midbrain tegmentum but also includes nuclear areas extending into the pons. Fibers from these tracts go to many areas, but ascending fibers are known to travel to the nonspecific nuclei and nucleus reticularis of the thalamus. The *ventral tegmental pathway* is centered in parts of the substantia nigra and ventral tegmental area of Tsai in the anterior midbrain. Ascending fibers go to lateral nuclei of the hypothalamus, the striatum, septal nuclei, and the hippocampus. As will be discussed later, there has been particular interest in the cholinergic cells of the gigantocellular tegmental field (FTG) of the pontine reticular formation, which have been postulated to play a role in REM sleep generation (Hobson, McCarley, and Wuzinski, 1975).

Neurotransmitters and Sleep

Once some sense of localization of neurons using these transmitters was obtained, it became possible to test the effects of lesions in these areas. It was found that damage to 80–90% of the raphe nuclei, for instance, acutely produced total lack of sleep. With somewhat smaller lesions, slow-wave sleep appeared; with lesions that allowed a minimal amount of slow-wave sleep to occur, REM sleep also appeared (Jouvet and Renault, 1966). Analysis of the tissue after such lesions revealed a decrease in cerebral serotonin, with no change in norepinephrine. Conversely, lesions of the locus ceruleus produced decreased REM sleep, with depletion of norepinephrine in the rostral part of the brain (Jouvet and Delorme, 1965). Studies such as these brought morphological, biochemical, and electrophysiological data together and aided in formulating hypotheses on the control of sleep. Jouvet (1972) combined these lines of evidence to suggest a control mechanism as follows: The caudal two-thirds of the locus ceruleus are responsible for inhibition of muscle tone during REM sleep. The medial one-third of the locus ceruleus deals with such *tonic* aspects of REM as cortical activation and such *phasic* events as eye movements and pontine-geniculate–occipital (PGO) spiking. Serotonergic neurons of the anterior part of the raphe system are related to behavioral and EEG aspects of slow-wave sleep. Fibers from the caudal raphe travel to the area of the locus ceruleus. Activity of such fibers both "primes" the initiation of REM sleep and inhibits the appearance of PGO spikes. An inhibitory pathway from the locus ceruleus, however, decreases firing in the raphe and allows PGO spikes to occur during REM sleep. In summary, Jouvet suggested that serotonergic activity may be related to the maintenance of slow-wave sleep and the priming of REM sleep. In this view, adrenergic activity may be related to both tonic and phasic aspects of REM sleep.

A number of studies suggested that the Jouvet (1972) model would have to be modified. Animals with lesions of the raphe system or whose serotonin concentrations were depleted pharmacologically by para-chlorophenylalanine (PCPA) eventually resumed normal amounts of sleep (e.g., see Dement et al., 1969; Morgane and Stern, 1972). Adrien (1978) found that after lesions of the raphe nuclei in young rats and cats, the animals grew up to have normal amounts of sleep. Rechtschaffen et al. (1969) reported that after depletion of serotonin by PCPA in rats, reductions in sleep were smaller than had previously been reported. Similarly, after lesions of the locus ceruleus, normal amounts of wakefulness reappeared after two days, and REM sleep returned to normal within two weeks (Jones, Harper, and Halaris, 1977). Tobler and Borbely (1982) demonstrated that following pretreatment with PCPA, normal sleep regulatory mechanisms continued to function in response to sleep deprivation (see Chapter 2). Drucker-Colin and Bernal-Pedraza (1983) found that following kainic acid lesions of the

FTG cholinergic neurons of cats, amounts of REM sleep returned to normal (Fig. 1-10). It became clear, then, that although these monoaminergic and cholinergic centers have some role in sleep regulation, the nature of this relationship is much more complex than was originally supposed.

One major contribution to understanding the role of monoaminergic activity in sleep regulation comes from electrophysiological studies of single cell firing patterns. From such studies, which have been reviewed in detail by Jacobs (1985), some patterns have emerged. Serotonergic, noradrenergic, and dopaminergic cells are autoactive; that is, they have a slow spontaneous firing rate during quiet wakefulness. In general, serotonergic neurons of the raphe nuclei and noradrenergic cells of the locus ceruleus fire most rapidly during waking and their activity progressively decreases in non-REM and REM sleep. In contrast, dopaminergic cells of the ventral mesencephalon have fairly stable rates across the states of consciousness. All these groups are sensitive to external stimuli, responding first with initial excitation followed by decreased firing. The response of noradrenergic neurons may habituate, however, whereas serotonergic neurons do not. All three groups are very sensitive to their own neurotransmitter. Both serotonergic and noradrenergic neurons project widely through-

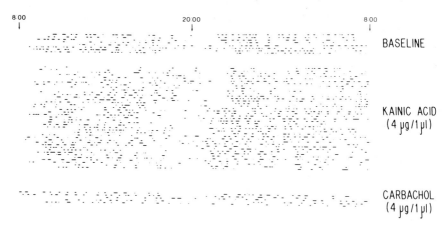

FIGURE 1-10. Frequency of REM sleep periods throughout 24-hr recording sessions in cats studied by Drucker-Colin and Bernal-Pedraza (1983). The kainic acid section represents the distribution of REM throughout the eight weeks after its administration (one recording/week). No changes in REM sleep distribution occurred following either kainic acid or carbachol administration. (From Drucker-Colin and Bernal-Pedraza, 1983. Reprinted by permission.)

out the nervous system, with overlapping though not identical projections; pathways of dopaminergic cells are more discrete. One implication may be that serotonergic and noradrenergic systems are involved in coordinating a wide variety of nervous system functions.

Since the original concepts of the role of the raphe nuclei and the locus ceruleus were formulated, there has been growing speculation that sleep regulation may be more diffusely controlled. We have already mentioned some evidence for this view; that is, lesions of these areas may induce transient changes in sleep, which eventually returns to normal. Similarly, metabolic mapping of monkey brains, using the 2-deoxyglucose technique (thought to reflect neuronal activity), showed relatively uniform decreases in glucose consumption when the animals went from waking to non-REM sleep, with no evidence of discrete changes in areas thought to be involved in sleep regulation (Nakamura et al., 1983). One major reinterpretation was offered by McGinty (1985) who suggested that these observed sleep phenomena result from complex interactions in the pontine and bulbar reticular formation involving mechanisms controlling sleep and other physiological processes (Fig. 1-11). It has been observed, for instance, that increased reticular formation neuron firing facilitates breathing and that, in turn, blood gas concentrations affect sleep. Such interactions may very well exist with other processes, including hormone secretion (see Chapter 5), cerebral blood flow, and blood pressure control. It is possible, then, that nuclei traditionally thought to be sleep centers may be loci mediating these complex interactions. Moreover, it has been hypothesized that the cyclic aspects of sleep may result from inherent rhythmic processes found in many cells. Llinas and Jahnsen (1982), for instance, found, in a brain slice preparation of thalamic cells, that there are two distinct firing patterns that may correspond to non-REM sleep (burst–pause) and waking (regular) activity (Fig. 1-12). If indeed the basic rhythmicity of a widespead network of neurons accounts for many sleep phenomena, then it would be reasonable to expect little lasting effect from lesions in discrete areas of the brain stem.

Models of Sleep Regulation

Not surprisingly, the number of models of sleep regulation grew side-by-side with the observations described above. In 1975, Hobson and colleagues presented the *reciprocal interaction model*. As originally described (Hobson, McCarley, and Wyzinski, 1975), the predominantly noradrenergic cells of the locus ceruleus fire more slowly in REM sleep compared with non-REM (''REM-off'' cells). In contrast, predomi-

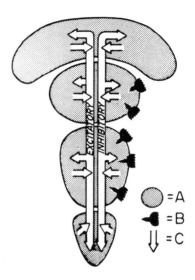

FIGURE 1-11. Scheme of the neural control of sleep without "sleep centers," as suggested by McGinty (1985). The fundamental capacity for cyclic quiescent and waking states may reside in individual cells at all levels of the neuraxis (A). These "oscillators" are synchronized by such diffuse interconnecting systems as the reticular formation (C). Many quantitative and temporal features of sleep state patterns may reflect the impact of physiological signals acting through specialized receptors and control systems, to modulate the multioscillator network (B). (From McGinty, 1985. Reprinted by permission.)

nantly cholinergic cells of the pontine FTG field fire more rapidly during the initiation of REM sleep ("REM-on" cells). The REM-off cells were thought to inhibit the REM-on cells and also to have a negative feedback; REM-on cells were thought to have feedforward and feedback excitation properties (Fig. 1-13). Thus, as an organism approaches REM sleep, REM-on cells become much more active as they are released from REM-off cell inhibition, whereas in the transition back to non-REM sleep, the REM-on cells once again reduce firing as REM-off cellular activity increases. In subsequent years, several reports appeared to question various aspects of the model (Mendelson, 1986e). They included observations that FTG firing is as great during certain movements in wakefulness as in REM (Siegel and McGinty, 1977) and that kainic acid lesions of the FTG cells do not abolish REM sleep (Sastre, Sakai, and Jouvet, 1981; Drucker-Colin and Bernal-Pedraza, 1983). In response to these and other findings, the model was revised (Hobson, Lydic, and Baghdoyan, 1986) to suggest that the REM-on and REM-off cells were not found in discrete nuclei but rather in wide-

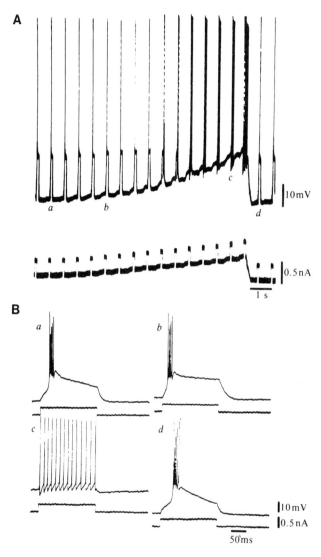

FIGURE 1-12. Voltage-dependent, burst-to-tonic switching of thalamic cell activity. A, response of a thalamic cell after short current pulses delivered from a slowly rising ramp depolarization pulse. The cell switched abruptly from a burst response to tonic firing as the DC potential decreased by about 10 mV from the initial value; B, records obtained at a higher sweep speed at the times indicated by *a* to *d* in A. Note the transition from burst response (*a* and *b*) to tonic response (*c*), followed by the abrupt return to a burst response (*d*). (From Llinas and Jahnsen, 1982. Reprinted by permission.)

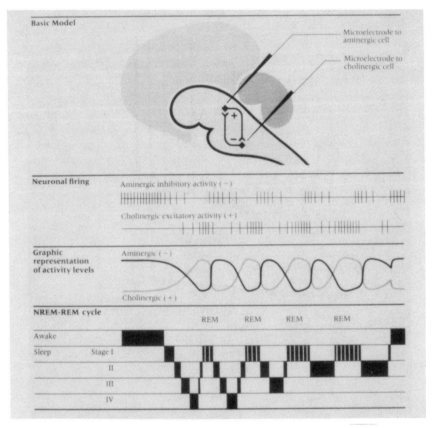

FIGURE 1-13. The reciprocal interaction model. (From Hobson, 1983. Reprinted by permission.)

ranging, interpenetrating fields. Serotonergic cells, with greatest density in the raphe nuclei, were also included among the REM-off cells. The model also evolved to include all three states of consciousness: waking, non-REM sleep, and REM sleep. Certainly one of its strengths is that it may be applied to clinical conditions, including depression (Chapter 9). Among its present limitations are that it does not seem to explain some observations, such as the acute lack of sleep after administration of the serotonin-depleting drug parachlorophenylalanine (Delorme, 1966) or following lesions of the raphe nuclei (Jouvet et al., 1966; Kostowski et al., 1968). In the context of the model, these manipulations might have been expected to increase sleep time. Similarly, it is hard to explain, in the context of the model, how the serotonin precursor L-tryptophan or the tricyclic antidepressants (which block re-uptake of amines) induce sleep (see Chapter 2). Nonetheless, the reciprocal interaction model does indeed fit well with many observed phenomena, as well as with other theories of sleep regulation.

A number of other models, which are not necessarily mutually exclusive, have also appeared. Two major views regard sleep regulation in the context of general body rhythms. Wever (1975) and Kronauer *et al.* (1982) presented a *two-oscillator model*, in which cyclic processes are regulated by a dominant pacemaker that controls body temperature, cortisol secretion, and REM sleep and a weaker pacemaker that affects sleep versus waking. Borbely (1982) presented the *two-process model*, which suggests that sleep results from the interaction of two regulatory mechanisms. One, a homeostatic princple referred to as process S, operates during wakefulness and dissipates during sleep. In contrast, process C is a circadian principle. These processes are discussed in detail in Chapter 10 and their implications for sleep in depression are presented in Chapter 9.

Circulating Humors and Sleep

Although the study of the monoamines has been fruitful, only a small fraction of neurons are monoaminergic. This and the general impression that monoaminergic neuron function may be necessary but perhaps not sufficient to explain sleep regulation (Morgane, 1982) led to investigations in other areas. There are, of course, a variety of other neurotransmitters, such as GABA and adenosine, and their possible role in sleep has also been examined (Chapter 2). The search for circulating substances (hypnotoxins) responsible for the regulation of sleep has also been emphasized. The first modern report of a possible hypnotoxin comes from Legendre and Pieron (1910), who found that a circulating substance from sleep-deprived dogs could induce sleep when injected into naive animals. Subsequently, a number of possible endogenous substances thought to have a role in sleep have been identified, including delta sleep-inducing peptide (DSIP), a muramyl dipeptide (MDP), sleep-promoting substance (SPS), arginine vasotocin (AVT), and an adrenal corticosteroid, 3-alpha, 5-alpha tetrahydrodroxycorticosterone. It is fair to say that although several of these substances have been shown to be present in mammals, and to influence sleep when administered, none have yet been convincingly shown to play a role in physiological sleep regulation. The importance of such circulating substances has also been questioned by studies of Siamese twins (Lenard and Schulte, 1972) and of dogs with both natural and surgically attached heads (Des Andres *et al.*, 1976). In both cases, although their circulations were interconnected, their patterns of sleep were relatively independent. A detailed discussion of several possible hypnotoxins will be found in Chapter 2.

Some hormones may influence sleep, as manifested either in patients with diseases of oversecretion (e.g., hyperthyroidism) or in studies involving exogenous hormone administration. The best evidence is that the release of several anterior pituitary hormones, including growth hormone, adrenocorticotropic hormone, and thyroid-stimulating hormone, is influenced by sleep and that, in turn, they may alter sleep (Chapter 5).

HYPNOTICS

As long as sleep was viewed as a passive process, it was simpler to speculate that hypnotics induced sleep by suppressing various CNS functions. As sleep came to be seen as an active, multifaceted process, it became harder to conceive how it might be induced by drugs. Work in this area has also been complicated by the recognition that a wide variety of pharmacological classes of compounds (e.g., barbiturates, benzodiazepines, chloral hydrate derivatives) may all induce or increase sleep. The multiplicity of endogenous and artificial substances that alter sleep points to an important characteristic of sleep regulation: that it is diffuse and involves feedback relationships with neurons employing many neurotransmitters in a variety of physiological systems. It has been known for some time that hypnotics alter the function of many of the transmitters thought to be involved in sleep regulation (Mendelson, 1980). Barbiturates, for instance, may inhibit release of acetylcholine (Carmichael and Israel, 1975; Crossland and Slater, 1968) and facilitate some effects of GABA (Nicoll, 1975a,b). Benzodiazepines may decrease turnover of norepinephrine, dopamine, and serotonin (Bartholini *et al.*, 1973; Wise, Berger, and Stein, 1972) and may facilitate GABA effects (Costa, Guidotti, and Mao, 1975; Haefley *et al.*, 1975). It is less clear whether these activities are the mechanisms by which they induce sleep. The discovery of the benzodiazepine receptor complex, groups of neuronal membrane proteins to which these compounds bind with high affinity (Squires and Braestrup, 1977; Mohler and Okada, 1977), has led to a new understanding of how some hypnotics may function. As will be seen in Chapter 4, evidence is accumulating that sedating drugs of several different types, including benzodiazepines, barbiturates, and ethanol, may produce pharmacological effects by changing the ion flux at this receptor complex.

SUMMARY

Human sleep is not a passive state occurring in the absence of stimulation; rather, it is an active process reflecting the interaction of complex structures in the diencephalon and brain stem. Electroencephalographically, it comprises four non-REM stages and REM sleep. Each of these stages, in turn, is probably not a unitary phenomenon but rather a combination of several simultaneously occurring processes (e.g., mechanisms controlling muscle relaxation, eye movements, and EEG activation occur together in REM sleep). The sleep stages do not appear randomly but rather are subject to definite rhythmic influences, including a non-REM–REM cycle of roughly a 90-min periodicity. Other influences include age, circadian rhythmic mechanisms, and the presence of disease and drugs. Some aspects of sleep regulation involve monoaminergic and cholinergic pathways from the brain stem that spread diffusely throughout the nervous system. Other neurotransmitters and neuromodulators, circulating hypnotoxins, and hormones may be involved in this process. It seems likely that what we observe is the result of a complex interaction in which sleep mechanisms influence other physiological processes (e.g., respiration, blood pressure, temperature) that, in turn, influence how sleep is manifested.

CHAPTER 2

Pharmacology and Neurotransmitters in Sleep

In Chapter 1 we outlined the development of the concept of "wet" neurophysiology, which emphasizes understanding neural systems by examining synaptic transmitters. As we discussed, initial experiments on animals seemed to indicate that serotonergic, noradrenergic, and cholingeric systems are involved in the regulation of sleep. In this chapter, we will describe human studies in which the activity of these systems has been pharmacologically altered. Several types of manipulations are usually employed. Chemical precursors of a transmitter are given to increase its concentration. Drugs that block a transmitter's metabolism may also raise its concentration, and, in addition, prevent the formation of metabolites that may be biologically active. The amount of available transmitter can be decreased by compounds that inhibit its synthesis. Drugs that bind to the neurotransmitter receptor may act as agonists or antagonists and, hence, may be used to characterize function.

The role of a neurotransmitter may be studied by observing the sleep of normal volunteers who have received the types of drugs outlined above. In some cases, however, a drug can have undesirable side effects, and ethical considerations prevent its use in normal subjects. Fortunately, some are used clinically for certain diseases, and sleep recordings are often obtained on patients receiving them. The problem, of course, is that patients with a particular disease may respond to a drug differently than a normal subject. In this chapter, we will stress pharmacological studies of normal volunteers; medical patients will be discussed only when data on normal subjects are not available. The emphasis, then, is on changes in normal sleep induced by drugs that modify neurotransmitters in a relatively specific manner. Drugs that may be less specific in their actions but that are important because of their clinical usefulness will be discussed in the chapters on specific diseases.

Neurotransmitters which will be discussed in most detail are the biogenic amines serotonin, norepinephrine, and dopamine. Although they are active at only a very small fraction of neurons, these amines are involved in many processes and behaviors, which include sleep, mood, appetite, pain and stress responses, thermoregulation, attentiveness, and aggression. These transmitters are often co-localized with peptides in nerve endings, and their functional relationships are a subject of much current research. Among the biogenic amines, sleep studies of serotonin are probably the most complete. As with all the biogenic amines, many pharmacological studies of serotonin and human sleep were done in the 1970s; there has been an apparent hiatus in such work in recent years. With the development of more specific agents and increased interest in receptor subtypes, it is hoped that more studies clarifying transmitter action in humans will start to appear. We will begin by examining studies of L-tryptophan, which is metabolized to serotonin and other substances.

SEROTONIN AND SLEEP

L-Tryptophan

Effects of Administration on Sleep

The metabolism of L-tryptophan is shown in Fig. 2-1. Although synthesis of serotonin accounts for only a small amount of the total tryptophan used by the body, this is the major metabolic route in the brain. Excess peripheral tryptophan is metabolized primarily in the liver via the kynurenine pathway to niacin, acetyl-CoA, and acetoacetyl-CoA (Trulson and Sampson, 1986). L-Tryptophan cannot be synthesized in humans but is found in the normal diet in amounts of 0.5–2 g/day.

Even before EEG studies were performed, it was observed that L-tryptophan had sedative qualities (Oates and Sjoerdsma, 1960). Subsequently, authors such as Greenwood *et al.* (1974) documented slowing of the clinical EEG and drowsiness (but not euphoria) following paren-

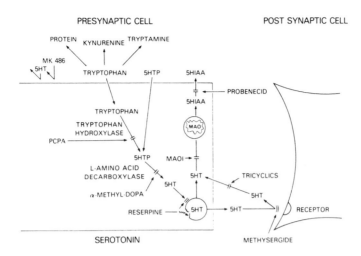

FIGURE 2-1. Synthesis and degradation of serotonin, showing hypothesized actions of drugs discussed in the text.

teral administration, and various clinical studies described subjective sleepiness (Fig. 2-2). A number of studies have examined its effects on nocturnal sleep (Table 2-1, Fig. 2-3). One (Schneider-Helmert, 1981) focused on the placebo nights immediately following L-tryptophan administration. In six of the studies, increased total sleep time was reported; in nine others, no effect was found. Reports on REM latency described either decreased (Oswald *et al.*, 1964; Schmidt, 1983) or increased values (Wyatt *et al.*, 1970a). Griffiths *et al.* (1972) reported variable changes at relatively low doses but a consistent decrease in REM latency at higher doses (12 g).

As in the case of REM latency, there are conflicting accounts of the effects of L-tryptophan on total REM sleep time. Eight studies reported no change; two found decreased, and two increased, REM sleep following moderate doses of less than 10 g. One study reported decreased (Hartmann, Cravens, and List, 1974a) or increased REM sleep (Griffiths *et al.*, 1972) at higher doses (10 and 12 g, respectively). Schmidt (1983) found that REM sleep increased in sleep apnea patients after 2.5 g of L-tryptophan. This, however, may have reflected better sleep as a result of improvement in the respiratory pathophysiology rather than a more direct effect of the drug on sleep. Thus, there seems to be no real agreement on the effects of L-tryptophan on REM sleep, and the differ-

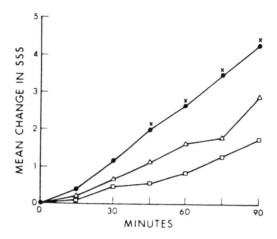

FIGURE 2-2. Sleepiness after 4 g L-tryptophan (•), 4 g L-leucine (△), or placebo (□) was given to 12 normal volunteers 3 hr before bedtime. SSS, Stanford Sleepiness Scale; X, significantly different from placebo. $p < 0.01$. (From Hartmann, 1982. Reprinted by permission.)

ences do not seem to be resolved by studies of possible dose-dependent effects.

Most of the studies indicated that L-tryptophan increases slow-wave sleep. There has been much interest in the possibility that L-tryptophan may, in fact, be a natural sedative (Wyatt *et al.*, 1970a; Hartmann *et al.*, 1971). This position is strengthened by the report by Hartmann *et al.* (1974a) that 1 g—roughly the amount in 0.5 kg of meat—can reduce sleep latency. Subjects in this study were men with prolonged sleep latencies but no subjective complaints about their sleep. This is the first example we will see of various attempts to deal with a methodological problem when assessing possible sedative effects of L-tryptophan—or any compound—in normal volunteers. Since the normal sleep latency is so short (perhaps 5 or 10 min), it is difficult to tell if a compound can reduce it further. For this reason, and because of the interest in L-tryptophan as a "natural" sedative, it has been given to insomniacs in several studies. The results have sometimes been disappointing. Hartmann, Lindsley, and Spinweber (1983), for instance, found no improvement in reported sleep latency of "serious outpatient insomniacs" given 1 g for a week. As mentioned earlier, L-tryptophan has also been used experimentally to treat sleep apnea syndrome patients (Schmidt, 1983; see Chapter 6).

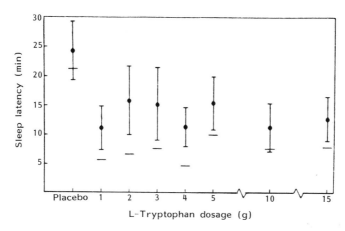

FIGURE 2-3. The sleep latency for placebo and L-tryptophan. ●, mean values for all subjects; |, standard error of the mean; and −, median values for each dose level are shown. Data represent 10 volunteers, each of whom had all eight treatments. (From Hartmann, 1982. Reprinted by permission.)

In two studies, L-tryptophan effectiveness in normal subjects was observed during the daytime. Nicholson and Stone (1979) found that the only significant change induced by 1–4 g was an increase in stage 3 sleep at the highest dose. In a much larger study, Spinweber *et al.* (1983) found that, at 4 g, there was a reduction in sleep latency, with no alteration in sleep stages. If confirmed, this suggests that L-tryptophan might be useful as a hypnotic at clock times not usually associated with sleep. Any recommendations for its use, however, should be tempered with the caution that animal studies have shown some association of high doses with bladder cancer (Bryan, 1971) and liver damage (Trulson and Sampson, 1986).

Dietary L-Tryptophan and Sleep

The biochemical consequences of altering dietary L-tryptophan are complex, insofar as different amino acids may compete for the same metabolic and transport mechanisms. Thus, a balanced diet may decrease, and a high carbohydrate diet may increase, brain tryptophan levels, compared to fasting conditions (Perez-Cruet, Chase, and Murphy, 1974). Special diets have also been used to change tryptophan concentrations. This has usually been done by administering an amino acid mixture without tryptophan, which has been shown to lower tryp-

TABLE 2-1. The Effect of L-Tryptophan on Human Nocturnal Sleep[a]

Study	Dosage (mg/kg)[b]	Subjects	Total sleep	Non-REM sleep	Delta sleep	REM sleep	REM (%)	REM latency	No. of eye movements	REM density
Oswald et al., 1964, 1966	70–140	16 normal males	0	NS	NS	NS	NS	+, 5 of 16	NS	NS
Evans and Oswald, 1966	70	7 narcoleptics	NS	NS	NS	↑ Length of 1st REM period	NS	NS	NS	NS
Cazzullo et al., 1969	NS	6 severe depressives	↑	↑	↑	↓	↓	NS	NS	NS
Williams et al., 1969	109	15 normals	NS	NS	↑	0	0	0	NS	NS
Wyatt et al., 1970a	109	5 normal females	↑	↑	↑	↓	↓	↑	↑	↓
	109	7 insomniacs (3 had affective disorders)	↑	↑	0	0	0	0	0	NS
Hartmann et al., 1971	120	10 normals	0	0	NS	0	0	0	NS	NS
Murri et al., 1971	100	7 chronic schizophrenics	0	0	0	0	0	0	NS	0
Griffiths et al., 1972	171	8 normals	NS	NS	↑, 6 of 8 subjects	↑	↑	↑	NS	0
Makipour, Iber, and Hartmann, 1972[c]	71	20 schizophrenics	↑	NS	0	0	NS	NS	NS	NS

Study	Dose (mg/kg)	Subjects								
Mendels and Chernick, 1972	107	4 psychiatric patients 4 normal controls	NS	NS	NS	NS	NS	NS	NS	↑
Hartmann et al., 1974a	14–214	10 normal men	↓	NS	NS	NS	↓ >140 mg/kg	↑ at 140 mg/kg	NS	NS
Moldofsky and Lue, 1980[d]	71	7 fibrositis patients	NS	NS	0	0	0	0	0	0
Nicholson and Stone, 1979	28–85	6 normal men	0	0	0	0	NS	NS	NS	0
Hartmann and Spinweber, 1979[e]	4–14	15 normal men	0	0	0	0	0	↑ Stage 4 (250 mg)	NS	0
Brown et al., 1979[f]	14–43	18 normal women	NS	NS	NS	NS	0	0	NS	0
Schneider, 1981[g]	28	8 insomniacs	NS	NS	NS	NS	↑	↑	↑	↑
Schmidt, 1983	36	15 apnea patients	NS	NS	↑	↑	↑	0	0	0

[a]NS, not stated.
[b]For dosages not reported as mg/kg, recalculations assumed a 70-kg subject.
[c]Decreased sleep latency at 5 g.
[d]Comparison to placebo condition.
[e]Decreased sleep latency at 250 mg and 1 g.
[f]Decreased sleep latency, some nights, with 3 g.
[g]Data from a four-night placebo period date, following three days of 2 g L-tryptophan.

tophan and serotonin concentrations in rat brain (Gessa *et al.*, 1974), as well as CSF tryptophan and 5-hydroxyindoleacetic acid (5-HIAA) levels in humans (Corsini *et al.*, 1977). The interpretation of such studies, however, is difficult because it is not clear whether these manipulations actually affect serotonin function. Trulson (1985), for instance, found that diets including tryptophan, or tryptophan-free diets, did indeed change brain serotonin and its metabolite 5-HIAA levels but did not modify the firing rate of serotonergic neurons.

Initially, an acute study in rats showed that a tryptophan-free diet decreased REM sleep, with a small "compensatory" increase in non-REM sleep, resulting in no change in total sleep (Moja *et al.*, 1977). A long-term (up to 16 weeks) study in rats indicated modest increases in wakefulness and small decreases in non-REM and REM sleep (Lanoir *et al.*, 1981). Later, the waking and non-REM time returned to normal, but REM sleep did not. Moja *et al.* (1984) administered this diet acutely to humans and found an increase in stage 4 sleep, with nonsignificant decreases in stage 2 and REM sleep. Given these mixed findings, it is fair to say that the results of such dietary manipulations are not clear. Whatever changes are induced might also be attributable to mechanisms other than changes in serotonin concentrations. A diet that acutely reduces available tryptophan, for instance, might well alter the synthesis of tryptophan-containing proteins.

5-Hydroxytryptophan

5-Hydroxytryptophan (5-HTP), the immediate precursor of serotonin (Fig. 2-1), has been used as a neuroendocrine challenge agent (Meltzer *et al.*, 1984; Murphy *et al.*, 1986; Koyama, Lowy, and Meltzer, 1987) and as an experimental treatment for depression (van Praag, 1984; Nolen *et al.*, 1985). It may also induce delirium (Irwin *et al.*, 1986). In human sleep studies, it has been given orally and intravenously in the racemate (D,L) and the L forms (Mendelson, Gillin, and Wyatt, 1977). In general, there has been no effect on total sleep (Hartmann, 1970; Wyatt *et al.*, 1971d; Gillin *et al.*, 1972b; Zarcone, Hoddes, and Smythe, 1973; Zarcone *et al.*, 1973), except in patients with brain lesions that greatly decrease sleep (Fischer-Perroudon, Mouret, and Jouvet, 1974; Guilleminault, Cathala, and Castaigne, 1973a). Low doses in normal subjects have produced either no change in (Hartmann, 1970) or have increased (Mandell *et al.*, 1964; Wyatt *et al.*, 1971d) REM sleep. In schizophrenics, low doses increased the amount of REM sleep in both children (Zarcone *et al.*, 1973) and adults (Murri *et al.*, 1972); high doses decreased both REM and delta sleep (Dawson *et al.*, 1974). Zarcone and Hoddes (1975) gave 5-HTP to abstinent alcoholics. They found that although it did not change the total amount of REM sleep, it decreased the fragmentation of REM periods (defined as two consecutive REM episodes separated by less than 25 min of non-REM sleep). This was taken to imply that 5-HTP may help correct disturbances in alcoholics that result from abnormal serotonergic regulation. These studies are difficult to interpret, however, because of uncertainty as to the degree to which exogenous 5-HTP acts as a precursor of serotonin, as well as other possible actions that might include functioning as a false neurotransmitter or interfering with catecholamine metabolism.

A related compound, alpha-methyl-5-HTP, is converted to alpha-methyl-serotonin, which is a poor substrate for monoamine oxidase (MAO). Wyatt (1972) administered it to three hypertensive patients. REM sleep increased by 4–50% with doses over 0.75 g.

Parachlorophenylalanine

As seen in Figure 2-1, parachlorophenylalanine (PCPA) interferes with serotonin synthesis by inhibiting the enzyme tryptophan hydroxylase (Valzelli, Bernasconi, and Dalessandro, 1983). Its physiological action is complex, however, as it has been reported not to change the raphe firing rate, although it decreases a measure of serotonin release by 82% (Trulson, 1985). A number of studies from the late 1960s and early 1970s reported that PCPA acutely decreases sleep in animals (Table 2-5). More recently, it has been reported to actually increase non-REM sleep in rats during the first 24 hr, followed by one or two days of decreased non-REM and REM sleep and a subsequent rebound increase. Administration of tryptophan during the period of decreased sleep resulted in increases in brain serotonin concentrations and temporary restoration of amounts of non-REM and REM sleep (Borbely, Neuhaus, and Tobler, 1981b). In analogous study in cats using 5-HTP, similar results were obtained (Petitjean et al., 1985).

Because of the relatively high incidence of toxic effects, PCPA studies have not been performed on normal volunteers, although PCPA has been studied in medical patients undergoing therapeutic trials of the drug. Wyatt (1972) gave PCPA to 17 patients, including those with carcinoid tumors, migraine headaches, Huntington's chorea, and dystonia musculorum deformans. Doses of 2–5 mg/24 hr were given for periods ranging from 14 days to three years; REM sleep was decreased by 20–70%, with a maximum effect occurring after two to three weeks of treatment (Fig. 2-4). In some patients, non-REM sleep

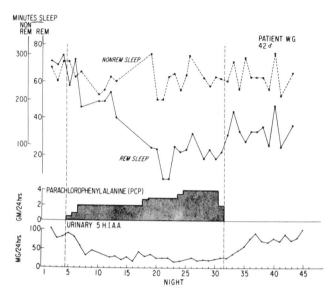

FIGURE 2-4. Effects of PCPA on sleep. (From Wyatt, 1972. Reprinted by permission.)

increased slightly, so that total sleep time was not disturbed. These patients had only small amounts of delta sleep, which usually did not change upon administration of the drug. Some, however, had small increases in delta sleep, an effect also noted by Chernik, Ramsey, and Mendels (1973) in a patient receiving both methadone and PCPA. In contrast to studies with many REM-sleep-suppressing drugs, there was no rebound increase in REM sleep above normal amounts upon withdrawal of PCPA. In fact, the amount of REM sleep did not return to normal levels for about three weeks. This might suggest that PCPA interferes with a fundamental aspect of REM sleep production rather than suppressing its occurrence.

The phasic aspects of REM sleep may also be affected by PCPA. The number of eye movements per minute of REM sleep (*REM density*) and the total number of eye movements in REM sleep over the whole night (*REM index*) decreased in the Wyatt (1972) study, but the number of isolated rapid eye movements increased in stage 2 sleep. Similarly, PCPA induced an increase in phasic integrated potentials (PIPs) in non-REM sleep in two patients [PIPs are a measure of the integrated potential of eye movement activity and may be analogous to the pontine–geniculate–occipital (PGO) spikes in cats]. These observations with rapid eye movements and PIPs have been taken to imply that one function of the serotonergic system is to confine such phasic events to REM sleep. It has been speculated, incidentally, that the escape of phasic REM events into waking and non-REM sleep might be a cause of psychosis (Dement et al., 1969). In a later study, however, it was found that schizophrenics did not differ from their controls in the incidence of PIPs appearing in non-REM sleep (Benson and Zarcone, 1985).

Since PCPA has been found to affect several biochemical systems (e.g., Pucilowski and Valzelli, 1985), the question arose as to whether its effects on REM sleep are, in fact, the result of serotonin synthesis inhibition. Wyatt (1972) approached this problem by giving 5-HTP to four carcinoid tumor patients who were being treated with PCPA. (The principle was that since 5-HTP is the immediate precursor of serotonin, the addition of 5-HTP might have made serotonin synthesis possible in the presence of PCPA.) In three of four patients, 400–800 mg of D,L-5-HTP resulted in partial or total recovery of REM sleep (Fig. 2-5). Total rapid eye movement activity also approached normal. Upon withdrawal of 5-HTP, the amount of REM sleep decreased to the lower level associated with PCPA treatment; non-REM sleep, however, was unaffected. This experiment seems to imply that PCPA affects REM sleep by inhibiting serotonin synthesis. The effects of PCPA and 5-HTP in animals (e.g., Petitjean et al., 1985) will be described later.

Methysergide

Methysergide, a serotonin receptor blocker, is used clinically to prevent migraine headaches (Douglas, 1980) and has been used experimentally as a treatment for narcolepsy (Chapter 7). Many of its actions are thought to be at the serotonin type-2 receptor, although it may bind at some type-1 receptors in nanomolar concentrations. It is inactive at beta-adrenergic sites (Hiner, Roth, and Peroutka, 1986). In 1966, Oswald et al. observed that pretreatment of normal volunteers with methysergide (3 mg/24 hr over 72 hr) could prevent the reduction in REM latency that is usually produced by a single dose of 5–10 g of L-tryptophan. Mendelson, Reichman, and Othmer (1975a) gave methysergide to normal volunteers, at a dose of 8 mg/24 hr, over a 48-hr period. There was no change in total sleep time, sleep latency, or REM latency. Stage 4 sleep decreased and stage 3 sleep increased, with no change in total slow-wave sleep. Total REM sleep time, however, was reduced by 36%, and there was a small, but significant increase in total non-REM sleep. This pattern—a decrease in REM, with a small "compensatory" increase in non-REM sleep and no change in total

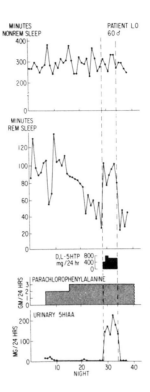

FIGURE 2-5. REM sleep response to 5-HTP in patient taking PCPA. (From Wyatt, 1972. Reprinted by permission.)

sleep time—is similar to that observed by Wyatt (1972) with PCPA in humans. In contrast, a study of rabbits found that PCPA or methysergide markedly decreased REM sleep, with a smaller decrease in non-REM sleep (Tabushi and Himwich, 1971). Thus, in rabbits and humans, these drugs have been reported to have different effects; within each species, however, their effects may be similar. In humans, the implication seems to be that both an inhibitor of serotonin synthesis and blockers of its receptors decrease the amount of REM sleep. The species-specific nature of these effects, however, is emphasized by a report that 5 mg/kg of methysergide did little beyond increasing REM latency in rats (Fornal and Radulovacki, 1982).

Lysergic Acid Diethylamide

The hallucinogen lysergic acid diethylamide (LSD) has profound effects on the serotonergic system (Douglas, 1980). Raphe nuclei neurons may have either an increased or a decreased firing rate in response to LSD, depending on the dose and the route of administration. Although LSD was originally thought to act by blocking serotonin receptors, later work suggested that, at psychoactive doses, it may mimic serotonin at central synapses. It binds to both serotonin type 1 and 2 receptors (Iverson, 1985). Muzio, Roffwarg, and Kaufman (1966) gave 0.13–0.31 μg/kg of LSD orally to normal volunteers either just before they went to bed or 1 hr after they had fallen asleep and found that the length of the first or the second REM period increased. Similarly, Torda (1968) observed that intravenous infusions of LSD 30–50 min after the onset of the third REM period of the night reduced the latency before the next REM period. Unlike methysergide, then, LSD may enhance REM sleep in humans.

Fluoxetine

Fluoxetine, which may have antidepressant (Fabre and Crismon, 1985) and anticataplectic (Langdon et al., 1986b) properties, is a relatively specific inhibitor of serotonin re-uptake. Hence, its effects on sleep might be expected to result from enhanced synaptic serotonin concentrations. In prepubertal boys, fluoxetine reduced REM latency and increased REM sleep time (Pavel et al., 1981); it was also found to potentiate the REM-enhancing effects of arginine vasotocin (to be discussed later). Like LSD, it seems to have some REM-enhancing properties in humans. In a cat study, however, REM sleep was suppressed, with some increase in non-REM sleep (Slater, Jones, and Moore, 1978).

Quipazine and Fenfluramine

These serotonergic agonists are thought to have anorexic properties, for which fenfluramine is used clinically. Quipazine is a direct receptor agonist (Peroutka, 1985; Green, Youdin, and Grahame-Smith, 1976), whereas fenfluramine may induce the release of serotonin from presynaptic terminals and prevent re-uptake (Garattini et al., 1986; Kannengiesser, Hunt, and Raynaud, 1976; Rowland and Carlton, 1986). As we will see later, some indirect evidence suggests that it may also be a postsynaptic receptor agonist (Fornal and Radulovacki, 1982a). Quipazine has been reported to decrease both non-REM and REM sleep in rats; the effects on non-REM sleep were greatly reduced by pretreatment with serotonin blockers metergoline (Fornal and Radulovacki, 1981) or methysergide (Fornal and Radulovacki, 1982b). Fenfluramine has been reported to decrease both non-REM and REM sleep in rats, and the effects on non-REM sleep were partially reversed

by metergoline (Fornal and Radulovacki, 1983). Because the effects on
sleep were not changed by pretreatment with fluoxetine or PCPA, the
authors suggested that its ability to reduce non-REM and REM sleep
may be related to postsynaptic receptor stimulation by the drug or a
metabolite (Fornal and Radulovacki, 1982). These animal studies were
taken to imply that serotonin receptor stimulation may decrease non-
REM sleep. In humans, fenfluramine caused more shifts to stage 1 or
to wakefulness (Lewis, Oswald, and Dunleavy, 1971). High doses suppressed REM sleep, but the effect on slow-wave sleep was inconsistent. Some caution is in order in interpreting these studies, insofar as
fenfluramine may also affect other biogenic amines (Rowland and
Carlton, 1986).

Ritanserin

Ritanserin, a relatively selective antagonist of serotonin type-2 receptors (Leysen et al., 1986), has been reported to improve depressed
mood, sleep difficulty, and anxiety in patients with dysthymic disorder
(Reyntjens et al., 1986). Idzikowski and Mills (1986a) found that 10 mg
of ritanserin enhances slow-wave sleep in normal volunteers and that
this effect persists for at least 14 days. Sleep latency and total sleep
were relatively unaffected. Ritanserin also blocks the reduction in slow-
wave sleep induced by nitrazepam (Idzikowski and Mills, 1986b).
Whether these effects are the result of a blockade of the serotonin-2
receptor, their down-regulation [which surprisingly has been reported
(Leysen et al., 1986)], or some other mechanism is not clear. This
represents some of the first clinical work examining the possible physiological significance of serotonin receptor subtypes.

Ventricular Fluid 5-HIAA

Another approach to understanding the relation of serotonergic activity to sleep is to determine the levels of 5-HIAA (a serotonin metabolite) in the cerebral ventricles. This is possible in dementia patients in
whom ventricular cannulas have been surgically inserted for therapeutic purposes. Traditionally, it has been thought that production of 5-
HIAA is proportional to serotonergic neuronal activity (Aghajanian,
Rosecrans, and Sheard, 1967), and hence that 5-HIAA concentrations
might indicate the relative activity of serotonergic neurons in different
stages of sleep. More recently, this has been questioned, and the exact
relation of 5-HIAA activity to serotonergic activity is still unclear (Fornal and Radulovacki, 1981; Kuhn, Wolf, and Youdim, 1986; Murphy,
1986).

Wyatt *et al.* (1974) found that 5-HIAA concentrations in the CSF of dementia patients were higher in non-REM sleep than in waking or in REM sleep. Levels during REM were lowest, being significantly less than those during waking. A study by Raffaele *et al.* (1983) of hydrocephalic patients found concentrations in non-REM sleep higher than in waking or in REM sleep, which had roughly similar values. Benson *et al.* (1981) found CSF 5-HIAA concentrations to be inversely proportional to the number of eye movements during REM sleep in psychiatric patients, and particularly, chronic schizophrenics. Serotonin and 5-HIAA have also been reported to be higher in the CSF of patients with the excessive sleepiness of Klein–Levin syndrome (Koerger *et al.*, 1984). In a study of cats, Radulovacki *et al.* (1977) reported that either tryptophan or natural sleep increased CSF 5-HIAA. In general, this work seems most compatible with the concepts—derived from animal studies—that serotonergic neurons initiate or sustain non-REM sleep (Jouvet, 1962) or that aminergic activity is lowest during REM sleep (Hobson, Lydic, and Baghdoyan, 1986). It seems less compatible with human studies, suggesting that drugs that increase serotonergic activity will enhance REM sleep.

DOPAMINE

L-Dihydroxyphenylalanine (L-DOPA)

L-DOPA, which may be converted to dopamine and norepinephrine (Fig. 2-6), has been used in many human sleep studies, although few in recent years (Mendelson, Gillin, and Wyatt, 1977). Primarily, these involve patients with Parkinson's disease, although L-DOPA has been studied in depressed and narcoleptic patients as well as in normal volunteers. Its effects on total sleep are inconsistent. Most commonly, there was no change in total sleep (Bricolo *et al.*, 1970; Greenberg and Pearlman, 1970; Kendel *et al.*, 1972; Gillin *et al.*, 1973; Nakazawa *et al.*, 1973), although Fram *et al.* (1970) and Zarcone, Hollister, and Dement (1970) found an increase, and Wyatt *et al.* (1970b) reported a decrease. The effects of L-DOPA seem most marked on REM sleep, although studies differ on the direction. One review found increases in REM sleep in seven, decreases in four, and no consistent changes in another four studies (Mendelson, Gillin, and Wyatt, 1977). These effects may be dose related (Bergonzi *et al.*, 1974) and may reflect differences between acute and chronic administration (Schneider *et al.*, 1974a). In a more recent study, Askenasy and Yahr (1985) gave L-DOPA/carbidopa to five parkinsonian patients who were already receiving the ergot

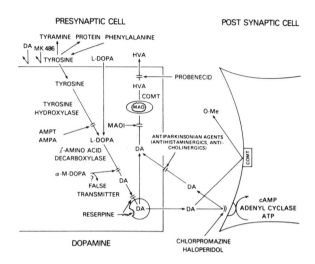

FIGURE 2-6. Synthesis and degradation of dopamine, showing hypothesized actions of drugs discussed in the text.

derivative pergolide; sleep efficiency improved, with an increase in stage 2 sleep and a decrease in the number of awakenings. There was little or no change in REM or slow-wave sleep.

Intravenous L-DOPA, in contrast to oral, clearly seems to affect REM sleep. Gillin *et al.* (1973) gave L-DOPA intravenously to sleeping recovered depressed patients. When infused 25 min after sleep onset, L-DOPA significantly delayed the onset of REM sleep from 44 to 71 min. When L-DOPA was given immediately after the onset of the first REM period, the length of the REM period was reduced by about one-half. The second REM episode was increased to about the same extent the first one had been reduced.

Dopamine Receptor Agonists and Antagonists

Post *et al.* (1978) gave the dopamine agonist piribedil (175 mg/day) to depressed patients and found that REM sleep decreased. Cianchetti *et al.* (1980), however, found that intravenous infusion of the agonist apomorphine in normal subjects decreased both REM and delta sleep. [It is possible that a decrease in delta sleep was not seen in the Post *et al.* study because, in general, depressed patients already have low levels of delta sleep (Chapter 9).] In rats, a dopamine receptor blocker, alpha-flupenthixol (0.2 mg/kg, intraperitoneally), increased non-REM sleep and decreased wakefulness when given either at the onset of a 12-hr light period or a 12-hr dark period (Fornal, Wojcik, and Radulovacki, 1982a).

Pimozide

Pimozide, a neuroleptic agent chemically related to haloperidol, is a central dopamine blocker used in the treatment of Tourette's syndrome (Colvin and Tankanow, 1985). Thus, it might help distinguish the roles played by dopamine and by norepinephrine. Pimozide may have biphasic effects on sleep in dogs, since at low doses it increases wakefulness and decreases both non-REM and REM sleep, whereas at high doses it has the opposite effect (Wauquier, 1983). Sagales and Erill (1975) gave 1–4 mg of pimozide to six normal subjects. During their first night, there was a small decrease in stage 1 sleep, but no change in the percentage of stage 2, 3, or 4 or of REM sleep. Although there was no change in REM latency, the mean duration of the first REM episode increased somewhat. In general, then, possible dopaminergic blockade with pimozide had dose-dependent effects in dogs, but in humans seemed to have little effect on sleep.

Other Studies of Dopamine and Sleep

The relationship of dopaminergic function to REM sleep regulation has also been examined in other types of studies. It has been variously reported that REM sleep deprivation in animals increases (Hernandez-Peon et al., 1969), or has no effect (Carlini, 1983) on, brain dopamine concentrations. Englen, Milon, and Wurzner (1980) gave caffeine to pregnant rats and found that, in the next two generations, REM sleep increased. In the first generation, dopamine concentrations in the locus ceruleus were markedly reduced, while norepinephrine concentrations remained unchanged. Lesion studies of dopaminergic areas in cats have also suggested that dopamine plays a role in the behavioral aspects of arousal (Jones et al., 1973).

NOREPINEPHRINE

Alpha-Methyl-Paratyrosine (AMPT)

AMPT decreases catecholamine synthesis by inhibiting tyrosine hydroxylase (Figs. 2-6 and 2-7). After administration in rats, CNS

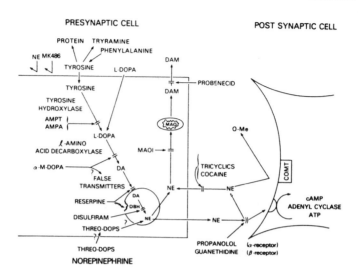

FIGURE 2-7. Synthesis and degradation of norepinephrine, showing hypothesized actions of drugs discussed in the text.

dopamine and norepinephrine decrease in a time-dependent, multiphasic manner (Hallman and Jonsson, 1984). As seen in Table 2-2, the effects of AMPT on sleep in humans have been examined in five medical or neurological patients (Wyatt *et al.*, 1971a) and five patients with nonpsychotic depression (Vaughn, Wyatt, and Green, 1972). During the first five nights, total REM sleep was increased by 3–52%. The return to baseline was variable when the drug was discontinued, but in general, REM sleep dropped below predrug values. There were no striking changes in non-REM sleep; since the patients were allowed to sleep for a limited period (8 hr), however, large changes in total sleep were not possible. In these studies, as well as a report on sleep time estimated by nursing observations (Brodie *et al.*, 1971), total sleep time decreased during the first few nights after AMPT was discontinued. A similar phenomenon was seen after discontinuing AMPT in 14 affective disorder patients; this was attributed to catecholamine receptor hypersensitivity induced during drug administration (Bunney, Kopanda, and Murphy, 1977). In normal volunteers, AMPT caused hypersomnia and decreased REM latency (Gillin *et al.*, 1984). This has been taken as evidence of a catecholaminergic role in depression (see Chapter 9).

Human studies with AMPT suggest that decreased catecholamine synthesis is related to increased total REM sleep. It should be noted, of course, that different monoamine systems are interrelated and that a

TABLE 2-2. Effects of Alpha-Methyl-Paratyrosine on Sleep

Study	Animal	Non-REM	REM	Dosage (mg/kg)[a]
Marantz and Rechtschaffen, 1967	Rat	0	0	150
Marantz et al., 1968	Rat	0	0	75
Torda, 1968	Rat	↑	↓	240
Weitzman et al., 1969	Monkey	↑	↓	110–260
Branchey and Kissin, 1970	Rat	↓	0	200
Hartmann and Bridwell, 1970	Rat	0	↑	50-75 (PO)
		0	↓	75 (IP)
Iskander and Kaebling, 1970	Cat	↑	↓	320
King and Jewett, 1971	Cat	Trend↑	↓	3.125–400
Wyatt et al., 1971a	Man	0	↑	29–43
Hendricksen et al., 1972	Cat	↑	↑	150 (IV over 24 hr)
Stern and Morgane, 1972	Cat	0	↑	75
Vaughan et al., 1972	Man	Trend↓	Trend↓	43
Gillin et al., 1984	Man	↑	↑	43
Gaillard and St. Hilaire-Kafi, 1985	Rat	0	0	150

[a]Key: PO, oral; IP, intraperitoneal; IV, intravenous.

decrease in synthesis in one system could act directly, or indirectly by influencing other biochemical systems. Stein, Jouvet, and Pujol (1974), for instance, showed that injections of AMPT in cats both decreased catecholamine and increased serotonin in different areas of the brain.

Alpha-Methyldopa

Alpha-methyldopa, which is used clinically to treat hypertension, inhibits aromatic-L-amino acid decarboxylase, which is involved in the synthesis of both norepinephrine and serotonin. When 1.25 g/24 hr was given to 10 normal adults, the total REM sleep for the night did not change (Baekeland and Lundwall, 1971). During the first 3 hr of sleep, however, REM sleep increased and stage 4 sleep decreased. Oswald et al. (1966) found that alpha-methyldopa did not block the ability of L-tryptophan to shorten REM latency.

Adrenergic Receptor Blockers

Propranolol, which is used as an antihypertensive agent, acts by blocking beta$_1$- and beta$_2$-adrenergic receptors. Dunleavy, MacLean, and Oswald (1971) gave 120 mg of propranolol before bedtime to three men for 13 days. There was no effect on total sleep time, percentage REM sleep, or other measures. Unpublished data from this laboratory also showed no effect of 100 mg/24 hr in normal volunteers. In contrast to these EEG studies, however, many clinicians have the impression that propranolol, as well as alpha-methyldopa, may induce subjectively poor sleep (Association of Sleep Disorder Centers, 1979).

Propranolol has been studied in animals as well. It was found to have no effect on sleep in dogs (Gordon and Lavie, 1984). In rats, propranolol given in the morning (a nocturnal animal's usual sleep period) had no effect on non-REM sleep, but elevated it when administration was at night. The percentage of REM sleep decreased at both times (Mendelson et al., 1980a). A cat study found increased drowsiness and decreased deep non-REM sleep and REM sleep (Hilakivi, 1983).

An alpha-adrenergic blocking agent, thymoxamine, has been reported to increase REM sleep (Oswald et al., 1974). This is consistent with the previously described studies of AMPT, in which this inhibitor of norepinephrine synthesis increased REM sleep.

Clonidine is a noradrenergic alpha-receptor agonist whose human pharmacologic effects appear primarily to be the result of activity at the presynaptic alpha$_2$ receptor, resulting in decreased noradrenergic activity. It is used clinically as an antihypertensive (Weiner, 1980) and causes sedation. When 225 μg of clonidine (Kanno and Clarenbach, 1985), or 300 μg of a sustained-release clonidine preparation (Dollery, Hamilton, and Maling, 1977), was given to normal volunteers, stage 2 sleep increased, while REM sleep declined; the total sleep time, however, was not significantly altered. In a study of clonidine in rats, changes in theta and delta activity and dose-related effects on sleep spindles were observed, but there were no major effects on sleep stages per se (Pastel and Fernstrom, 1984). In cats, clonidine increased drowsiness and deep non-REM sleep and decreased REM sleep (Hilakivi, 1983).

Several relatively selective alpha$_1$ and alpha$_2$ agonists and antagonists have been studied in animals, but not yet in humans. Methoxamine, an alpha$_1$ agonist, has been reported to increase wakefulness while decreasing the number of REM sleep periods in the cat (Hilakivi and Leppavour, 1984) or to decrease both non-REM and REM sleep in the rat (Pellejero et al., 1984). In the latter study, yohimbine, which blocks alpha$_2$ receptors, had similar effects to the alpha$_1$ agonist methoxamine. Similar doses of prazosin, an alpha$_1$ antagonist, have been reported to increase (Hilakivi and Leppavouri, 1984) or decrease (Pellejero et al., 1984) REM sleep in the cat and the rat, respectively.

The relation of noradrenergic activity to the REM sleep rebound process in rats has also been studied. Radulovacki et al. (1981a,b) reported that the alpha blocker phentolamine or the dopamine receptor agonist bromocriptine will prevent the appearance of a REM rebound after REM sleep deprivation by the "flower pot method" (see Mendelson et al., 1974). They hypothesized that these two agents fulfilled the need for REM sleep and, hence, abolished a buildup of REM sleep pressure.

OTHER DRUGS INFLUENCING AMINES

Reserpine

Reserpine depletes stores of catecholamines and serotonin (Weiner, 1980) without altering acetylcholine concentrations (Palfai et al., 1986). It is used clinically as an antihypertensive and may induce depressive symptoms in some patients. In humans, reserpine is one of the few agents known to increase REM sleep (Tissot, 1965; Hartmann, 1966; Hoffman and Domino, 1969; Coulter, Lester, and Williams, 1971), and decrease REM latency. In a number of studies, shortened REM latencies in depressed patients have been reported, and this particular effect of reserpine is taken by some as evidence for decreased aminergic function in depression (Chapter 9).

Amphetamines

Amphetamines, which are thought to enhance catecholaminergic activity, have been reported to decrease percentage REM sleep (Gillin et al., 1975b; Baekeland, 1967; Rechtschaffen and Maron, 1964). The D- and L-isomers may have somewhat different effects. Gillin et al. (1975b) gave single, 30-mg doses of each isomer to seven depressed patients in the morning. Although both decreased percentage REM sleep, only the D-isomer delayed sleep onset and reduced total sleep time and non-REM sleep. Gillin et al. (1975b) and Feinberg et al. (1974a) found that D-amphetamine did not change REM density. The latter authors suggested that this property may differentiate its effects from the effects of the sedative–hypnotics.

Withdrawal after chronic administration has been associated with large "rebound" increases in REM sleep that may last for some weeks (Watson, Hartmann, and Schildkraut, 1972; Oswald and Thacore, 1963). Feinberg et al. (1974a), studying the effects of chronic amphetamine administration on hyperactive children, suggested that the REM rebound is not necessarily a constant finding and may be related to changes in dosage before the drug is discontinued. Gillin et al. (1975b)

noted no rebound during the first night following a single amphetamine night. Earlier we referred to evidence that there is no REM rebound following suppression by PCPA (Wyatt, 1972), so this once
again demonstrates the complexity of REM sleep regulation.

Amphetamine is an important drug in the management of narcolepsy; it will be discussed in Chapter 7.

Chlorpromazine

Chlorpromazine, a phenothiazine used to treat schizophrenia, has
central dopaminergic-blocking activity as well as other actions, including anticholinergic and membrane permeability effects. Three studies
describe the effects of single doses of chlorpromazine (100–150 mg
orally and 0.4 mg/kg intramuscularly) on normal subjects (Lester and
Guerrero-Figueroa, 1966; Lester et al., 1971; Sagales, Erill, and
Domino, 1969). Total sleep or REM sleep time did not change. Several
studies of repeated administration of chlorpromazine (25–100 mg) in
normal subjects found an increase in total sleep time (Okuma, Hata,
and Fugii, 1975; Hartmann and Cravens, 1973c; Naiman, Poitras, and
Engelsmann, 1972; Lewis and Evans, 1969). Okuma et al. (1975) and
Lewis and Evans (1969) reported some increase in REM sleep at 25 mg,
whereas Hartmann and Cravens (1973c) reported no change at 50 mg.
The study of Naiman et al. (1972) was oriented to the effects of chlorpromazine on REM rebound after REM deprivation. Predeprivation
nights with no medication, however, were indistinguishable from
predeprivation nights in which the subjects received 1 mg/kg of chlorpromazine. Thus, multiple low doses of chlorpromazine in normal subjects may have some effect on the duration of sleep, but little effect on
other parameters.

Chlorpromazine studies in normal subjects differ somewhat from
the reported effects in schizophrenics, which include decreases in percentage REM sleep (Feinberg et al., 1969) and increases in REM density
and REM index (Kaplan et al., 1974). Changes in the latter studies may
reflect higher dosages as well as the more disturbed sleep of such patients. The relative lack of actions of low doses of chlorpromazine on
normal sleep is similar to that seen with the more specific dopamine-
blocker pimozide (Sagales and Erill, 1975); the failure to alter REM
sleep with either of these agents contrasts with the increased REM
sleep seen after AMPT administration, which may decrease both dopamine and norepinephrine synthesis. It is also possible that this difference may be accounted for by the low doses of chlorpromazine used in
the normal volunteer studies.

Hartmann and Cravens (1973c) have suggested that the increased sleep time observed with chlorpromazine is consistent with the view that a certain amount of dopaminergic activity is necessary for wakefulness, a view strengthened by some animal study results [see Jones (1969) and discussion in Chapter 1].

Tricyclic Antidepressants

The tricyclic antidepressants are thought to increase noradrenergic and serotonergic activity by blocking re-uptake. In addition, they possess anticholinergic alpha-blocking and antihistaminic properties to varying degrees. The tricyclics have been studied by a number of investigators (Dunleavy et al., 1972; Hartmann, 1969; Zung, 1969; Ritvo et al., 1967; Toyoda, 1964). Dunleavy et al. (1972) gave six different tricyclics to normal volunteers over a period of four weeks. All decreased total REM sleep to varying degrees, with some increase in stage 2 sleep. With time, recovery toward normal occurred. Following discontinuation, a REM sleep rebound occurred, which lasted up to a month. Some authors have suggested that the REM-suppressing property of tricyclics is an integral part of their antidepressant effect (Chapter 9).

The effects of tricyclics on slow-wave sleep are unclear. Dunleavy et al. (1972), for instance, found no systematic effect, although Zung (1969) found increases with desmethylimipramine. Dunleavy et al. (1972) found that intrasleep restlessness (as determined by frequency of spontaneous shifts into stage 1 sleep or wakefulness) increased with imipramine, desipramine, and chlorimipramine and did not go down during chronic administration.

Of particular interest is chlorimipramine, a halogenated form of imipramine that is five times more potent than the parent compound in its ability to block serotonin re-uptake (Carlsson et al., 1969a). Compared to such tricyclics as protriptyline and desipramine, it is a relatively weak blocker of norepinephrine re-uptake (Carlsson et al., 1969b). It, too, is a powerful inhibitor of REM sleep, which moves toward normal during chronic use (Dunleavy et al., 1972). Chlorimipramine has also been found useful in the treatment of cataplexy, sleep paralysis, and hypnogogic hallucinations in narcoleptic patients (Shapiro, 1975; Guilleminault, Carskadon, and Dement, 1974), as discussed in Chapter 7.

Monoamine Oxidase Inhibitors

Monoamine oxidase inhibitors (MAOIs) block the breakdown of serotonin and norepinephrine by oxidative pathways (Figs. 2-1 and 2-7).

There is some evidence that their therapeutic activity is more closely associated with changes in noradrenergic function (Murphy, Sunderland, and Cohen, 1984). High doses of the hydrazine MAOI phenelzine (60–105 mg), as well as isocarboxazid (60 mg), mebamazine (15 mg), and the nonhydrazine MAOI pargyline (60–100 mg), markedly decreased REM sleep when given for 10 days to depressed or narcoleptic patients (Wyatt et al., 1971b; Wyatt, 1972). Non-REM sleep was either unchanged or showed a small "compensatory" increase. The observation that the non-MAOI isoniazid (400 mg) did not suppress REM sleep suggests that the sleep-related effects of these drugs are, in fact, the result of their inhibition of MAO and not some other property (Wyatt, 1972). Akindale, Evans, and Oswald (1970) reported decreases in REM sleep following the administration of 60–90 mg of phenelzine but not nialamide.

Kupfer and Bowers (1972) measured monoamine metabolite levels in the cerebrospinal fluid of nine psychotic patients and found that phenelzine in relatively high doses (45–60 mg/day) decreased levels of the dopamine metabolite homovanillic acid (HVA) to a greater extent than 5-HIAA (a metabolite of serotonin). During a REM rebound following discontinuation, spinal fluid HVA levels increased in four patients; in one patient who showed no rebound, HVA levels remained unchanged. Concentrations of 5-HIAA were not significantly changed during REM suppression or a later REM rebound. These results seem to suggest a role for dopamine in the control of REM sleep.

Monoamine oxidase in the CNS exists in two forms, depending on the preferred substrate (Neff and Yang, 1974). The type A enzyme preferentially metabolizes serotonin, norepinephrine, and normetanephrine, whereas the type B enzyme metabolizes benzylamine and beta-phenylethylamine. Histological studies indicate that type A is found primarily in regions of high catecholamine content, as in the locus ceruleus, whereas type B is found in regions high in serotonin, as in the raphe dorsalis (Westlund et al., 1985; Fig. 2-8). Some of the MAOIs preferentially inhibit type A or B enzymes, and thus it might be possible that they have different effects on sleep-related phenomena. Most of the MAOIs used in sleep studies are the "mixed" type and inhibit both type A and B enzymes. Exceptions include pargyline and deprenyl, which may preferentially inhibit the type B enzyme. Limited experience with these agents in the author's laboratory, however, suggests that their effects on sleep are no different from those of other MAOIs.

In order to examine the effects of MAO inhibition on sleep in the developing brain, Mendelson et al. (1982b) exposed fetal rats to clorgyline, a type A inhibitor, and continued treatment postnatally at a dose

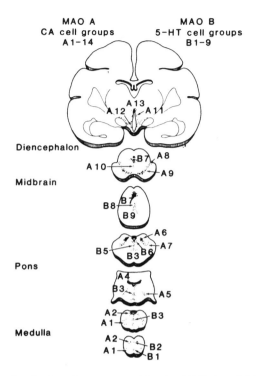

FIGURE 2-8. The distribution of neurons positive for MAO A and MAO B throughout the brain stem of the monkey, schematically illustrated in coronal tissue sections. Amine-containing cell groups of Dahlstrom and Fuxe (1964) are indicated. Catecholamine (CA) cell groups are denoted A 1–14 and serotonin (5-HT) cell groups are denoted B 1–9. (From Westlund *et al.*, 1985. Reprinted by permission.)

of 1 mg/kg a day for six weeks. At that time, type A MAO was inhibited by 99%, but there was no change in REM sleep. In contrast, subacute clorgyline administration to six-week-old rats of 2 mg/kg a day for 60 hr resulted in a decrease of type A MAO activity and of REM sleep (Table 2-3). Thus, the effects of clorgyline on MAO activity and on sleep may be dissociated, at least in the developing brain.

Endogenous MAO and Biogenic Amines

Platelet MAO Activity

In platelets, which contain primarily type B MAO, there is an over 20-fold range of activity in the general population (Murphy *et al.*, 1976). Platelet MAO activity may be decreased in depression and schizophre-

TABLE 2-3. Effects of Subacute Administration of
Clorgyline on Sleep in Rats

	Clorgyline (N = 12)		Saline (N = 10)	
	Mean	SE	Mean	SE
Total recording period	483.0	3.1	487.0	1.7
Total sleep time	265.0	11.2	294.0	13.6
Non-REM time	243.5	9.9	260.4	13.1
REM time	21.5	3.0	33.6	2.7 ($p<0.01$)
Intermittent waking time	171.8	12.3	151.0	12.4
Disconnect time	5.2	2.2	5.4	2.5
Non-REM (%)	92.0	1.0	88.4	1.1 ($p<0.02$)
REM (%)	8.0	1.0	11.6	1.1 ($p<0.02$)
Intermittent waking (%)	39.2	2.5	34.0	2.9
Sleep latency	41.8	8.8	53.2	14.4
REM latency	159.0	32.6	100.8	20.0
REM episodes (N)	8.2	1.1	15.7	1.2 ($p<0.001$)
REM episode length	2.5	0.2	2.1	0.1
REM efficiency	91.6	2.4	94.8	0.6
REM–non-REM cycle length	39.0	6.2	24.2	2.2 ($p<0.05$)
Intermittent waking episodes (N)	19.8	1.7	18.3	1.8

(From Mendelson et al., 1982b. Reprinted by permission.)

nia (Wyatt and Murphy, 1976). There has been some interest in the "high-risk paradigm" of following normal subjects in the highest and lowest deciles of platelet MAO, and it has been postulated that those with very low MAO may be more likely to develop psychiatric illness (Buchsbaum, Coursey, and Murphy, 1976). Mendelson et al. (1978a) studied sleep in these normal subjects and found that those with high MAO had less REM sleep time, as well as lower REM density and fewer total eye movements (Fig. 2-9). The values for the low MAO group tended to be similar to those seen in the general population. Kupfer et al. (1979) examined platelet MAO and sleep in 56 hospitalized affective disorder patients. In the group as a whole and in the unipolar patients, there were no clear associations; in the bipolar patients, there was an inverse relationship between MAO activity and percent REM sleep. Interpretation of these studies is difficult, insofar as MAOIs at therapeutic doses usually decrease REM sleep, although as mentioned, very low doses of phenelzine may increase REM sleep (Wyatt, 1972). Perhaps the main point is that this is one of the few cases in which levels of an endogenous substance have correlated with sleep parameters.

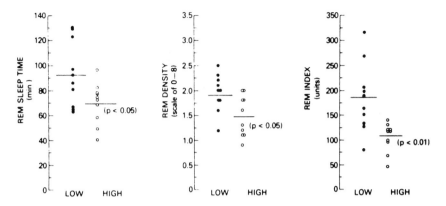

FIGURE 2-9. REM sleep parameters in normal subjects with high and low platelet MAO activity. (From Mendelson *et al.*, 1978a. Reprinted by permission.)

Metabolites of Norepinephrine and Dopamine in the CSF

Wyatt *et al.* (1976) examined metabolites in the CSF of patients who had ventriculoatrial shunts as a treatment for normal pressure hydrocephalus and dementia. 3-Methoxy-4-hydroxyphenylglycol (MHPG), a metabolite of norepinephrine, was measured during waking and non-REM and REM sleep in five patients. Concentrations were highest in REM sleep, followed by waking and non-REM sleep. Homovanillic acid, a metabolite of dopamine (Fig. 2-6), showed a similar pattern in six patients. It should be recalled that these were seriously ill patients, whose sleep was disturbed. Twenty-four–hour urinary and cerebrospinal fluid MHPGs have also been examined in seven depressed patients (Benson, Berger, and Zarcone, 1981). There was no significant correlation with amounts of REM sleep, although there was a tendency toward an inverse relationship. The relation of CSF MHPG to sleep is, thus, unclear.

Plasma Norepinephrine and Sleep

Several studies have examined the relationship of sleep to plasma norepinephrine, for which there is a circadian rhythm, with a peak in the late morning, and lowest concentrations at night (Prinz *et al.*, 1979). An acute 180° reversal of sleep–wake times had little effect on 24-hr plasma norephinephrine (Prinz *et al.*, 1984). There is no obvious relation to sleep stage (Dollery, Hamilton, and Maling, 1977; Prinz *et al.*, 1979), and no increase is associated with spontaneous or experimentally induced awakenings (Prinz *et al.*, 1984). Elderly subjects have elevated plasma norephinephrine concentrations, particularly at night (Prinz *et al.*, 1979), and it has been suggested that this is related to their disturbed sleep (decreased stage 4 and REM sleep and increased wakefulness; see Chapter 1). This view has been strengthened by a study of sodium-restricted diets in young men (Vitiello *et al.*, 1983). This diet, which is thought to lead to mild volume depletion and sympathetic activation, elevated the plasma norepinephrine. Sleep was disturbed, with decreased slow-wave and REM sleep and increased wakefulness.

THE CHOLINERGIC SYSTEM

Muscarinic

There is surprisingly little information available on the role of acetylcholine in human sleep, although until recently, many over-the-counter sleeping medications contained the anticholingeric agent scopolamine. Scopolamine has been reported to decrease REM sleep in normal subjects, although the total sleep time remains unchanged (Sagales *et al.*, 1969). Methscopolamine, which is not thought to cross the blood–brain barrier, has no effect on sleep (Sagales *et al.*, 1969). Toyoda, Saraki, and Kurihara (1966) observed that atropine resulted in decreased REM sleep in the first 2 hr of sleep and increased the REM latency.

In contrast to the anticholinergic agents, anticholinesterases (which increase acetylcholine by inhibiting its metabolism) increase REM sleep. These agents have been associated with nightmares and increased dreaming (Holmes and Gaon, 1956; Grob and Harvey, 1958). Industrial workers exposed to organophosphates, which have anticholinesterase properties, have been reported to have unusually long REM periods of particularly rapid onset (Stoyva and Metcalf, 1968).

Sitaram *et al.* (1976, 1977, 1982) demonstrated that the anticholinesterase physostigmine, or the muscarinic cholinergic receptor agonist arecoline, induces REM sleep in normal subjects if given during the first or second non-REM period (Fig. 2-10). This was a time-dependent effect, with a more potent action noted when given 35 min (compared to 5 min) after sleep onset. Similarly, the dose of physostigmine (0.5 mg) that would induce REM periods in the first non-REM period would often produce arousals when given in the second non-

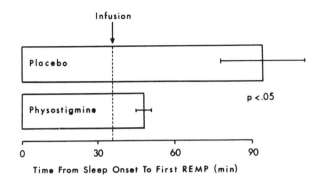

FIGURE 2-10. The effect of physostigmine infusion during non-REM sleep on REM latency. Physostigmine (0.5 mg), or placebo, was given 35 to 40 min after the onset of stage 2 sleep. (From Sitaram *et al.*, 1976. Reprinted by permission.)

REM period. A lower dose (0.25 mg) would induce REM periods at that time. This may imply that sensitivity to cholingergic effects changes throughout sleep. Interestingly, these compounds seemed to bring on REM periods without altering their duration. Similarly, a 1-hr slow drip of physostigmine did not change the duration of REM sleep (Gillin *et al.*, 1978b). This suggests that induction and maintenance of REM sleep are regulated separately. It has been reported that depressed patients are more sensitive to REM sleep induction (Gillin, Sitaram, and Mendelson, 1982), a topic discussed in more detail in Chapter 9. In general, these studies are consistent with the view put forth by Moruzzi (1972) that non-REM and REM sleep and the awake state form a continuum of progressively higher levels of arousal and that the shift between these levels may be mediated by cholinergic mechanisms. A general review linking cholinergic mechanisms to various aspects of REM sleep is found in *Psychological Medicine* (Editorial, 1984). There has also been a great deal of interest in a possible cholinergic role in memory function (Heise, 1987).

Animal studies going back many years have shown that intracerebral acetylcholine or cholinergic agonists may induce states similar to REM sleep. Hernandez-Peon *et al.* (1963, 1967), for instance, showed that acetylcholine crystals placed in the limbic midbrain and forebrain induce REM sleep. More recently, a series of elegant studies using microinjection of the cholinesterase inhibitor neostigmine have helped define the cholinergic role in REM generation in the cat (Baghdoyan, McCarley, and Hobson, 1985; Baghdoyan *et al.*, in press). Thus, REM-like states were induced by injection of neostigmine into the pontine reticular formation; injection into the medullary or midbrain reticular formation seemed to suppress REM. Both the amount and latency of REM sleep could be altered by injection at various sites in the pontine reticular formation. At different sites, various components of REM sleep might be induced, for example, PGO waves or eye movements. These studies suggest that what is observed as REM sleep is the result of a complex orchestration of a number of physiological processes, with a major role apparently being played by cholinergic mechanisms. These observations are consistent with the reciprocal interaction model of sleep regulation (Hobson *et al.*, 1975; Hobson, Lydic, and Baghdoyan, 1986).

Nicotinic Agonists

Relatively little is known about the role of the nicotinic cholinergic system and sleep. Mendelson *et al.* (1981c) found that intravenous infusion of 100 mg of piperidine, a nicotinic agonist, had no effect on the sleep of normal volunteers, although it enhanced sleep-related growth hormone secretion (see Chapter 5).

GAMMA-AMINOBUTYRIC ACID

Gamma-aminobutyric acid is the major inhibitory neurotransitter in the central nervous system. One aspect of GABA function that has received attention is the location of GABA recognition sites as part of the benzodiazepine receptor complex, which is discussed at length in Chapter 4. Benzodiazepines are potent anticonvulsants, and substantial data show that this property derives from a facilitation of GABA. In contrast, there have been relatively little data relating GABA agonists and antagonists to sleep. In humans, for instance, the GABA agonist progabide may increase responsiveness of schizophrenics to the environment and elevate mood in depression, properties not usually associated with a sedative (Lloyd *et al.*, 1983). In rats, intraperitoneal progabide (300 mg/kg) decreased REM sleep and slightly decreased total sleep (Lloyd *et al.*, 1982). Gamma-acetylenic GABA and gamma-vinyl GABA, which inhibit GABA transaminase, as well as the indirect GABA antagonist picrotoxin, produced behavioral quiescence along with epileptiform activity in rats (Myslobodsky and Mansour, 1979). Similarly, Mendelson *et al.* (unpublished data) found that both picrotoxin and the agonist imidazole-4-acetic acid (IMA) produced behavioral quiescence, but the only effect on sleep was a modest increase in total sleep in the first 2 hr at the highest dose (164 mg/kg) of IMA, and nonsignificant trends toward decreased sleep with picrotoxin. Monti, Altier, and D'Angelo (1979) found that the GABA$_B$ agonist baclofen had no effect on the sleep of rats, except for increasing REM latency at doses of 2.5–5.0 mg/kg. The GABA transaminase inhibitor aminooxyacetic acid (AOAA) actually delayed sleep onset, although higher doses increased total sleep time (Wambebe, 1983).

Some animal data, however, do suggest sedative effects in terms of EEG-defined sleep. Gamma-hydroxybutyrate (GHB), which has been used to treat narcolepsy (Chapter 7), may decrease latency to deep non-REM sleep and, at a higher dose (25 mg/kg), may increase the total amount of sleep. Noneffective doses of baclofen, or GHB combined with diazepam, increased deep non-REM sleep; this effect was prevented by pretreatment with the GABA blocker bicuculline (Monti et al., 1979). In young chicks (1–28 days old) lacking a significant blood–brain barrier, GABA itself potentiated, and bicuculline blocked, nitrazepam-induced sleep (Wambebe, 1983). In summary, GABA agonists and antagonists seem to show behavioral sedation, but evidence regarding EEG-defined sleep is less clear. It seems likely that GABA plays an important role in some (e.g., anticonvulsant) effects of systemically administered benzodiazepines, but the degree to which it plays a direct role in sleep, other than by altering the affinity of benzodiazepines for the recognition site, remains to be determined.

ADENOSINE

Purines interest sleep researchers for a variety of reasons. Inosine and hypoxanthine are among the endogenous substances with the highest affinity to the benzodiazepine recognition site, although their affinity is relatively low (IC$_{50}$ values of 10^{-3} M) compared to benzodiazepines (Marangos et al., 1983). It has been suggested that inosine may be involved in anxiety-related behaviors, insofar as it may reverse diazepam-induced exploratory activity in mice (Crawley et al., 1981). Centrally (Feldberg and Sherwood, 1954) and peripherally (Maitre et al., 1974) administered adenosine has been reported to produce behavioral sedation. Although the affinity of adenosine is lower, it has been studied extensively because there is substantial evidence that it is involved in central neurotransmission (Phillis and Wu, 1981). Benzodiazepines may block adenosine uptake, possibly resulting in increased adenosine concentrations and downregulation of receptors (Hawkins, Pravica, and Radulovacki, 1986). It has been speculated that uptake inhibition may be one of the mechanisms of action of these compounds (Phillis and Wu, 1981). This seems less likely, however, since the affinity of benzodiazepines for their own recognition site is much greater than for the adenosine uptake site (Skolnick, Paul, and Marangos, 1979). There has also been a great deal of interest in adenosine receptors, which, in turn, have been subtyped A_1 and A_2 (Daly, 1982).

A number of sleep studies of adenosine receptor agonists or metabolism blockers have been performed in animals. Berman et al. (1982) found that 100 and 200 $\mu g/kg$ of the A_1 agonist L-phenylisopropyl adenosine (L-PIA), intraperitoneally, greatly reduced motor activity in rats. Through EEG recordings, however, it was found that the lower dose did not alter sleep, but the higher dose actually disrupted sleep, with increased sleep latency and decreased total sleep time during the first 2 hr. Erythro-9-(2-hydroxy-3-nonyl)-adenine (EHNA), an adenosine deaminase inhibitor that might be expected to increase available adenosine, was also found to decrease motor activity. Once again, lower doses had no effect on sleep, whereas higher doses reduced total sleep and percent REM sleep (Mendelson et al., 1983d; Table 2-4). The authors speculated that the sedative actions of adenosine were more evident in terms of motor activity than of sleep and that agents that enhance adenosine activity lead to a state of "quiescent waking." Other work on L-PIA has suggested that it increases deep slow-wave sleep (S_2); lower doses did not alter total sleep, but higher doses decreased it (Radulovacki et al., 1984). Deoxycoformycin, another adenosine deaminase inhibitor, was reported to increase S_2 at the expense of S_1. As with L-PIA, the lower dose had no effect on total sleep, whereas the higher dose actually decreased it during hours 3–6 (Radulovakci et al., 1983). Adenosine-5'-N-ethylcarboxamide (NECA), a primarily A_2 agonist, also enhanced S_2, with a small increase in total sleep during the first 3 hr at the highest dose (Radulovacki et al., 1984). Withdrawal from chronically administered NECA has also been associated with decreased wakefulness and enhanced S_2 and REM sleep (Porter et al., 1986). The effect of pharmacological alteration of adenosine activity is not entirely clear, then, but a general impression is that blockade of metabolism, or A_1 stimulation, induces behavioral sedation and may enhance deep slow-wave sleep. During this period of decreased motor activity, total sleep may be unaffected or it may actually decrease.

CIRCULATING SLEEP FACTORS

Many endogenous substances have been identified as possible natural sleep-inducing materials or hypnotoxins (Mendelson, Gillin, and

TABLE 2-4. Effects of Erythro-9-(2-Hydroxy-3-Nonyl-Adenine) on Sleep in the Rat

	Placebo (N=10)	EHNA (37.5 mg/kg) (N=10)	Placebo (N=8)	EHNA (75 mg/kg)	Placebo	EHNA (200 mg/kg)
Total sleep	296.1	270.4	278.9	239.5[a]	294.3	183.8[a]
Non-REM sleep (%)	87.0	87.9	91.3	92.9	90.5	98.5[a]
REM sleep (%)	13.4	12.1	8.7	7.1	9.5	1.5[a]
Intermittent waking (%)	33.2	37.4	36.3	41.7	36.8	56.9[a]
Sleep latency	32.4	44.5	22.8	44.8	19.0	47.8
REM latency	94.2	107.6	150.8	180.3	126.0	278.0[a]
REM episodes (N)	16.5	13.1	11.5	7.5	14.6	1.5[a]
REM episode duration	2.4	2.5	2.1	2.2	1.9	1.8
REM efficiency[b]	97.1	97.0	93.5	94.8	96.7	94.0
REM cycle duration	22.6	31.0	27.6	32.7	31.4	42.8
Waking episodes (N)	23.2	25.6	22.0	28.8[a]	28.1	25.4

[a]Differs from placebo by at least $p < 0.05$
[b]Actual minutes of REM divided by total duration of REM episode.
(From Mendelson et al., 1983e. Reprinted by permission.)

Wyatt, 1983f). In general, most have been obtained by experiments in which extracts of blood, urine, or cerebrospinal fluid from sleep-deprived animals have been found to induce sleep upon injection into naive animals. Since very little human work has been done with these substances, they will be reviewed only briefly, and the reader may pursue specific topics in the reviews cited. One study of particular interest is that of Inoue et al. (1984), in which five different possible sleep factors were studied in the same laboratory.

Arginine Vasotocin (AVT)

First described in the pineal gland by Milcu et al. (1963), AVT has been reported to have several properties, including inhibition of gonadotropin release, modification of conditioned behavior, and enhancement of slow-wave sleep. The sleep-enhancing effects were of particular interest because of the extremely low concentrations (e.g., 10^{-6} pg, intraventricularly) reported to be active in the cat (Pavel, Psatta, and Goldstein, 1977). AVT was also thought to be effective when higher doses were given intraperitoneally in the cat. Intraperitoneal administration of 50 μg/kg of AVT to rats had no effect, other than shortening REM latency and lowering REM efficiency (Mendelson et al., 1980). A higher dose (500 μg/kg) was very toxic. The mechanism of action of AVT is not understood, although some data suggest that its effects are mediated by an inhibitory GABAergic habenula-raphe pathway (Pavel, Goldstein, and Petrescu, 1980; Pavel and Eisner, 1984) involving serotonergic neurons (Pavel et al., 1980).

Studies of AVT in human cerebrospinal fluid suggest that it may be released during sleep (Pavel et al., 1979). In a study of normal humans, 2–23 μg of AVT given subcutaneously was found to increase REM sleep, whereas intravenous infusions over 30 min did not produce clinical signs of sleep (Coculescu, Serbanescu, and Temeli, 1979). When given intranasally to narcoleptics and symptomatic hypersomniacs, 1.5 μg of AVT often induced sleep with REM onsets and increased the amount of REM sleep in 180-min recordings (Popoviciu et al., 1982). The implications of both animal and human pharmacological studies, then, is that AVT affects REM sleep regulation; whether its role is physiological is not yet clear.

Delta Sleep-Inducing Peptide (DSIP)

Delta sleep-inducing peptide (DSIP) was first described in an ultradialysate of blood from rabbits in whom a sleeplike state had been induced by electrical stimulation of the thalamus (Monnier and Hosli, 1964). The synthetic nonapeptide may increase delta activity in rabbits (Schoenenberger et al., 1978). Studies in rats using conventional sleep staging, however, have been largely negative (Mendelson et al., 1982a; Tobler and Borbely, 1980). In the latter study, motor activity was found to be decreased one to two days after administration. Intravenous infusions given for seven nights to human insomniacs have been reported to increase total sleep by a mean of 72 min (Schneider-Helmert, 1984). The onset of sleep-promoting effects began after 1 hr of infusion, analogously, perhaps, to the delay in effects that has also been described with muramyl dipeptide. Daytime infusions were thought to improve the level of arousal and to increase various performance measures, which differs from experiences with daytime administration of most traditional hypnotics. In two case studies, DSIP was thought to ameliorate symptoms of withdrawal from benzodiazepines and to improve wakefulness in a narcoleptic patient (Schneider-Helmert, 1984, 1985).

Muramyl Dipeptide (MDP)

In 1967, Pappenheimer, Miller, and Goodrich described factor S, a low-molecular-weight (100-dalton) substance from sleep-deprived rabbit brains which, when infused into the cerebrospinal fluid of rabbits or rats, increased non-REM sleep for several hours. Later a similar substance, SPU, was obtained from human urine (Krueger, Bacsik, and Garcia-Arraras, 1980). Although not all studies in animals have been positive (Mendelson et al., 1982a), there has been continued interest in this substance, leading to the finding that it closely resembles the muramyl dipeptides found in bacterial cell walls (Krueger, Pappenheimer, and Karnovsky, 1982; Krueger, 1986). In rats, 2 nmole of MDP infused intraventricularly increased non-REM sleep in the middle of the infusion period, and increased body temperature as well. In at least one study in rats, MDP did not alter temperature or slow-wave sleep (Fornal, Markus, and Radulovacki, 1984). Further studies seem indicated, then, before the significance of earlier MDP findings can be determined. Work with MDP may be pointing to an intriguing relationship between the immune system and sleep. Preliminary studies, for instance, have claimed that interleukin 1 and interleukin 2 increase during human sleep (Moldofsky, 1986) and that various lymphokines enhance slow-wave sleep in animals.

Since the mid-1970s Uchizono's group has described a sleep-enhancing substance from the brain stem of sleep-deprived rats (Uchizono et al., 1975, 1978). Original reports described decreased motor activity and enhanced delta wave activity; later studies found increases in both non-REM and REM sleep (Nagasaki et al., 1980; Inoue et al., 1984). Mendelson, Gillin, and Wyatt (1983f) were unable to find sleep-promoting effects from a substance prepared in a similar manner. Issues of dose, time of sacrifice of animals, and similar factors seem necessary to further clarify the possible effects of SPS.

Steroids

It has been known for some time that certain steroids may have sedative properties, and some have been used as anesthetics. 3 Alpha, 5 alpha-tetrahydrodeoxycorticosterone (THDOC), a potent hypnotic in rats, is discussed in detail in Chapter 4.

Cholecystokinin (CCK)

CCK is an example of the series of peptides found in both gut and brain. The biological activity of CCK is centered around the C-terminal octapeptide (CCK-8), which decreases motor activity (Zetler, 1980) and food consumption (Crawley, Rojas-Ramirez, and Mendelson, 1982). CCK is thought to coexist with dopamine in mesolimbic neurons (Hokfelt et al., 1980), and its effects on satiety may be mediated by peripheral receptors, with feedback to the CNS via the vagus nerve, insofar as vagotomy greatly reduces these effects. In one study, 10 μg/kg of CCK was given intraperitoneally to rats. A decrease in sleep latency was observed (Crawley, Rojas-Ramirez, and Mendelson, 1982). Other actions, such as those on satiety, occur at much lower doses. The tentative implication seems to be that CCK-8 is a very active peptide in terms of behavioral quiescence but may have little effect in terms of sleep.

In summary, a number of circulating endogenous substances appear to alter various aspects of sleep. It is uncertain if their mechanisms of action relate to traditional structures and neurotransmitters thought to be involved in sleep regulation. Among the few associations noted to date is the possibility that AVT may involve serotonergic mechanisms and that CCK-8 (which is probably associated more with behavioral sedation than with sleep) may coexist with dopamine in certain neurons. Muramyl-dipeptide is of particular interest in that it relates sleep regulation to immunological mechanisms.

DISCUSSION

The human studies described here are necessarily indirect and open to varying interpretations. Some common themes, however, may be found throughout the data. We will now examine these and suggest some hypotheses that may explain a number of the observations.

Serotonin

We have presented a variety of studies in which drugs that modify serotonergic activity were found to influence sleep. This brings a number of questions to mind:

1. What is the nature of the relation of serotonin to REM and non-REM sleep?
2. Do current electrophysiological or receptor studies shed light on the seeming contradictions of serotonin-related pharmacological studies?
3. How necessary is serotonergic function to sleep regulation?

Serotonin and REM Sleep

Parachlorophenylalanine, which decreases synthesis of serotonin, reduces the amount of REM sleep in humans with little change in non-REM sleep (Wyatt, 1972). Since this effect can be reversed by giving the serotonin precursor 5-HTP, it seems likely that decreases in serotonergic activity were, in fact, related to reductions in REM sleep. The effects of PCPA are all the more striking in that (1) REM sleep is decreased as long as PCPA is given (in contrast to the experience with such REM-suppressing drugs as the sedative–hypnotics) and (2) when PCPA is discontinued, REM sleep gradually returns to normal, with no "rebound" increase. These findings imply that PCPA interferes with the genesis of REM sleep in some very fundamental way. Conversely, raising serotonergic activity with low doses of 5-HTP or alpha-methyl-5-HTP increases REM sleep. Fluoxetine, which may enhance serotonergic activity, has been reported to increase REM sleep in prepubertal boys (Pavel *et al.*, 1981); the receptor blocker methysergide, however, decreases REM sleep (Mendelson *et al.*, 1975a). Within limits, then, in humans there seems to be a positive correlation between drug effects that might alter serotonin function and the total amount of REM sleep.

Animal studies have given mixed results with regard to REM sleep. Such agents as fluoxetine, quipazine, or fenfluramine, which might be expected to enhance serotonergic activity, tend to decrease REM sleep. The classical PCPA studies in animals, however, indicate that this serotonin-depleting agent acutely decreases REM sleep. Another suggestion growing out of PCPA studies has been that serotonin may act as a releasing agent for a nonindoleamine endogenous factor that induces REM sleep (Sallanon *et al.*, 1985); this will be addressed later in the chapter.

Serotonin and Non-REM Sleep

In contrast to human studies, animal studies have emphasized the relationship of serotonin to both non-REM and REM sleep. The two foundations of this viewpoint are observations of the acute effects of lesions of the raphe nuclei and on the administration of doses of PCPA that are much higher than those given to humans. Under these conditions (and with the possible exception of the rat), PCPA markedly decreases non-REM sleep and less strikingly, decreases REM sleep (Table 2-5). In the cat, for instance, a sleepless state develops within 24–48 hr of a large acute dose of PCPA and persists for about a week. This may be reversed by giving 5-HTP (Petitjean *et al.*, 1985). Analogously, a reduction in sleep is induced by injecting the benzodiazepine triazolam into the dorsal raphe nuclei, presumably by facilitating GABAergic

TABLE 2-5. Effects of Parachlorophenylalanine on Sleep

Study	Animal	Non-REM	REM	Dosage (mg/kg)
Delorme, 1986	Cat	↓	↓	100–300
Torda, 1967	Rat	↓	?	510
Crowley *et al.*, 1969	Monkey	↓	?	1,000
Florio *et al.*, 1968	Cat, rat, rabbit	↓	↓	300
Koella, Feldstein, and Czieman, 1968; Koella, 1969	Cat	↓	↓	50–200
Mouret, Bobillier, and Jouvet, 1968	Rat	↓	↓	500
Weitzman *et al.*, 1968b	Monkey	↓	0	600–1,000
Dement, 1969	Cat	↓	↓	75–300
Rechtschaffen *et al.*, 1969	Rat	↓	↓	500
Wyatt, 1972	Man	0	↓	50
Pujol *et al.*, 1971	Cat	↓	↓	500
Bert, 1972	Baboon	↓	↓	150–300
Ursin, 1972	Cat	↓	0	200
Chernik *et al.*, 1973	Man	0	0[a]	30
Cohen, Dement, and Barchas, 1973	Cat	↓	↓	150
Kaufman, 1983	Albino rat	↓	↓	376
Borbely *et al.*, 1981b	Rat	↓[b]	↓	300
Petitjean *et al.*, 1985	Cat	↓[c]	↓[c]	400
Gaillaird and St. Hilaire-Kafi, 1985	Rat	↓	↓	200

[a]Patient on methadone and PCPA; although REM sleep did not change, other REM measures diminished.
[b]Initial increase in non-REM, followed by decrease.
[c]Reversed by parenteral administration of D,L 5-HTP.

inhibition of serotonergic neuronal activity (Mendelson *et al.*, 1987a; Fig. 2-11).

A similar discrepancy between clinical and animal studies appears with serotonin receptor blockers. While a human study of methysergide found a relatively discrete suppression of REM sleep (Mendelson *et al.*, 1975a), a rabbit study reported decreases in both REM and non-REM sleep (Tabushi and Himwich, 1971). Yet another source of data suggesting a role for serotonin in non-REM sleep came from studies in which raphe nuclei lesions, which lower serotonin concentration acutely, induced a state in which very little non-REM or REM sleep occurred.

In summary, human pharmacological studies have tended to emphasize the relation of serotonin to REM sleep, whereas animal studies have pointed to a role for serotonin in both non-REM and REM sleep.

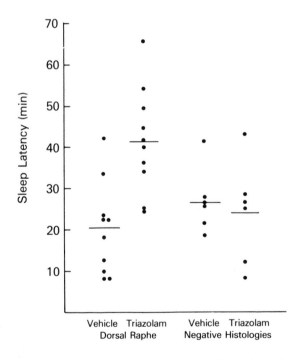

FIGURE 2-11. Sleep latencies in rats in which vehicle or 0.5 μg of triazolam were injected into the dorsal raphe nuclei (left) or surrounding areas ("negative histologies," right). It can be seen that triazolam significantly ($p < 0.002$) increased sleep latency when injected into the dorsal raphe nuclei. During an 8-hr recording it also decreased non-REM ($p < 0.01$) and total sleep ($p < 0.01$). Benzodiazepines may facilitate GABA function (e.g., Costa *et al.*, 1982), and it is possible that the arousing effect seen here is the result of facilitation of GABAergic inhibition of neuronal firing rate in the dorsal raphe nuclei.

These discrepancies may merely reflect differences in dosage. Another possibility is that decreases in non-REM sleep in animal studies are the result of a rapid rate of change in serotonin concentrations. One suggestion that this is the case comes from human studies, in which acute discontinuation of 5-HTP or phenelzine (that presumably produce a sudden decline from pharmacologically induced high serotonin concentrations) led to severe loss of sleep (Wyatt and Gillin, 1975; Wyatt, Kaplan, and Vaughan, 1973; Wyatt et al., 1972a).

Yet another approach to explain some of the apparent differences between human and animal studies has been the *phasic event suppression hypothesis*. This view derives from the observations of Dement et al. (1969), who noted that PGO spikes, which are normally confined to REM sleep, appeared in non-REM sleep and in waking in PCPA-treated cats. They suggested that a function of serotonergic neurons is to confine such phasic events as PGO spikes to REM sleep. It follows that when serotonin concentrations decrease, PGO waves enter non-REM sleep, where they might serve as a disruptive influence to reduce non-REM sleep. Perhaps the low doses of PCPA given to humans lead to a more gradual release of PGO waves into non-REM sleep, with time for habituation and, hence, less sleep disruption.

One challenge to the PGO suppression hypothesis comes from the observation that, in albino rats, PCPA does not seem to affect PGO waves, yet it still decreases sleep greatly (Kaufman, 1983). This hypothesis might be tested further by giving low doses of PCPA to cats, but such data are not yet available. Another difficulty with this hypothesis comes from studies of rhesus monkeys, in which PCPA decreased non-REM sleep without altering REM sleep (Weitzman et al., 1968b; Crowley, Pegram, and Smith, 1969).

Other lines of evidence argue against interpreting the animal PCPA and raphe lesion studies as showing a critical role for serotonin in the maintenance of non-REM sleep. The first is that the time-course of sleep enhancement by 5-HTP in PCPA-treated animals, which may be up to 10 hr, is difficult to explain on the basis of restoration of serotonergic activity (Sallanon et al., 1985). The second is that during chronic administration of PCPA, total sleep time has been reported to return to normal after about a week, although serotonin concentrations remain suppressed (Dement et al., 1969). Similarly, the decrease in the amount of sleep produced by lesions of the dorsal raphe nuclei in cats is only temporary, later returning to normal (Morgane and Stern, 1972). Children with phenylketonuria, in whom blood and CNS serotonin concentrations are low, have sleep similar to that of controls (Schulte et al., 1973). These observations suggest that acute perturbations of serotonin do alter non-REM sleep, but that, in time, compensatory mechanisms will return sleep to normal. This implies that the role of serotonin in non-REM sleep is much less critical than was originally supposed.

Electrophysiological Studies

Electrophysiological data have also altered concepts of the role of serotonin in sleep. As discussed in Chapter 1, a widely accepted view is that serotonergic and noradrenergic neurons may fire most rapidly in the waking state, with a progressive decline in non-REM and REM sleep (McGinty and Harper, 1976; Jacobs, 1985). If this is so, and if this association is causal and not merely correlative, then the implication might be that increased serotonergic or noradrenergic activity would cause a decline in non-REM sleep, in favor of wakefulness. The observation that many clinically used stimulants facilitate aminergic activity is consistent with this view.

The nature of aminergic neurons, as observed in the electrophysiology laboratory, may also influence the interpretation of pharmacological observations. Jacobs (1985), in describing serotonergic and noradrenergic neurons, emphasizes that they are autoactive and are also exquisitely sensitive to inhibition by their own neurotransmitters through their autoreceptors. When a serotonin agonist has a given effect on sleep, then, it is difficult to know whether to attibute this effect to enhanced serotonergic activity on postsynaptic target neurons or to autoinhibition of serotonergic neurons.

Another outgrowth of electrophysiological work has been broader hypotheses that attempt to describe the role of neurotransmitters in the regulation of all three states of consciousness (waking, non-REM sleep, and REM sleep), rather than taking the traditional view in which investigators attempted to relate specific neurotransmitters to specific stages of sleep. In the "reciprocal interaction hypothesis," for instance, the state of consciousness depends on the relative activity of largely aminergic "REM-off" cells and primarily cholinergic "REM-on" cells (Chapter 1). This suggests that drug-induced increases in aminergic activity relative to cholinergic activity might lead progressively from REM sleep to non-REM sleep to waking. It seems likely that views that try to explain neurotransmitter function both in relation to other transmitters and to all states of consciousness will be more fruitful than views that do not offer such explanations.

A Releasing Agent for Sleep Factors?

One response to both the electrophysiological findings of decreased serotonergic activity in sleep and to the discrepant timing of biochemical and hypnogenic effects of 5-HTP in PCPA-pretreated animals has been to explore alternative relationships of serotonin to sleep. Sallanon *et al.* (1983) found that administration of PCPA at the end of 48 hr of sleep deprivation in cats resulted in a loss of rebound of deep slow-wave sleep (SWS₂) and a great decrease in light slow-wave sleep (SWS₁). Interestingly, episodes suggestive of REM sleep still appeared, accompanied by "narcolepticlike attacks" (see Chapter 7). This was taken to imply that release of serotonin in waking or during sleep deprivation may be necessary for the expression of a possible SWS₂ factor (Sallanon *et al.*, 1985). As we will see later, a study using a slightly different approach was not consistent with the basic observation on which this hypothesis is based (Tobler and Borbely, 1982), so some caution regarding this view is appropriate. It was also observed that infusion of CSF from REM sleep-deprived cats into PCPA-treated cats produced a slight increase in slow-wave sleep and a large increase in REM. The cerebrospinal fluid from both control and REM-deprived animals contained total indoleamines (5-HTP, 5-HIAA, serotonin) in quantities at least 1000 times less than the minimal amount of 5-HTP needed to restore sleep in PCPA-pretreated animals. This implies that

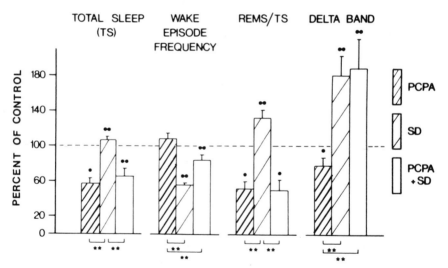

FIGURE 2-12. The effect of treatment with PCPA, sleep deprivation (SD), and a combined treatment (PCPA and SD) on sleep. Mean values with SEM are expressed as a percentage of the control day (100%, ---). Control-day values for group 1 (PCPA; $n=9$) and group 2 (SD and PCPA+SD; $n=6$) are, respectively: TS, 76.8 and 76.2%; (REM/TS) × 100, 21.1, and 18.9%; wake episode frequency per hour, 21.6 and 21.0. The power density of the delta band in non-REM sleep was expressed in arbitrary units. •, Significant differences from control; *, significant differences between the values marked by brackets (• and *, $p < 0.05$; •• and **, $p < 0.01$; Wilcoxon paired and unpaired signed rank test, two-tailed). (From Tobler and Borbely, 1982. Reprinted by permission.)

a substance independent of serotonergic mechanisms can induce REM sleep.

Receptor Subtypes

As mentioned in the discussion of ritanserin, it now appears that subtypes of serotonin receptors exist (Iverson, 1985). Types 1 and 2 have been defined by binding of serotonin and ketanserin, respectively, and are found both in the central nervous system, and peripherally. The traditional serotonin blockers discussed such as methysergide, cyproheptadine, and methergoline, may bind primarily at type 2; LSD may bind at both types. A new class of serotonin blockers, typified by ICS 205-903, shares structural similarities to both serotonin and cocaine. These agents bind to type M receptors, which may be associated with peripheral nervous tissue. So far, receptors for these new antagonists have not been reported in the CNS, but if they should be found there, then the effects of these compounds on sleep would be of interest. For purposes of the immediate discussion, however, the point is that subtypes of serotonin receptors exist and that they could conceivably have different actions on sleep and waking. If this were so, then it is possible that apparent contradictions between different pharmacological studies might involve effects on different receptor subtypes.

How Necessary Is Serotonergic Activity to Sleep Regulation?

Another approach to determining the role of serotonin in sleep regulation would be to observe which processes still occur after acute serotonin depletion. Tobler and Borbely (1982) gave PCPA to rats 2 hr before 24-hr sleep deprivation. The latter procedure, alone, was followed by recovery sleep with increased energy in the delta EEG band and decreased incidence of waking episodes. After pretreatment with PCPA, sleep deprivation was still followed by both these occurrences (Fig. 2-12). These data should be considered tentative, since they contradict those of Sallanon *et al.* (1983), whose study differed in dose, number of injections of PCPA, and method and duration of sleep deprivation. They suggest, however, that even acutely some basic regulatory processes of non-REM sleep continue to function after serotonin depletion.

Dopamine

The most striking feature of agents that affect dopamine is the inconsistency of results. L-DOPA has variable effects on REM sleep;

reports have also been mixed with regard to non-REM sleep, although high doses tend to reduce it. Receptor agonists (piribedil, apomorphine) have been found to decrease REM sleep, whereas some antagonists (pimozide, chlorpromazine) have relatively little effect in normal subjects. Agents with mixed catecholaminergic effects but which tend to predominantly enhance dopamine activity (D-amphetamine, methylphenidate, high doses of L-DOPA, cocaine) decrease total sleep time (Gillin et al., 1978a). Also, like many noradrenergic agonists, they decrease REM sleep time. The stimulating effects of these agents seem consistent with studies of lesions in the ventral mesencephalic tegmentum, which extensively destroy dopamine-containing neurons and lead to a state of lack of behavioral arousal with no evident change in the EEG (Jones et al., 1973). This suggests that behavioral aspects of arousal are separable from EEG markers of waking and that dopamine may play a role particularly in the former.

One challenge to the pharmacologist will be to relate the observations with regard to stimulants that are largely noradrenergic and dopaminergic agonists to the results of electrophysiological studies of dopamine-rich areas. The substantia nigra and the ventral tegmental area have fairly slow, regular firing patterns, with virtually no change between waking, non-REM-sleep, and REM sleep (Jacobs, 1985). The method by which mixed dopamine agonists might induce wakefulness is, thus, not clear.

Norepinephrine

In general, changes in catecholaminergic activity seem to affect REM sleep in the opposite direction as changes in serotonergic activity. Inhibition of tyrosine hydroxylase with AMPT, which may lower functional levels of norepinephrine, usually has led to increases in REM sleep (Table 2-2). The alpha blocker thymoxamine may also enhance REM sleep. The observation that amphetamines, which enhance catecholaminergic activity, decrease REM would be consistent with this view. Propranolol, however, has been reported to have little effect on REM sleep in humans, and clonidine (which because of its $alpha_2$ agonist properties might be expected to decrease alpha noradrenergic activity) may reduce REM sleep. The literature on human studies, then, is not entirely consistent; perhaps studies with the newer $alpha_1$ and $alpha_2$ agonists or antagonists will clarify some of these issues. Interesting leads from the animal literature include the observation that phentolamine and bromocriptine may prevent a REM rebound after REM deprivation; this suggests a critical role of catecholamines in the "need" for REM sleep.

Acetylcholine

Less information is available about the role of the cholinergic system in humans, although in general it appears to be facilitative to REM sleep. Atropine and scopolamine suppress REM sleep; it is increased by anticholinesterases. These findings seem consistent with the results of animal studies, in which the systemic administration of atropine (Jouvet, 1969) and the intraventricular administration of hemicholinium-3 (Hazara, 1970) reduce REM sleep. Acetylcholine is known to be released from the cerebral cortex of cats at a higher rate during REM than during slow-wave sleep (Jasper and Tessier, 1971). Physostigmine induces REM sleep in the pontine cat (Jouvet, 1969). Similarly, Sitaram et al. (1976) found that intravenous physostigmine can induce episodes of REM sleep in humans without affecting total REM sleep for the night or the length of the first REM period. This suggests that cholinergic systems are related to initiation, rather than duration, of REM sleep episodes. In animal studies, however, when neostigmine is infused into the pontine reticular formation, the timing and duration of REM sleep episodes can be altered, and individual components of REM sleep can be induced (Baghdoyan, McCarley, and Hobson, 1985). This implies that acetylcholine plays a role in orchestrating a series of mechanisms that, in their totality, appear as REM sleep.

Circulating Sleep Factors

In the last few years, work on possible circulating sleep factors has increased greatly. The administration of AVT and DSIP in humans has been of particular interest. The former appears to be more associated with aspects of REM sleep; it has been claimed that the latter promotes sleep, when given under conditions conducive to sleep, and enhances wakefulness, when given during the day. Little is known about whether these possible sleep factors act via classic neurotransmitters, although it has been suggested that AVT acts by an inhibitory GABAergic action on the serotonergic system.

Gamma-Aminobutyric Acid

Sleep studies in animals with drugs that increase or decrease GABAergic activity have been very inconsistent. These range from enhancing (GHB, baclofen, GABA), decreasing (progabide, possibly picrotoxin), or inducing dose-dependent biphasic (AOAA) effects on sleep. Although the major role played by GABA in some actions of systemically administered benzodiazepines (e.g., anticonvulsant ef-

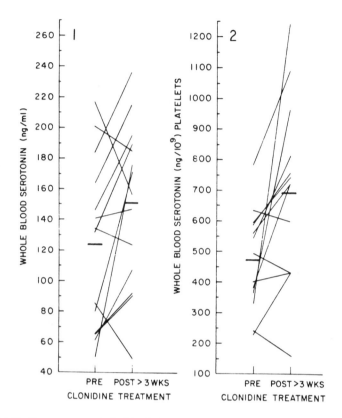

FIGURE 2-13. Pretreatment whole blood 5-HT levels (ng/ml) and ng/10⁹ platelets versus whole blood 5-HT post three week clonidine (3–6 μg/kg a day, orally). Bars, mean whole blood 5-HT levels. (From Leckman *et al.*, 1984. Reprinted by permission.)

fects) is clear, the role of GABA in sleep processes appears to be uncertain.

Interaction between Transmitters

Many inconsistencies and unpredicted responses to drugs have been presented here. We have attempted to reconcile differences and find common trends by noting that responses to drugs may depend on dose, duration, and administration route. Another factor that may aid in the understanding of the effects of drugs on sleep is interactions between neurotransmitters. It has been observed, for instance, that in some cases cholinesterase inhibitors may not only raise levels of acetylcholine, but may also increase serotonin and decrease norepinephrine (Karczmar, 1975). In the Englen *et al.* (1980) study, caffeine (which might be expected to affect adenosine and cyclic AMP function) changed REM sleep and dopamine concentrations in subsequent generations of rats. Neuroanatomical and iontophoretic studies also suggested interactions between serotonergic and noradrenergic systems (Bunney and de Reimer, 1982). Raphe lesions may lead to an increased turnover of norepinephrine (Pujol *et al.*, 1973), whereas destruction of the rostral one-third of the locus ceruleus increases tryptophan and 5-HIAA (Petitjean and Jouvet, 1970). Serotonergic fibers appear in the area of the locus ceruleus (Pickel, Joh, and Reis, 1978) and noradrenergic terminals are found in the dorsal raphe nuclei (Aghajanian, 1981). Such interactions also appear in clinical pharmacological studies. For instance, clonidine, an alpha$_2$ adrenergic receptor agonist, may cause elevations in plasma serotonin in patients with Tourette's syndrome (Leckman *et al.*, 1984; Fig. 2-13). Fenfluramine, which may enhance release and block re-uptake of serotonin, lowers plasma norepinephrine in depressed patients (Lake *et al.*, 1979). Thus, it is clear that neurotransmitters cannot be studied in isolation; an understanding of their effects must include recognition of their actions on other transmitters. Finally, it should be remembered that, for all their complexity, the serotonergic, adrenergic, and cholinergic systems make up less than 1% of the synaptic connections in the brain. It seems likely that a more complete understanding of the regulation of sleep will await knowledge of other neurotransmitter systems.

CHAPTER 3

Pharmacological Treatment of Insomnia

About 35% of the American population complain of difficulty going to sleep or maintaining sleep, and perhaps half of this group consider it a major problem (Mellinger and Balter, 1983). As a consequence, many persons consult a physician, and 4.3% of them receive a prescription for a sleep medication each year. (About 60% of these persons receive a traditional hypnotic; the remainder receive anxiolytics and antidepressants.) Of those who obtain medication, roughly three-fourths take it for less than two weeks; 11%, however, use it nightly for over a year. Although the utilization of hypnotics is widespread, the total number of prescriptions is less than in past years. Since careful data were first collected in 1964, the number of prescriptions rose from 32.5 million to a peak of 42 million in 1971 and gradually declined to 23 million in 1982. In 1985, there were approximately 24 million prescriptions for barbiturates (excluding long-acting forms), chloral hydrate, and other nonbarbiturate hypnotics combined.* Of the nonbarbiturate prescriptions (21 million), 94% were for benzodiazepines.

The type of hypnotics prescribed has also changed over the years. Flurazepam (Table 3-1) was introduced into the marketplace in 1970. From 1971, when it made up 7% of hypnotic prescriptions, it rose to 53% by 1977 (Institute of Medicine, 1979b). In 1982, it amounted to

---

*Data kindly supplied by National Prescription Audit, IMS American, Ltd., Ambler, PA 19002.
Portions of this chapter are taken from Mendelson (1985). Reprinted by permission.

TABLE 3-1. Generic and Trade Names of
Common Anxiolytics and Hypnotics

Generic name	Registered trade name
Chloral hydrate	Noctec
Chlordiazepoxide	Librium
Diazepam	Valium
Ethinamate	Valmid
Flurazepam	Dalmane
Glutethimide	Doriden
Lorazepam	Ativan
Methyprylon	Noludar
Oxazepam	Serax
Temazepam	Restoril
Triazolam	Halcion

two-thirds of all such prescriptions. By 1985, with the growing use of short-acting benzodiazepines, the three most widely prescribed non-barbiturate agents were flurazepam, triazolam, and temazepam.

A survey of more than 4000 physicians indicates that about 17% of their patients complained of insomnia; the specialists to whom such comments were most frequent were psychiatrists, who reported insomnia in 32.4% (Bixler et al., 1979). Of the prescriptions given in response to these complaints in 1985, only about 64% were traditional sedative–hypnotics. Other classes of medications included benzodiazepine minor tranquilizers (13%), antidepressants (7%), phenothiazines (5%), and antihistamines (3%).* Physicians also tended to view sleep difficulty in the context of some other medical or psychiatric illness. In 1985, only 12% of nonbarbiturate sedative prescriptions were given to patients with an isolated "diagnosis" of sleep disturbance.*

This chapter will examine the role of hypnotics in the treatment of sleep disturbance. After a few comments on some aspects of insomnia and the pharmacology of these agents, possible benefits and disadvantages will be considered. Among the latter are residual daytime effects, reliance, alterations in respiration, interactions with alcohol, and special problems of the elderly.

ASPECTS OF INSOMNIA

Perhaps the major movement in sleep research in recent years has been the growing recognition that insomnia may be a manifestation of

*National Disease and Therapeutic Index, IMS America, Ltd., Ambler, PA 19002.

a variety of disorders. This viewpoint is best represented in a systematic nosology of sleep disorders (Association of Sleep Disorders Centers, 1979), which describes a variety of pathophysiological and psychological conditions that result in the sensation of disturbed sleep. Relatively specific treatments are available for many of them, such as tricyclic antidepressants for patients with sleep disturbance resulting from affective disorders, or surgical procedures for obstructive sleep apnea. In most of these cases, hypnotics are unlikely to help; under some conditions, they may conceivably be dangerous, as in patients with sleep apnea (Mendelson, Garnett, and Gillin, 1981a). With a few special exceptions, then, it seems reasonable to suggest that the use of hypnotics be directed to acute situational difficulties and to those chronic disorders in which no major pathophysiology has been found. In terms of the current nosology, many of the latter fall into such categories as "persistent psychophysiological disorders of initiating and maintaining sleep" (DIMS), "subjective DIMS complaint without objective findings," and "not otherwise specified complaints" (see Chapter 12). Possible exceptions to this rule of thumb might be the adjunctive use of hypnotics in major affective disorders, the benefits of which have not been well established, and the use of hypnotics after acute phase shift of the sleep–waking cycle, an area currently under investigation.

PHARMACOLOGY OF HYPNOTICS

Prescription hypnotics may conveniently be grouped into three classes, the pharmacology of which has been reviewed in detail (Mendelson, 1980).

Barbiturates

From the time that Veronal was introduced by Fischer and von Mering in 1903, barbiturates were widely used as sedatives and hypnotics; their use declined only after the introduction of the benzodiazepines in the early 1960s. In 1985, barbiturates represented only 9% of hypnotic prescriptions. However, there is a continuing concern about the lethality of overdoses (death often results from about 10 therapeutic doses), abuse potential, interaction with alcohol, and the stimulation of hepatic microsomal oxidizing systems responsible for metabolizing a variety of drugs. This latter property may enhance the breakdown of concomitantly administered drugs that are metabolized by cytochrome

P-450. Thus drugs that are metabolized by P-450 to inactive compounds might be expected to have less therapeutic effect when given with barbiturates. In the case of the anticonvulsant valproic acid, which is metabolized by P-450 to a hepatotoxic compound, the potential for liver damage may be increased if the two drugs are given together (Rettie *et al.*, 1987).

The biturates most often used as hypnotics are secobarbital, amobarbital, and pentobarbital, which are considered short- to intermediate-acting, with plasma half-lives of 14 to 48 hr. They are rapidly distributed in body tissues, metabolized primarily in the liver, and excreted as conjugated hydroxyl compounds by the kidney.

Benzodiazepines

These compounds were introduced as the anxiolytics chlordiazepoxide and diazepam in the 1960s, and flurazepam was marketed as a hypnotic in 1970. More recently, short-acting benzodiazepines recommended for anxiety (lorazepam) and sleep (temazepam) have become available, as has the traizolobenzodiazepine hypnotic triazolam. Benzodiazepines are relatively benign compared to other drug classes when taken alone in acute overdose by medically healthy persons. Although at low doses and with relatively subtle measures, there may be no interaction (or even antagonism) of some alcohol effects, toxicity is clearly potentiated by alcohol in clinical overdose. There has been little "street" drug abuse with these agents, in contrast to other classes of hypnotics. However, at least one study suggests that patients are as likely to develop reliance (prolonged use of prescribed doses) with benzodiazepines as with barbiturates (Clift, 1975).

Benzodiazepines are not thought to stimulate hepatic microsomal oxidizing systems, but their own metabolism may be altered by drugs that do affect hepatic function. Flurazepam is absorbed relatively rapidly; it is, however, a relatively long-acting agent, the active metabolite (desalkylflurazepam) having a plasma half-life of 47 to 100 hr. After hepatic transformation, metabolites are excreted primarily in the urine, in which approximately 81% of the dose can be found after 98 hr (Schwartz and Postma, 1970). Among the short-acting benzodiazepines, temazepam decreases in the plasma in a biphasic manner, with half-lives of 0.6 and 9 hr; after ingestion, peak levels are not achieved for 2 to 3 hr. Triazolam and lorazepam, with half-lives of 1.5 to 5 and 10 to 20 hr, respectively, attain peak-blood levels in 1 to 2 hr. In contrast to such long-acting benzodiazepines such as flurazepam, all are metabolized to inactive compounds before excretion.

Nonbarbiturate, Nonbenzodiazepine Hypnotics

These include compounds from a variety of pharmacological classes, such as chloral hydrate, methaqualone, the piperidinedione compounds glutethimide and methyprylon, ethchlorvynol, and ethinamate. Because of the heterogeneity of this group, generalizations are difficult. Most are very toxic in acute overdose, have enhanced toxicity when combined with alcohol, and are associated with varying degrees of abuse potential. With the possible exception of ethchlorvynol, they tend to stimulate hepatic microsomal oxidizing systems.

EFFICACY STUDIES OF HYPNOTICS

The issues of how best to assess the efficacy of hypnotics are complex. Insofar as the ultimate goal is the patient's sense of having slept well, nonlaboratory clinical studies ot subjective response are important. On the other hand, EEG studies provide objective measures and guard against the possibility that patients prefer a particular agent for some other property than sleep induction, such as euphoriant qualities. Thus, at this time it seems wise to assess hypnotics by both means. Problems in testing hypnotics have been reviewed by Mendelson et al. (1980), and basic standards for studies have been discussed by a number of authors, including Kay et al. A review of the literature suggests that few efficacy studies of barbiturates or other nonbenzodiazepine hypnotics have been conducted since that time. The following sections discuss efficacy studies of flurazepam, triazolam, and temazepam, the three most commonly prescribed benzodiazepines. The material is a fairly detailed account of individual studies, and is intended for reference. *The reader who wishes more generalized information will find a brief summary at the end of the review of each drug.*

Flurazepam

Clinical Studies

A variety of studies summarized by Mendelson (1980), as well as more recent work (Fillingim, 1982; Roehrs et al., 1982; Hartmann, Lindsley, and Spinweber, 1983; Murphy and Ankier, 1984) indicate that flurazepam, given for a week or less, is clearly beneficial. Little difference in efficacy between 15 and 30 mg was brought out in these subjective reports. In the Murphy and Ankier (1984) study, 15-

mg doses given to 85 insomniacs for five nights improved the ease of going to sleep, as well as sleep quality, depth, and duration. In one of the few negative studies, Linnoila, Erwin, and Logue (1980) found that 30 mg flurazepam given for 14 days was not more effective than a placebo in inducing sleep. One study in geriatric outpatients (Reeves, 1977), and one in younger insomniacs (Dement et al., 1978), found that 30 mg flurazepam helped in sleep induction for a period of 28 nights. Mendelson et al. (1982c) found a nonsignificant trend toward decreased sleep latency on the first two nights of administration; subjective total sleep time was not significantly altered but tended to increase over the 28 nights studied. Leibowitz and Feldman (1978) found that both 30 mg flurazepam and 0.6 mg triazolam benefited sleep over 12 weeks, although triazolam had a more rapid onset of action. In the Boston Collaborative Drug Surveillance Program (1972), physicians who made a judgment about efficacy felt that 85.7% of patients taking 15 mg and 91.4% taking 30 mg flurazepam had a "satisfactory" response.

EEG Studies

Reports of one (Hartmann, 1968), four (Vogel et al., 1976), five (Kales et al., 1971), seven (Roehrs et al., 1982), and nine (Roehrs et al., 1986) nights of flurazepam administration demonstrated increased total sleep time as well as decreased sleep latency and intermittent wakefulness. In the Roehrs et al. (1982, 1986) studies, the reduction in latency to persistent sleep reached statistical significance only on the first (1982) or first and second (1986) drug nights.

There have been at least four studies of four-weeks and one study of five-weeks administration of flurazepam. Kales et al. (1975c) gave 30 mg of flurazepam to four subjects and reported that total sleep time rose by 6 to 8%, whereas intermittent waking decreased by 14 to 17 min. Sleep latency was significantly decreased only on nights 11 through 13. When these data were later combined with shorter-term studies (Kales et al., 1976d), sleep latency was not significantly decreased until the second night. Dement et al. (1978) gave 30 mg flurazepam to five insomniacs and reported that total sleep time was increased by 1–2 hr over the 28 nights; decreases in sleep latency and intermittent waking time were not statistically significant. Mendelson and colleagues (1982c) gave 30 mg of flurazepam to 10 insomniacs and found total sleep to be increased by over 1 hr during the second and fourth weeks (Fig. 3-1). Both sleep latency and intermittent waking time tended to decrease but did not reach statistical significance. Kales and colleagues (1982c) reported that in six insomniacs given 30 mg of

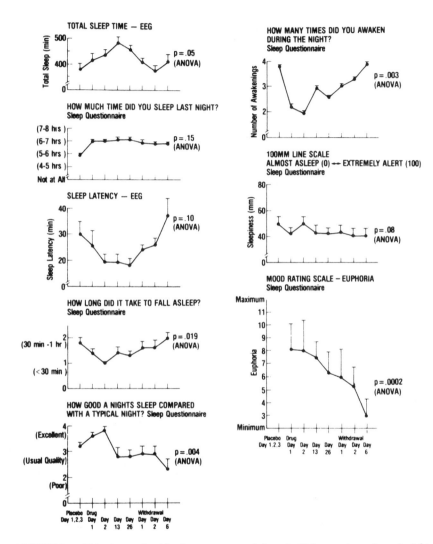

FIGURE 3-1. Objective and subjective measures of sleep in 10 insomniacs given 4 nights of placebo, 28 nights of 30 mg of flurazepam, and 7 nights of placebo. (From Mendelson et al., 1981. Reprinted by permission.)

flurazepam for 28 nights, the percent of sleep time was enhanced. Improvement in sleep latency was no longer evident by the fourth week. Mitler *et al.* (1984) found improvement in sleep latency only during the first week of administration of 30 mg flurazepam; total sleep was significantly increased for the first three weeks of the five-week study.

Summary

In summary, clinical studies of flurazepam have described improvement in some measures of sleep for as long as 12 weeks. Short-term polygraphic studies of flurazepam have shown significant improvement in sleep maintenance. Studies of four or five weeks of administration have tended to show enhanced total sleep for at least four weeks. Effects on sleep latency have been inconsistent. In some cases improved sleep latency has not been evident until the second night of administration, an observation consistent with the long half-life of flurazepam.

Temazepam

Clinical Studies

Fowler (1977) reported that of 147 general practice outpatients who had already responded well to temazepam for one week, 90% reported a "good" or "very good" response over a 12-week period. Generalization from this study is difficult, however, since the patients were selected on the basis of a good acute response. A study of eight psychiatric patients by Maggini, Murri, and Sacchatti (1969) described patient reports of quieter and more restful sleep. Bixler *et al.* (1978), in a 28-night study of 30-mg temazepam in six insomniacs, found consistent benefits only in terms of a decreased number of awakenings. Mitler, Phillips, and Billiard (1975) gave 30 mg temazepam for 35 nights to seven insomniacs and reported an estimated increase in total sleep but no change in sleep latency. Bailie *et al.* (1980) found that medical inpatients preferred 20 mg temazepam over placebo but not over 5 mg nitrazepam. Lehmann and Liljenberg (1981) gave 20 mg for two nights to five normal volunteers and found no statistically significant change in subjective measures of sleep. Fisher and Dean (1985), in a large multicenter study of 246 patients, found that 1 mg of flunitrazepam was more effective than 20 mg of temazepam.

EEG Studies

In the Maggini *et al.* (1969) study, temazepam decreased sleep latency and increased total sleep. Bixler *et al.* (1978) found no effects on sleep latency or percentage sleep. The number of waking episodes decreased, however. Studies of 20 mg for two nights (Beary *et al.*, 1984) and 30 mg for nine nights (Roehrs *et al.*, 1984) reported significant decreases in sleep latency and increases in total sleep time. Mitler *et al.* (1975) found that 30 mg of temazepam increased total sleep for five weeks. Sleep latency was not significantly reduced, although there was a trend toward reduction in the first week. This may have been related to the relatively short sleep latencies of these patients (20.8 min under baseline conditions). Two studies of normal volunteers found no significant changes in sleep latency with 20 mg (Lehmann and Liljenberg, 1981) or 10 to 30 mg (Nicholson and Stone, 1979), although in the latter study, 30 mg of temazepam decreased the number of waking episodes. Roehrs *et al.* (1986) found that 30 mg reduced latency to persistent sleep and increased total sleep of normal volunteers on the first two drug nights, but not on nights eight and nine. Temazepam has been marketed in relatively soft capsules in Europe and in hard capsules in the United States. The Mitler *et al.* (1975) and Roehrs *et al.* (1984) studies, which showed increased total sleep, but differed with respect to sleep latency, were performed with the hard capsules. The Roehrs (1986c) study used a tablet preparation.

Summary

In summary, clinical and polygraphic studies of patient groups have generally shown benefits of temazepam in increasing total sleep over at least 5 weeks. Studies of normal volunteers have had mixed findings, possibly as the result of their more normal baseline values.

Triazolam

Clinical Studies

A variety of studies have compared triazolam with flurazepam (Nair and Schwartz, 1978; Fabre *et al.*, 1977; Reeves *et al.*, 1977; Sunshine, 1975; Vogel *et al.*, 1976; Leibowitz and Sunshine, 1978), nitrazepam (Ellingsen, 1983), secobarbital and placebo (Rickels *et al.*, 1975), or placebo (Kales *et al.*, 1976c; Vogel *et al.*, 1975c) in various patient groups. In most cases, 0.5 mg triazolam was preferred by patients (or in some manner showed better ratings) than 30 mg flurazepam, 5 mg nitrazepam, or 100 mg secobarbital. [In the Vogel *et al.* (1976) study and in the 12-week study of Leibowitz and Sunshine (1978), ratings of the two drugs were roughly comparable.] When 0.4 and 0.8 mg triazolam were studied, only 0.8 mg of the drug was consistently better than placebo (Sunshine, 1975). Roth, Kramer, and Lutz (1977), however, found dose-dependent benefits with 0.25 and 0.5 mg in comparison to placebo. In the Reeves (1977) study, 0.25 mg triazolam was rated during 28 nights and found to be better than placebo, but it differed from 15 mg flurazepam on only one of six measures (duration of sleep). Similarly, Okawa (1978) found that among elderly insomniacs, triazolam (0.5 mg) was of benefit on the several measures but was considered more effective than 15 mg flurazepam on only one of five scales. Ellingsen (1983) found that 0.5 mg triazolam given for one night to 40 insomniacs was rated better than 5 mg nitrazepam on several scales, including rapidity of falling asleep and sleep duration. Mamelak, Csima, and Price (1984) found that 0.5 mg given to 12 insomniacs for 14 nights significantly increased perceived total sleep for 3 nights and soundness of sleep for all 14 nights but showed only a trend toward decreasing sleep latency. Cordingley, Dean, and Harris (1984) found that 0.25 mg given to 312 general practice outpatients for 7 to 14 nights was generally similar to 1 mg flunitrazepam.

EEG Studies

Kales *et al.* (1976c), in a two-week study of 0.5 mg triazolam in insomniacs, found increased percentage of sleep and decreased waking time in the first week. Sleep latency tended to decrease, but this change did not reach statistical significance. A two-week study of 0.5 mg by Roth *et al.* (1976a) reported decreased sleep latency and awake time. In a comparison of 0.5 mg triazolam and 30 mg flurazepam for four nights, Vogel *et al.* (1976) found both drugs equally effective and better than placebo on a variety of measures. In a seven-night dose-response study, Vogel *et al.* (1975c) found that 0.5 mg triazolam decreased sleep latency, increased total sleep time, and decreased waking time; 0.25 mg had less effect. A six-night study of poor sleepers found that 0.5 mg triazolam reduced sleep latency and increased total sleep time and sleep efficiency (Spinweber and Johnson, 1982). Mamelak *et al.* (1984), as mentioned earlier, reported that 0.5 mg triazolam increased total sleep time and decreased wakefulness over 14 nights, although the trend to decrease sleep latency did not reach significance. Mitler *et al.* (1984) found that 0.5 mg triazolam increased total sleep over the five weeks of the study, although it had little effect on sleep latency during administration.

Summary

In summary, benefits of triazolam have been documented in clinical studies for at least 12 weeks and in EEG studies for at least 5 weeks. These effects are dose-dependent. As we will see later, acute use of triazolam may have some potential benefits during rapid shifts of time of sleep.

RESIDUAL DAYTIME EFFECTS

General Issues

At least two different therapeutic goals may lead a physician to prescribe hypnotics. One of these, as just discussed, is better sleep at night. The second is improved daytime alertness and functioning. The distinction between these goals is important because the relative efficacy of hypnotics differs greatly in the two situations. Although most prescription hypnotics appear to improve some aspects of nocturnal sleep (at least in the short term), the evidence for benefits by day is slight. Detailed reviews by Mendelson (1980) and Johnson and Chernik (1982) describe a host of studies documenting decrements in daytime performance in subjects taking a variety of hypnotics. Some hypnotics have not been associated with daytime impairment, and in one case (to be discussed later), improvement in some measures was noted.

Several studies suggest that hypnotic-induced daytime impairment of performance is not merely of academic interest. In a Finnish study, Linnoila (1978) found diazepam in blood samples from 5% of injured drivers, compared to 2% of controls. Binnie (1983) pointed out that among patients in a general practice in Britain, those taking benzodiazepines had a higher incidence of automobile accidents when they were on medication but not when they were drug free. (Patients taking antidepressants or phenothiazines did not have more accidents.) Although these data are associational and do not necessarily imply causality, other studies suggest that the drugs may be responsible for this effect. Betts and Birtle (1982) had 12 female volunteers drive a Datsun through a test course on the morning after taking 15 mg flurazepam, 20 mg temazepam, or a placebo. On the test in which the cars had to be driven on a weaving course, the drivers who had previously taken flurazepam hit the ballards that defined the course significantly more often. When going through a narrow gap, drivers hit the side more often after having taken either drug, compared to placebo. A variety of other studies have documented such effects in the laboratory, both in terms of motor performance and cognitive function. It has sometimes been argued that although decrements in daytime performance are well described in normal subjects, such findings do not necessarily apply to insomniacs, in whom the benefits from a good night's sleep will outweigh any detrimental pharmacological effect. This does not seem to be the case, for several reasons. First, the sense of discomfort of the insomniac is apparent, but actual deficits in daytime performance are subtle and probably occur in narrow, specific areas. Church and Johnson (1979) found no difference in performance between insomniacs and good sleepers on such tasks as digit-symbol substitution, choice reaction time, and digit span. Linnoila, Seppola, and Mattila (1980), studying patients chosen by case history but without confirmatory EEG studies, found greater variability in performance measures over time and some decrements in tracking and reaction time. Mendelson et al. (1984d) compared insomniacs and controls on a wide variety of measures, including tracking tasks thought to have some relevance to driving skills. Deficits were found in only one area, the quantitative Romberg task. Mendelson et al. (1984c) also found that although insomniacs did not differ from controls on a variety of performance measures such as pegboard speed, finger tapping rate, and letter cancellation, some difficulties with semantic memory were present. As will be discussed in Chapter 12, the impression from the current literature seems to be that although a few subtle deficits have been described (and clearly need further exploration), by and large the few performance decrements of insomniacs are small compared to the host of drug-induced deficits.

A second problem with the view that benefits from improved nighttime sleep may outweigh deficits resulting from daytime pharmacological sedation is that many studies, described in the reviews mentioned above, have documented hypnotic-induced residual daytime impairment in insomniacs. Mendelson et al. (1982c), for instance, found that when insomniacs took 30 mg flurazepam for 28 nights, there were very potent detrimental effects on cognitive performance during the first few days, with scores comparable to those of subjects taking alcohol or scopolamine. Other studies in which vigilance or various performance measures of insomniacs were impaired by flurazepam include those of Tansella, Zimmermann-Tansella, and Lader (1974), Oswald et al. (1978), and Carskadon et al. (1982).

Occasionally, sedative–hypnotics do produce small improvements in performance in normal subjects when given by day, probably by reducing anxiety. Linnoila *et al.* (1974), for example, showed that chronic diazepam administration improved reaction time and slightly improved coordination on a simulated driving task performed at a fixed speed. On the other hand, subjects taking diazepam "drove" faster and made more errors when they were allowed to set their own speed. Thus, improvements in performance after daytime administration are usually selective. It has been suggested that such effects are most noticeably manifest in untrained subjects, in whom anxiety may be playing a relatively larger role, and that this confounding effect may be minimized by using well-trained subjects (Linnoila, 1978).

Data on Performance and Wakefulness

Studies of daytime effects of hypnotics since 1980 have focused on the short-acting benzodiazepines. Ogura *et al.* (1980) examined EEGs of normal volunteers kept in bed for 24 hr after administration of 0.25 and 0.5 mg triazolam, 15 and 30 mg flurazepam, and 5 and 10 mg nitrazepam. Daytime sedation (usually in terms of percentage sleep time or sleep latency) was noted with both flurazepam and nitrazepam; the only major effect of triazolam was some shortening of sleep latency in the morning recording. Spinweber and Johnson (1982) gave 0.5 mg triazolam for six nights to 20 poor sleepers. Morning testing 8.25 hr postdrug showed no decrements on a variety of mood and performance measures, although there was a small decrement on morning six in terms of long-term memory assessed by a recognition task. Pishkin *et al.* (1980) gave a single nighttime dose of 30 mg temazepam, 30 mg flurazepam, or 200 mg secobarbital–amobarbital to 50 normal male volunteers. The barbiturate and (to a lesser degree) flurazepam decreased performance on a variety of motor and cognitive tasks; performance had not decreased on the morning after temazepam administration. Mitler *et al.* (1984) found that 30 mg flurazepam reduced daytime performance on the Wilkinson Addition Test, whereas 0.5 mg triazolam improved it. de Jonghe *et al.* (1984) found no effects of flurazepam or triazolam on a daytime vigilance task. Roehrs *et al.* (1986b) reported that flurazepam (30 mg) significantly increased reaction time and reduced symbol substitution accuracy after the first two nights of administration, but not after nights eight and nine in normal volunteers. The Multiple Sleep Latency Test (MSLT; see Chapter 7) showed increased daytime sleepiness at both times. Temazepam (30 mg) did not significantly alter performance measures. After nights one and two, it induced some daytime sleepiness on the MSLT, which returned to normal on the days following nights eight and nine. Hindmarch (1984a,b) found that 30 mg temazepam impaired performance on choice reaction time and critical flicker fusion tests after single or repeated administration.

The notable exception to the studies showing daytime impairment from nighttime use of hypnotics is a series of studies of triazolam from Stanford University. Dement, Seidel, and Carskadon (1982) reported that 0.5 mg triazolam increased, and 30 mg flurazepam decreased, alertness as measured by the MSLT in normal subjects; they found similar results in a multilaboratory study of insomniacs. Interestingly in the normal group, these alterations occurred without changes in nocturnal sleep. Carskadon et al. (1982) found similar results with 0.25 mg triazolam and 15 mg flurazepam on the MSLT of elderly insomniacs. Again, the correlations between daytime wakefulness and nocturnal sleep were not significant. These findings comprise the first systematic claim of actual improvements in daytime functioning from a hypnotic. In evaluating this possibility, one should recall that Ogura et al. (1980) did not find increased wakefulness during the morning in a 24-hr EEG recording and that Mitler et al. (1984) found only a nonsignificant trend toward increased wakefulness on the MSLT in middle-aged insomniacs. Perhaps the most conservative reading is that this short-acting benzodiazepine, at least, does not appear to have a major sedative effect the next day.

One other possible daytime effect of 0.5 mg triazolam that has been raised, however, is enhanced daytime anxiety (Morgan and Oswald, 1982). Other authors, such as Carskadon et al. (1982) have described relative absence of mood changes after 0.25 mg triazolam in elderly insomniacs. Similarly, Mamelak et al. (1984) found no evidence of increased daytime anxiety after 0.5 mg triazolam was given to middle-age insomniacs for two weeks. Certainly the issue deserves further clarification.

THE ELDERLY

Persons over 65, who compose 12% of the American population, present a number of special problems. Complaints of poor sleep increase with age. Sleep difficulties and disruptive behavior at night among elderly invalids may be the most common reason cited by relatives for bringing them for chronic care in institutions (Sanford, 1975). Hypnotics are prescribed for older persons greatly out of proportion to their numbers. In nursing homes, usage is substantial, ranging in different studies from 26% (Martilla *et al.*, 1977) to 100% (Derbez and Grauer, 1967).

The disproportionate use of hypnotics by the elderly takes on greater significance in light of their increased incidence of adverse side effects from virtually all classes of drugs. Hurwitz (1969), for instance, found that persons over 60 were two and one-half times more likely to experience drug reactions in the hospital than were younger patients. There are probably several reasons, including altered drug kinetics and possible changes in nervous system sensitivity. In terms of kinetics, the half-life of many psychotropic drugs goes up with age, leading to increased accumulation. Although it is often assumed that this is due to decreased hepatic clearance, each drug must be considered separately. For diazepam, for instance, the half-life increases with age, but the clearance is unaltered (Klotz *et al.*, 1975), at least in women (Greenblatt *et al.*, 1980). Gender clearly plays a role; the half-life of flurazepam may increase with age in men but not women (Greenblatt *et al.*, 1981). In general, low-clearance drugs that are oxidized (e.g., chlordiazepoxide, desalkylflurazepam) have reduced clearance and increased half-lives in the elderly (Greenblatt, 1983). Triazolam, which has an intermediate degree of hepatic extraction and is oxidized, has reduced clearance and an increased area under the curve in a plot of plasma concentration versus time, without an increased half-life. Drugs of low clearance that are primarily conjugated (oxazepam, lorazepam, temazepam) have little or no reduction in clearance and little or no increase in half-life in the elderly (Greenblatt, 1983; Ghabrial *et al.*, 1986).

Sometimes the increased half-life of the drug in the elderly reflects a larger volume of distribution consequent to an increased amount of body fat. Other factors include decreased serum albumin levels (Greenblatt, 1979), which can allow larger amounts of unbound drug to enter tissues. Although the reasons are complex, the end result of enhanced side effects of long-acting agents such as flurazepam seems real. Estimates of the degree, however, vary. In a study of hospitalized medical patients in Boston, adverse reactions from flurazepam occurred in 1.9% of patients under 60 and rose to 7.1% of patients over 60. Of patients over 70 who received 30 mg of flurazepam, 39% experienced adverse reactions (Greenblatt and Shader, 1977). In a study of five nursing facilities, Martilla *et al.* (1977) found such adverse reactions as ataxia, confusion, and hallucinations in 26% of medicated patients.

A second issue concerning the use of hypnotics in the elderly is their substantially higher incidence of sleep apnea and nocturnal myoclonus. The limited longitudinal data available demonstrate an increase in number of apneas and hypopneas in middle-aged and elderly persons who were followed for several years (Bliwise *et al.*, 1984). Cross-sectional studies of elderly subjects who do not complain about poor sleep have reported a significant degree of apneas or hypopneas (greater than five an hour) in 44 to 67% (Smallwood *et al.*, 1983; Ancoli-Israel *et al.*, 1981; Krieger, Mangin, and Kurtz, 1980; Block *et al.*, 1979; Carskadon and Dement, 1981). Roehrs *et al.* (1983) found nocturnal myoclonus or sleep apnea in 50% of elderly patients complaining of poor sleep or hypersomnolence. In another study, six out of seven elderly patients complaining of poor sleep had such disorders as sleep apnea or narcolepsy (Reynolds *et al.*, 1980). The concern here is that prescribing hypnotics would not only be unhelpful if one of these disorders is overlooked, it might also be dangerous in the case of an undiagnosed sleep apnea. This possibility emphasizes the need for careful evaluation of sleep disturbance in the elderly, as well as the consideration of nonpharmacological treatment. In chronic patients in whom sleep pathophysiology has been ruled out, it is also reasonable to consider the moderate use of wine. Mishara and Kastenbaum (1974), in a study of long-term geriatric patients in a psychiatric hospital, found that when wine was made available, chloral hydrate use decreased significantly.

BENZODIAZEPINES AND RESPIRATION

In the preceding section, we raised the possibility that hypnotic use in patients with undiagnosed sleep apnea might result in significant respiratory suppression. Although this has long been a concern with barbiturates and other hypnotics, there is evidence that long-acting benzodiazepines may (to a lesser degree) also significantly affect respiration in susceptible individuals (Mendelson, in press, e). Nitrazepam, for instance, has been reported to increase pCO_2 and decrease respiratory drive in patients with chronic bronchitis (Rudolf *et al.*, 1978) and obstructive lung disease (Model, 1973). Diazepam may suppress respiration during endoscopy (Rao *et al.*, 1973). Therapeutic doses of chlordiazepoxide have been shown to increase mixed venous CO_2 tension in chronic bronchitis patients (Model and Berry, 1974).

There is some evidence that this process is not confined to persons with lung disease. Mendelson *et al.* (1981a) described a 38-year-old insomniac who had 2 to 18 apneas on placebo nights (well below the usual definition of sleep apnea syndrome), in whom apneas rose to 100 on the second night of 30 mg flurazepam, and returned to basal levels upon discontinuation of the drug (Fig. 3-2). In subsequent studies, Carskadon et al. (1982) found no effect of a lower dose (15 mg) of flurazepam on elderly insomniacs who had previously been screened to eliminate those with apnea. Dolly and Block (1982), however, reported that the number of apneas almost doubled in 20 normal volunteers (mean age 49) given 30 mg flurazepam. Similarly, Guilleminault et al. (1984) found that one night of 30 mg flurazepam increased the mean number of apneas and lowered oxygen saturation in a group of 10 elderly volunteers.

Kripke and Garfinkel (1984) addressed the possible interaction of hypnotic use and sleep apnea syndrome using data from the American Cancer Society's 1959 health survey. A previous analysis of these data had shown that persons who take hypnotics (usually barbiturates) had a 50% increased risk of dying in the next six years (Kripke et al., 1979). Since sleep apnea is one of the more common causes of excessive sleepiness, the hour of death in persons who reported relatively long (9 hr) sleep times was examined. In this group, which might be more likely to contain persons with undiagnosed sleep apnea, persons taking hypnotics were much more likely to die during the hours of sleep than persons who did not. Although the data from this particular study are associational and may not necessarily be causal, the weight of the studies described here suggests that the potential for respiratory suppression is real and should be considered when prescribing hypnotics, including long-acting benzodiazepines. The effect of short-acting benzodiazepines on respiration has not yet been clarified.

In passing, it should also be mentioned that 0.5 mg triazolam and 30 mg flurazepam have been associated with increased heart rate during sleep (Muzet, Johnson, and Spinweber, 1982). Whether this is clinically significant is not clear.

RELIANCE AND DEPENDENCE

The overt abuse of hypnotics has been well described and is put in good historical perspective by Allgulander (1978). Of more recent concern are the twin issues of *reliance* (a continuing need for recommended doses) and *dependence* (the occurrence of a withdrawal syndrome). As mentioned earlier, perhaps 11% of persons currently taking sleeping pills have been taking them for at least a year (Mellinger and Balter, 1983). Although the various pharmacological classes of hypnotics differ greatly in potential for overt abuse, it is not clear whether they vary in terms of reliance. A study by Clift (1975) of a British general practice

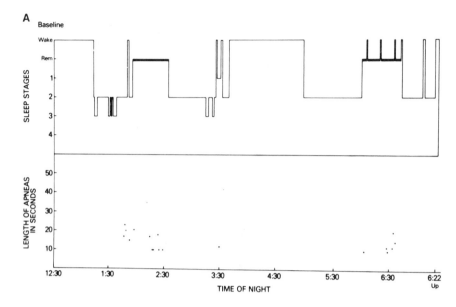

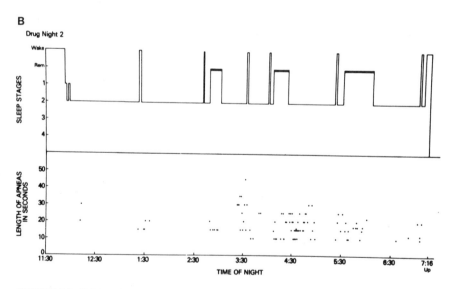

FIGURE 3-2. Schematic representation of sleep and number of apneas (•) in a 38-year-old insomniac before receiving drug (A), on the second night of 30 mg flurazepam (B), and six nights after flurazepam was discontinued (C). (From Mendelson *et al.*, 1981a. Reprinted by permission.)

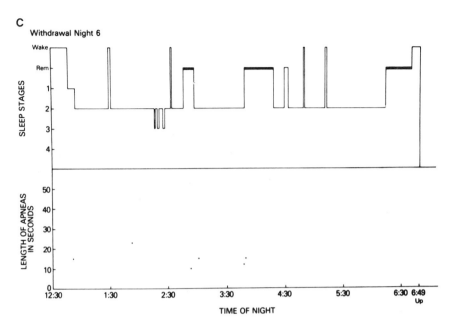

FIGURE 3-2. (*Continued*)

group found that patients started on nitrazepam or amobarbital were equally likely to be taking their medication six weeks later. Two years later, despite encouragement to discontinue medication, 8% had been on hypnotics continuously and 7% more were currently taking them after some drug-free period. Although the frequency of reliance upon individual compounds needs much more study, it is clear that one consequence of starting patients on hypnotics is that a certain percentage will continue to use them for prolonged periods.

The last few years have seen a growing concern about possible withdrawal disturbances from recommended doses of hypnotics. This has long been recognized as a problem with barbiturates and nonbarbiturate, nonbenzodiazepine hypnotics (e.g., Kales *et al.*, 1974) and was later raised with regard to the newer, short-acting benzodiazepines (Kales *et al.*, 1983). In the short-acting agents, withdrawal sleep disturbance may be dose-related (Roehrs *et al.*, 1986d). It has been claimed that such long-acting benzodiazepines as flurazepam do not cause withdrawal disturbance (Kales *et al.*, 1982). There is evidence, however, that withdrawal sleep disturbance or daytime dysphoria do indeed occur after flurazepam is stopped, albeit after several days and perhaps somewhat more mildly. Berlin and Conell (1983), for instance, found initial insomnia, dizziness, blurred vision, and other symptoms three days after a 37-year-old man was changed from 30 mg flurazepam to 30 mg temazepam. Mendelson et al. (1982c) described patient reports of poor sleep and dysphoria by the sixth day of withdrawal from flurazepam. Mitler et al. (1984) found that although decreases in sleep during withdrawal from flurazepam did not reach significance at any one time, six of the seven subjects had a sleep disturbance during the two-week withdrawal period. Hartmann et al. (1983) found increased scores on the SCL-71 withdrawal cluster during the week following a seven-night course of 30 mg flurazepam. Withdrawal symptoms, including anxiety (Fontaine, Chouinard, and Annable, 1984) or even hallucinations and psychosis (Greenblatt and Shader, 1977; Haskell, 1975; Nutt, 1986), have been described after withdrawal from therapeutic doses of diazepam. Such data have led several groups, including the authors of The Medical Letter (1981) and a National Institute of Mental Health Consensus Development Conference (1983), to conclude that all benzodiazepines may induce withdrawal reactions, although these might be milder with long-acting agents.

Another intriguing question is the mechanism by which benzodiazepine dependence is produced. There is some evidence that the alpha$_2$ antagonist yohimbine (which might be expected to enhance noradrenergic function) will induce symptoms of benzodiazepine withdrawal in normal volunteers (Goldberg, Hollister, and Robertson, 1983). On the other hand, there are conflicting accounts of whether the alpha$_2$ agonist clonidine does (Keshavan and Cramer, 1985) or does not (Goodman et al., 1986) ameliorate withdrawal. The possible role of noradrenergic hyperactivity in dependence is thus in need of further clarification.

HYPNOTICS AND ALCOHOL

In practice, hypnotics are frequently combined with alcohol. This may happen intentionally. Guilleminault, Spiegel, and Dement (1977), for instance, found that 21% of insomniacs in a Los Angeles survey took alcohol and sleeping pills together "frequently" in order to aid sleep. The two are often combined in overdoses. Ruedy (1973), for instance, found that 23% of drug poisoning patients had also taken alcohol. Ragno, Dumont, and Sitar (1982) reported that 33% of overdose patients admitted to a medical intensive care unit had measurable blood levels of a benzodiazepine and alcohol. The two may also be combined unintentionally—when a person receiving a long-acting hypnotic at night takes a drink the next day while the drug is still present in the blood.

Studies of the interaction of hypnotics and alcohol are reviewed in detail by Mendelson (1980) and Chan (1984). The potentiation of barbiturates and nonbarbiturate, nonbenzodiazepine hypnotics is well described. The situation with benzodiazepines is more complex. Several studies suggest that low doses of benzodiazepines in combination with moderate amounts of alcohol have little effect on performance measures (Lawton and Cahn, 1961; Miller, D'Agostino, and Minsky, 1963). There is even one report of inhibition of ethanol effects by a benzodiazepine, in which pretreatment with chlordiazepoxide made it more difficult to subsequently induce sleep with ethanol (Dundee, Howard, and Isaac, 1971). On the other hand, many studies show potentiation of sedative effects and decrements in performance (Linnoila and Mattila, 1973; Molander and Duvhok, 1976; Morland et al., 1974; Willumeit, Ott, and Neubert, 1984). It is very important, then, to caution patients taking hypnotics to abstain from alcohol.

HYPNOTICS AND ACUTE TIME SHIFTS

Acute shifts in work hours and transmeridian air travel frequently result in disturbed sleep (see Chapter 10) for which the physician is often called upon to prescribe hypnotics. Little work has been done to assess their effectiveness in this situation. Pollak, McGregor, and Weitzman (1975) acutely shifted sleep in normal volunteers so that they went to bed at 11:00 AM. Flurazepam (30 mg) aided the daytime sleep, primarily by reducing wakefulness toward the end of the sleep period. The following night, during which the volunteers were kept up, there was no difference in subjective sleepiness between those who had taken the active drug or a placebo. The implication seemed to be that a hypnotic would aid sleep at the new "nighttime," without improving wakefulness at the new "daytime." A subsequent study by Seidel et al. (1984) also found that 30 mg flurazepam increased sleepiness as measured on a MSLT during the new "daytime" after a 180° sleep–wake reversal; in contrast, 0.5 mg triazolam improved wakefulness relative to placebo (Fig. 3-3). A similar pattern was found with various performance measures. Bonnet et al. (1986), using a 12-hour, sleep–wake phase advance paradigm, found that triazolam improved wakefulness

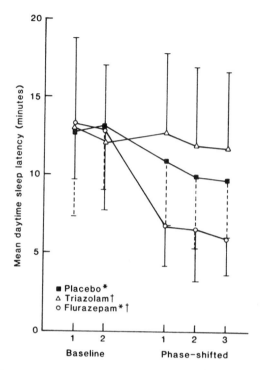

FIGURE 3-3. Daily mean of sleep latency on the Multiple Sleep Latency Test in normal volunteers receiving placebo, 0.5 mg triazolam, or 30 mg flurazepam after an acute 12-hr phase shift. *, Significant within-group change from baseline sleep tendency ($p<0.05$); +, significant between-group difference ($p<0.05$). (From Seidel et al., 1984. Reprinted by permission.)

on the MSLT and performance on a vigilance task, with generally best results after 0.25 mg. Although the magnitude was relatively small, this work was carried out in a situation of little or no sleep loss. It may be possible that benefits would be greater under more realistic conditions. Schweitzer, Sugarman, and Walsh (1986) and Walsh et al. (1986), however, phase-delayed the sleep of 10 volunteers by 8 hr and then had them sleep in the daytime for four days while performing MSLTs starting at 10:00 PM. Although triazolam (0.5 mg) enhanced daytime sleep, a preliminary analysis suggests that nighttime alertness was not significantly enhanced. Whether the discrepancies between these studies result from different alterations in schedule, or other factors, remains to be seen. They seem to raise the possibility, though, that short-acting benzodiazepines may be useful after some types of acute phase shifts.

The mechanism by which hypnotics might improve wakefulness at a new "daytime" after an acute phase shift is not clear. Before hastily attributing this to improved sleep, it should be remembered that in a study without a phase shift, triazolam given at night improved daytime wakefulness without altering nighttime total sleep or sleep efficiency (Dement, Seidel, and Carskadon, 1982). There is some evidence that triazolam may actually induce phase shifts of the circadian clock of hamsters (Turek and Losee-Olsen, 1986). The general topic of pharmacologically induced phase shifts is discussed in Chapter 10.

CLINICAL RECOMMENDATIONS

With these conclusions in mind, what considerations should guide the clinician treating a patient suffering from a sleep disorder? Some general approaches are summarized by Mendelson (1980) and an NIMH Consensus Development Conference (1983) (referred to earlier), from which some of the following thoughts come.

Certainly, the basic principle in treatment is to deal with insomnia as a complaint resulting from a variety of disorders, such as nocturnal myoclonus and sleep apnea, among others. Thus, the fundamental approach to the patient with insomnia should be first to look for such illnesses and, when they are found, to provide specific treatment. In those patients in whom such illnesses are not found, one may then consider psychological and pharmacological therapies. The selection of a specific hypnotic should be based on its pharmacological properties in conjunction with the clinical situation and the needs of the patient. Physicians should educate patients about the use of the drug and should monitor them to evaluate and reduce the risks of dependence, side effects, and possible withdrawal difficulties.

If a benzodiazepine is selected for an individual patient, pharmacological factors to be considered include: dose, rate of absorption, lipophilicity, rate of tissue distribution, elimination half-life, presence or absence of active metabolites, and presence or absence of drug interactions. Although low lethality gives the physician considerable leeway in individualizing the dose for each patient, the principle of using the lowest effective dose to achieve the desired result is still a good guide to avoid unwanted side effects. This applies especially to the elderly. The most common risk associated with some benzodiazepines is diminished daytime performance as a result of carryover effects from the previous evening's medication. This problem can be reduced by using lower doses or more rapidly eliminated drugs.

For transient insomnia related to minor situational stress usually lasting only a few days (for example, hospitalization, jet lag), drug treatment may or may not be necessary. When elected, the treatment should be a small dose of a rapidly eliminated hypnotic, usually a benzodiazepine; treatment should last only a few nights.

In short-term insomnia lasting only a few weeks (such as that related to stress from work or family life) the problem may, in part, be ameliorated by educating the patient in the principles of sleep hygiene (Chapter 12). If drug treatment is also required, the smallest effective dose should be used, with titration if necessary, and for a treatment period usually of not more than three weeks. The drug may be used intermittently, with the patient skipping the nightly dosage after one or two nights of good sleep. Therapy should be discontinued gradually.

The use of medication for long-term insomnia lasting several months or longer is controversial. Insomniacs who have failed to respond to nondrug strategies, and for whom major psychiatric and medical disorders have been ruled out, may be referred to a sleep disorders center. Long-term insomnia is often attributable to medical and psychiatric disorders or to such specific sleep disturbances as sleep apnea or nocturnal myoclonus. Patients in whom such conditions are ruled out may be treated following the principles of sleep hygiene and behaviorally oriented therapeutic techniques, with possible adjunctive use of hypnotics. Although not well documented by formal studies, the clinical impression of many physicians is that occasional, intermittent use of a hypnotic may be suitable in this situation. If benzodiazepines are not appropriate for the individual patient, the physician may consider a sedative antidepressant, such as amitriptyline (25–100 mg), at bedtime (see Ware, 1983). For patients who respond to this program, therapy should be discontinued gradually after three to four months.

CONCLUSIONS

In summary, hypnotics continue to be used widely, although in somewhat decreasing amounts. A small but persistent group of patients is likely to continue taking them for prolonged periods. The benzodiazepines have come to be the predominant agents prescribed for sleep, and in recent years the interest in short-acting agents has increased. There are many issues to consider in evaluating the efficacy of hypnotics, and at this point it seems wise to consider both subjective and polygraphic studies. In general, most prescription hypnotics have been shown to have some benefits for nocturnal sleep for a few weeks, with few data available for nightly use longer than four weeks. In contrast, and with the exception of one short-acting benzodiazepine, studies of hypnotics have not shown improvement in daytime mood, functioning, or alertness. (These daytime changes, incidentally, do not necessarily correlate with drug-induced alterations in the previous night's sleep.) On the contrary, many agents may adversely affect daytime cognition and performance in such crucial areas as driving skills. There is little evidence that such performance decrements are somehow compensated for by the benefit of improved sleep for insomniacs. Objective measures of performance show few, relatively subtle deficits to begin with, and in several studies of insomniacs, various hypnotics impaired rather than helped vigilance and other measures. The few cases of improved daytime performance after nighttime administration of hypnotics are often very selective and tend to occur in untrained subjects.

The elderly have a higher incidence of complaints of poor sleep and use hypnotics in disproportionately large numbers. Prescribing hypnotics for persons over 60 should be done with caution, both because of a higher likelihood of side effects and a higher incidence of such primary sleep disorders as sleep apnea syndromes. All hypnotics are respiratory suppressants, and the long-acting benzodiazepines are no exception. Withdrawal sleep disturbance and daytime dysphoria are apparent for virtually all hypnotics, although these may be delayed and less severe with long-acting benzodiazepines.

CHAPTER 4

The Benzodiazepine Receptor and Sleep

The benzodiazepines (BZs) are among the most widely prescribed drugs in the United States. Although therapeutic doses are measured in milligrams, annual consumption is measured in thousands of tons. Benzodiazepines are used as minor tranquilizers, anticonvulsants, muscle relaxants, and (of particular concern here) hypnotics. Indeed, for a decade or more, a single BZ, flurazepam, has been the most widely prescribed agent for sleep, comprising about two-thirds of hypnotic prescriptions in 1982 (Mellinger and Balter, 1983). Recent years have also seen the development of several short-acting BZs, currently the subject of a great deal of clinical interest (Mendelson, 1987e).

In 1977, a major step in understanding the mechanism of action of these compounds occurred with the discovery that labeled diazepam binds to high affinity ($K_d \sim 10^{-9}$M), saturable, stereoselective sites in the central nervous system (Squires and Braestrup, 1977; Mohler and Okada, 1977; Skolnick, Mendelson, and Paul, 1981a). Another receptor with affinity for some BZs has been found in liver, lung, and brain tissue (Benavides *et al.*, 1983; Bolger *et al.*, 1985; Mestre *et al.*, 1985; Basile and Skolnick, 1986). These "peripheral BZ receptors," which have a different pharmacological specificity and have been hypothesized to be involved in cellular differentiation (Curran and Morgan, 1985), will not be considered here. There may also be a BZ receptor of much lower af-

Portions of this chapter are taken from Mendelson (1984). Reprinted by permission.

finity ($K_d \sim 10^{-5} M$) linked to the calcium–calmodulin protein kinase system (DeLorenzo, Burdette, and Holderness, 1981), which is of uncertain physiological significance. The high affinity central receptors, on which this chapter focuses, are found in greatest density in the synaptosomal fraction of neurons, a location consistent with the possibility that they are involved in neurotransmission. The highest concentrations are found in phylogenetically "newer" portions of the brain such as the cerebral cortex, with lesser density in "older" areas such as the pons and medulla. In terms of evolution they are found in the more recently appearing vertebrates back through the bony fish, implying, perhaps, a role in more elaborate forms of behavior (Nielsen, Braestrup, and Squires, 1978). In molecular terms, they are thought to be macromolecular complexes with three or more components: a BZ recognition site, a GABA recognition site, and a chloride ionophore (Skolnick, Mendelson, and Paul, 1981a). The functional significance of these observations is suggested by the close correlation between the affinities of various BZs for these central sites and their potencies as anxiolytics, anticonvulsants, and muscle relaxants (Squires and Braestrup, 1977). Until recently, however, there has been little evidence linking the BZ receptor with the sleep-inducing qualities of these compounds. In this chapter, we will present studies indicating that the hypnotic properties of BZs are mediated by this receptor, and then describe pharmacological work implying that this action may involve changes in calcium flow across neuronal membranes.

PHARMACOLOGICAL PROBES OF THE BZ RECOGNITION SITE

Studies with Beta-Carbolines

The beta-carbolines, condensation products of aromatic amino acids and aldehydes, bind with various degrees of affinity to the BZ recognition site and have been useful in exploring its function. 3-Carboethoxy-β-carboline (β-CCE), first detected in human urine, was thought to be a possible endogenous ligand for the BZ receptor (Braestrup, Nielsen, and Oslen, 1980). It was later found to be artifactually formed during extraction procedures (Squires, 1981). β-CCE remains a valuable pharmacological probe, however, because it binds to the BZ recognition site with relatively high affinity ($K_i \sim 1$ nM), antagonizes the anticonvulsant effects of diazepam (Tenen and Hirsch, 1980), and in animals has anxiogenic effects that are blocked by diazepam (Corda *et al.*, 1983). It also has proconvulsant properties (Oakley and Jones, 1980) and may induce an anxietylike state in primates (Ninan *et al.*, 1982).

The sleep studies described here involve 3-hydroxymethyl-β-carboline (3-HMC), which binds less strongly to the receptor ($K_i \sim 1470$ nM), but which, in contrast to β-CCE, has a long enough half-life to persist during a 2-hr sleep study in rats. A previous study had suggested that 3-HMC blocks both the anticonvulsant and the anxiolytic actions of diazepam (Skolnick et al., 1981a). 3-HMC (7.5–50 mg/kg, intraperitoneally) produced a dose-dependent arousing effect in rats, measured in terms of increased sleep latency (Fig. 4-1) and decreased total sleep (Fig. 4-2; Mendelson et al., 1983a). Thus, a compound that binds to the BZ recognition site and belongs to a class of compounds which has actions opposite to BZs was found to reduce sleep.

Receptor Mediation of Beta-Carboline Effects

The arousing effect of 3-HMC has led to further questions: Is this activity mediated by the interaction of 3-HMC and the BZ recognition site or by some other (unknown) mechanism? Is the decrease in sleep a specific effect on sleep per se, or a nonspecific response to a more generalized behavioral arousal? A partial answer to the first question comes from studies of CGS 8216 (2-phenyl-pyrazolo [4,3-C] quinolone-3 (5H)-one, which binds to the BZ recognition site (Czernik et al., 1982), but (at least at relatively low doses) has little pharmacological activity of its own. (Also see the discussion of specificity of this compound in

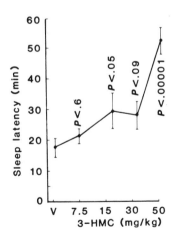

FIGURE 4-1. Effects of 3-HMC on sleep latency. The rats were given 3-HMC at 0900 hr, and 5 min later, EEGs were recorded for 2 hr. The overall significance by ANOVA was $p < 0.0001$. (From Mendelson et al., 1983a. Reprinted by permission.)

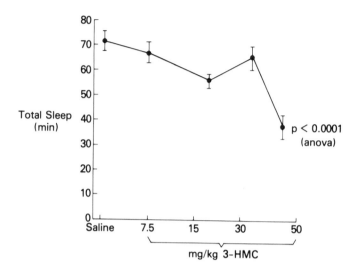

FIGURE 4-2. Effects of 3-HMC on total sleep in the rat (same study as that of Fig. 4-1). The overall significance by ANOVA was $p < 0.0001$. (From Mendelson *et al.*, 1983a. Reprinted by permission.)

the later section "Anxiolytic Effects of Pentobarbital.") If CGS 8216 could block the arousing properties of 3-HMC, the implication would be that these effects are due to interaction at the BZ recognition site. As can be seen in Fig. 4-3, this is indeed what appears to happen (Mendelson *et al.*, 1983a).

In a second approach to the question of whether the effects of β-carbolines on sleep are mediated by the BZ receptor, Mendelson *et al.* (1983e) studied receptor occupancy and the effect on sleep of 3-carbo-*t*-butoxy-β-carboline (β-CCT). This compound has a relatively high affinity ($K_i \sim 10$ nM) and is poorly metabolized, as demonstrated by *in vitro* plasma studies. Intraperitoneal β-CCT (30 mg/kg) significantly decreased total sleep in rats during the first 2 hr (20.8 ± 2.2 min vs. 48.1 ± 2.4 min control; $p < 0.002$). Similarly, sleep latency was increased (40.6 ± 7.4 min vs. 16.6 ± 3.6 min control; $p < 0.01$). Parallel studies of *in vivo* [³H]diazepam binding using the method of Williamson, Paul, and Skolnick (1978) showed relatively little binding 1 hr after β-CCT administration, when the awakening effect was maximal, presumably indicating that β-CCT was occupying the sites. At 6 hr, when the pharmacological effect was no longer present, significant [³H]diazepam binding occurred, indicating the presence of large amounts of free receptors. Thus, the effects of β-CCT on sleep had a parallel time course to receptor occupancy.

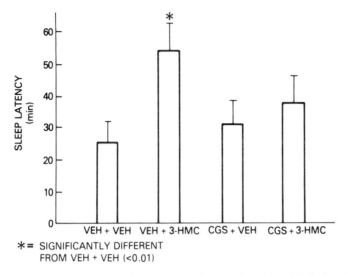

FIGURE 4-3. Effects of 5 mg/kg of CGS 8216 and 50 mg/kg of 3-HMC, both injected intraperitoneally, on sleep latencies in the rat. The overall ANOVA for all four groups was $p < 0.04$. *, $p < 0.01$ compared to the group receiving vehicle of both drugs. (From Mendelson, 1984. Reprinted by permission.)

Specificity of Effect for Sleep

The next question—the specificity of the arousing properties of 3-HMC—was explored by examining the effects of 3-HMC on motor activity in rats (Mendelson *et al.*, 1983a). As can be seen in Fig. 4-4, even the highest dose of 3-HMC had a relatively small effect on motor activity relative to its awakening properties, and as compared with traditional analeptics. It seems unlikely, then, that the arousing effect of 3-HMC is a nonspecific response to general behavioral activation, and instead is relatively specific for sleep. This raises the interesting possibility that a drug from this family might be clinically useful in treating disorders of excessive sleepiness without producing excessive motor agitation.

Beta-Carbolines and BZs

The CGS 8216 and β-CCT studies, which indicated that β-carbolines alter sleep consequent to interaction with the BZ receptor, made it possible to explore the mechanism of action of flurazepam. Mendelson *et al.* (1983a) gave rats a very low dose of 3-HMC (7.5 mg/kg), which by itself had no effect on sleep. It was reasoned that if

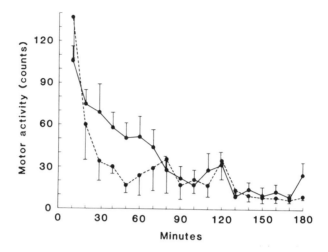

FIGURE 4-4. Effects of 3-HMC on motor activity. Rats were given vehicle (— — —) or 3-HMC (50 mg/kg; ————) and their motor activity was measured by a Motron Produkter apparatus. The ANOVA revealed no overall drug effect, but there was a significant drug × time interaction ($p<0.03$). (From Mendelson *et al.*, 1983a. Reprinted by permission.)

this pretreatment prevented sleep induction by flurazepam, then its hypnotic effects must be mediated by interaction with the BZ recognition site. As seen in Fig. 4-5, the low dose of 3-HMC had no effect on sleep by itself, but it did indeed prevent sleep induction by flurazepam.

The B_{10} Enantiomers

Another approach to the question of whether BZ effects on sleep are mediated by interaction with the BZ recognition site would be to examine whether the effect is stereospecific (a classic quality of a receptor). Although diazepam and flurazepam do not have asymmetrically arranged carbon atoms, several BZs do. Among these are the ''B_{10}'' enantiomers: $(+)B_{10}$ (RO 11-6896) binds to the receptor with an affinity approximately twice that of flurazepam ($K_i \sim 4.8$ nM), whereas $(-)B_{10}$ (RO 11-6893) is approximately two orders of magnitude less potent (Mohler and Okada, 1977). The apparent affinities of both compounds for the BZ receptor are enhanced in the presence of GABA, a quality usually associated with receptor agonists (Skolnick *et al.*, 1982). One might speculate, then, that if the hypnotic actions of BZ are consequent to binding at the recognition site, these two enantiomers would have very different effects on sleep.

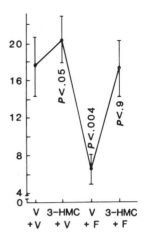

FIGURE 4-5. Effects of 3-HMC on hypnotic action or flurazepam. Rats were given vehicle or 3-HMC (7.5 mg/kg) 5 min before receiving vehicle or flurazepam (40 mg/kg). The EEGs were recorded for 2 hr after the last injection, beginning at 0905. The overall significance by ANOVA was $p<0.003$. (From Mendelson et al., 1983a. Reprinted by permission.)

Mendelson, Paul, and Skolnick (1982e), administered 20 mg/kg of $(+)B_{10}$ to rats, an intraperitoneal dose which was estimated to be roughly equipotent to a known hypnotic dose (40 mg/kg) of flurazepam (Mendelson et al., 1983a). As expected, $(+)B_{10}$ significantly reduced sleep latency ($p<0.02$), from 16.0 ± 2.7 min to 4.6 ± 2.4 min (Fig. 4-6). In contrast, 20 mg/kg $(-)B_{10}$ tended ($p<0.06$) to increase sleep latency, from 18.1 ± 3.1 min to 47.9 ± 12.2 min. This effect was dose-related, since 40 mg/kg raised sleep latency much further, from 27.0 ± 5.9 min to 169.0 ± 56.4 min ($p<0.02$). In a second experiment (Mendelson et al., 1985d), animals were pretreated with 5 mg/kg of intraperitoneal CGS 8216, and then given 40 mg/kg of $(-)B_{10}$. Once again, $(-)B_{10}$ alone raised sleep latency, from 24.2 ± 2.7 min to 74.1 ± 13.3 min ($p<0.001$). Pretreatment with CGS 8216 substantially blocked the increase in sleep latency, to 50.0 ± 11.2 min ($p<0.07$ compared to the control).

In summary, these experiments showed that two BZ enantiomers had opposite effects on sleep: $(+)B_{10}$, with a relatively high affinity for the BZ recognition site, had clear hypnotic properties; $(-)B_{10}$, which might be expected to be a much less potent hypnotic, was found instead to produce a dose-dependent arousal. This effect appears to be mediated by the BZ receptor, insofar as it was blocked by CGS 8216.

Whether this quality of having opposite effects can be generalized to other BZ properties is not clear. It has been shown that diazepam induces increased Ca^{2+} uptake into brain synaptosomes under depolarized conditions (Paul, Luu, and Skolnick, 1982; Paul and Skolnick, 1982). A preliminary study suggests that while $(+)B_{10}$ has this action, $(-)B_{10}$ may actually reduce uptake (Fig. 4-7). On the other hand,

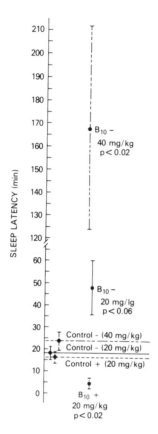

FIGURE 4-6. Effects of B_{10} enantiomers on sleep latency in the rat.

$(-)B_{10}$, at a twofold greater dose than $(+)B_{10}$, did not antagonize the anticonvulsant actions of the latter compound against pentylenetetrazole-induced seizures (Skolnick, personal communication).

The stereospecificity of sedative effects is not unique to BZs. The two enantiomers of 5-(1,3-dimethylbutyl)-5-ethyl barbituric acid (DMBB) have opposite properties, the $(+)$ enantiomer being convulsant, whereas the $(-)$ enantiomer is anticonvulsant and depressant (Downes et al., 1970). Similarly, $(+)$ pentobarbital and $(-)$ pentobarbital (PB) have predominantly excitatory and inhibitory properties, respectively, on cultured spinal neurons (Huang and Barker, 1980).

In summary, the observation that two BZ enantiomers have different effects on sleep is further evidence that the hypnotic property of BZs is receptor mediated and corresponds to the known stereospecificity of the binding site. These observations raise the interesting possibil-

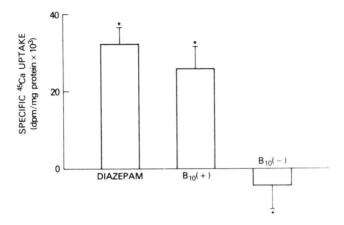

FIGURE 4-7. Effects of diazepam and B_{10} enantiomers on calcium uptake into synaptosomes under depolarized conditions.

ity that $(-)B_{10}$ might be a clinically useful agent to treat disorders characterized by excessive sleepiness.

DO ALTERATIONS IN CALCIUM FLUX MEDIATE SOME PHARMACOLOGICAL EFFECTS OF BZs?

Thus far, this chapter has been oriented to the question of whether the BZ receptor mediates the effects of BZs, and a variety of evidence has been presented suggesting that this is the case. We turn now to a second question: What cellular events occur in relation to BZ receptor stimulation? It is well known that BZs act postsynaptically by enhancing GABA-mediated inhibitory events (Haefely *et al.*, 1975). They are also known to alter such presynaptic events as GABA-mediated inhibition in the spinal cord (Polc, Mohler, and Haefely, 1974) and depolarization-induced release of GABA from cortical slices (Mitchell and Martin, 1978). As mentioned earlier, there is also some evidence that BZs may enhance $^{45}Ca^{2+}$ flux in depolarized synaptosome preparations (Paul *et al.*, 1982; Paul and Skolnick, 1982). This effect occurs at BZ concentrations that might be expected *in vivo* ($< 1\ \mu M$), and is blocked by CGS 8216. Substantially higher concentrations of BZs have been reported to reduce $^{45}Ca^{2+}$ flux (Chandler *et al.*, 1984). Possible calcium channels in brain have been described and may resemble those found in peripheral tissues (Murphy and Snyder, 1982). It has been suggested that such putative calcium channels are linked to central BZ receptors (Hirsch and Kochman, 1982). In terms of BZ receptor subtyping (to be discussed later), there are indications that fluctuations in calcium concentrations change the affinity of labeled flunitrazepam for the "DE" receptor, which corresponds to type II (Lo, Trifiletti, and Snyder, 1983). A calcium–calmodulin protein kinase system may be involved with a low-affinity receptor responsive to micromolar-range BZ concentrations (DeLorenzo et al., 1981). Peripheral BZ receptors in the heart may be associated with calcium channels (Mestre et al., 1985). These observations raise the possibility that at least some pharmacological effects of BZs might be mediated by alterations in cellular calcium. In order to explore this possibility with regard to central BZ receptors, a series of experiments on the effects of nifedipine and nitrendipine, which are dihydropyridine calcium channel antagonists (Vanhoutte and Paoletti, 1987), on BZ activity were performed. These involved both uptake of labeled calcium into synaptosomes in vitro and animal sleep studies.

Dihydropyridines and Diazepam-Stimulated Calcium Uptake into Synaptosomes

In the first study (Mendelson et al., 1984a), nifedipine or nitrendipine (1 μM) was added to an incubation mixture designed to measure the effect of 1 μM diazepam on $^{45}Ca^{2+}$ uptake into synaptosomes, as previously described (Paul et al., 1982). Nifedipine alone had no effect on basal uptake, whereas nitrendipine reduced it. As expected, diazepam consistently stimulated $^{45}Ca^{2+}$ uptake by 75–78% above control values, respectively. Addition of nifedipine or nitrendipine completely reversed the increased $^{45}Ca^{2+}$ uptake induced by diazepam. With nifedipine alone, $^{45}Ca^{2+}$ uptake was approximately 119% of control; in the presence of diazepam (which had increased the uptake to 175%), the uptake was only 74%.

Nifedipine Blocks Sleep Induction by Flurazepam

In the next study Mendelson et al. (1984b) examined the effects of pretreatment with 20 μg/kg of intraventricular nifedipine on sleep induction by 40 mg/kg intraperitoneal flurazepam. As seen in Fig. 4-8, sleep latency under the control conditions was 26.5 ± 5.1 min, which was unchanged by nifedipine alone (25.7 ± 2.9 min; NS). Flurazepam significantly reduced sleep latency ($p < 0.01$) to 12.6 ± 1.3 min. Pretreatment with nifedipine completely blocked this effect (25.6 ± 5.0 min; NS compared to control).

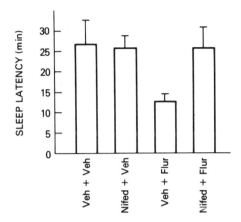

FIGURE 4-8. Effects of 20 μg/kg of intraventricular nifedipine (Nifed) and 40 mg/kg intraperitoneal flurazepam (Flur) on sleep latency in the rat. The overall ANOVA for all treatments was $p<0.03$. The least significant difference test showed that the "vehicle nifedipine + flurazepam" (Veh+Flur) treatment differed from the "vehicle nifedipine + vehicle flurazepam" (Veh+Veh) treatment by $p<0.01$. (From Mendelson *et al.*, 1984. Reprinted by permission.)

BAY K 8644 Enhances Hypnotic Effect of Flurazepam

In contrast to nifedipine, the dihydropyridine BAY K 8644 is thought to enhance calcium flux at potential-sensitive calcium channels (Schramm *et al.*, 1983; Greenberg, Cooper, and Carpenter, 1984). Mendelson, Martin, and Wagner (1986a) gave rats 100 μg/kg BAY K 8644 intraventricularly, alone and in combination with 40 mg/kg flurazepam intraperitoneally. As seen in Fig. 4-9, BAY K 8644 had little effect by itself on sleep latency, but it potentiated the effect of flurazepam.

In summary, putative calcium channels have been found in central nervous system tissue, and it has been suggested that some subclass of these channels may be linked to BZ receptors. Dihydropyridine calcium channel blockers prevent BZ-stimulated uptake of calcium in depolarized synaptosome preparations *in vitro* and prevent sleep induction by flurazepam *in vivo*. Because of the multiplicity of roles of calcium and the probable heterogeneous nature of calcium channels, these data might well be interpreted cautiously. The physiological significance of dihydropyridine binding sites in the CNS is still uncertain (Miller and Freedman, 1984). On the other hand, BAY K 8644 has been reported to augment K^+-stimulated release of serotonin from rat frontal cortex slices, and this effect can be inhibited by calcium antagonists (Middlemiss and Spedding, 1985). The implication is that the di-

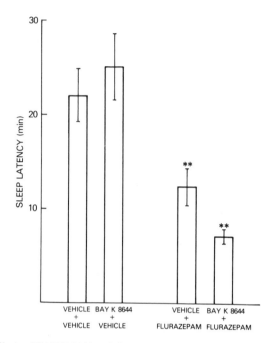

FIGURE 4-9. Effects of BAY K 8644 and flurazepam on sleep latency in the rat. **, Differs from "vehicle + vehicle" condition by $p < 0.01$. (Mendelson *et al.*, 1986a.)

hydropyridine sites may well be functionally related to calcium regulation. The present studies suggest, then, that alterations in calcium ion flux may be part of the effector mechanism for sleep induction after stimulation of the BZ recognition site. Benzodiazepines have many pharmacological properties, and it is not clear whether alterations in calcium ion flux are relevant to actions other than those on sleep. Preliminary animal studies suggest that intraventricular nifedipine does not block the anticonvulsant effect of flurazepam against pentylenetetrazole (Mendelson *et al.*, 1984a) or the anticonflict effect of diazepam (Mendelson *et al.*, unpublished). Thus, alterations in nifedipine-sensitive calcium channels may be involved to different degrees in the various pharmacological actions of BZs.

THE RELATION OF BARBITURATES AND ETHANOL TO THE BZ RECEPTOR COMPLEX

Until now we have dealt primarily with the role of the BZ recognition site in the sleep-inducing properties of BZs. This begs the broader question of whether the recognition site—or other portions of the receptor complex—might also be involved in the actions of other sedative–hypnotics. If this were the case, it would help explain a long-standing puzzle: the apparently similar effects of sedatives of diverse pharmacological classes. The barbiturates are of particular interest because of their potent hypnotic properties and because they may interact with part of the BZ receptor complex. Pentobarbital (PB) induces stereospecific anion-dependent enhancement of BZ binding at pharmacologically relevant doses (Leeb-Lundberg, Snowman, and Olsen, 1980; Skolnick et al., 1981). Similarly, the ability of various barbiturates to enhance BZ receptor affinity in vitro is correlated with their anesthetic potencies (Leeb-Lundberg, Snowman, and Olsen, 1980). The interaction of PB with the BZ receptor complex may be the result of binding at or near the dihydropicrotoxinin site (Skolnick, Paul, and Barker, 1980; Ticku and Olsen, 1978), which is associated with the chloride ionophore. As we will see in the next section, a growing body of evidence indicates that both PB and ethanol may profoundly alter chloride channel function.

Effects of PB and Ethanol on Ion Channels

Schwartz et al. (1984, 1985), using an in vitro synaptoneurosome preparation, demonstrated that low concentrations of PB enhance GABA-stimulated chloride transport and higher concentrations directly enhance it. The degree of increased chloride shift induced by various barbiturates parallels their anesthetic potencies in mice. This property, which is blocked by picrotoxin and bicuculline, is consistent with earlier electrophysiological studies (Barker and Ransom, 1978a,b) and seems to suggest a mechanism by which barbiturates might induce neuronal hyperpolarization.

Ethanol may act on chloride channels in a manner similar to that of barbiturates, with enhancement of GABA-stimulated chloride flux at low concentrations and direct enhancement at higher concentrations (Suzdak et al., 1986). Again, as with PB, these effects may be blocked by picrotoxin and bicuculline. It is possible that the action of ethanol on chloride flux is mediated by alterations of membrane fluidity, which has been considered a possible mechanism for some time (Chin and Goldstein, 1977; Goldstein and Chin, 1981; Strong and Wood, 1984; Hunt, 1985). This suggests that barbiturates and ethanol may have certain neurophysiological effects in common, which could conceivably mediate some of their pharmacological actions.

Barbiturates and ethanol also alter the movement of calcium across membranes. Pentobarbital may decrease depolarization-induced cal-

cium influx into synaptosomes (Leslie *et al.*, 1980). 80 mM ethanol has
been reported to increase calcium uptake (Friedman, Erickson, and
Leslie, 1980), while concentrations as low as 45 mM ethanol may inhibit it (Harris and Hood, 1980; Stokes and Harris, 1982). We have already discussed possible evidence that alterations in calcium flux may
play a role in the hypnotic actions of BZs. A preliminary study found
that nifedipine does not modify the hypnotic or anticonvulsant effects
of PB in rats (Mendelson *et al.*, 1986f; Fig. 4-10), suggesting that
changes in calcium flux may not play a significant role in these properties of barbiturates.

Chloride Channel Function: Ethanol and PB Toxicity

In order to assess whether the barbiturate-induced alterations in
chloride flux observed *in vitro* are functionally significant, Mendelson *et*

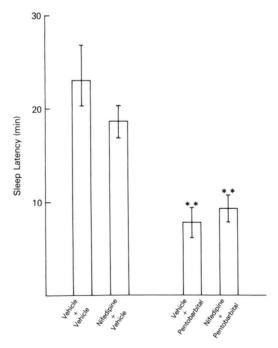

FIGURE 4-10. Effects of nifedipine and PB on sleep latency in the rat. (From Mendelson
et al., 1986b. Reprinted by permission.)

al. (1986b) studied the effects of isopropylbicyclophosphate (IPPO) on various barbiturate actions. IPPO, which binds at the dihydropicrotoxinin site associated with the chloride ionophore, did not alter hypnotic properties of PB in rats. On the other hand, IPPO did ameliorate the toxic properties of barbiturates and ethanol (Mendelson *et al.*, 1985a). In studies of 20-g male mice, it was found that 170 mg/kg intraperitoneal PB would cause deaths in 97% of the animals, with a mean latency to death of 24.8 ± 3.0 min. Five minutes after PB injection, progressive doses of intraperitoneal IPPO (125, 250, and 500 µg/kg) reduced death rates to 87% (NS), 70% ($p < 0.05$), and 58% ($p < 0.02$). The lower two doses also lengthened the time until death (45.4 ± 9.2 min at 125 µg/kg; 62.5 ± 16.2 min at 250 µg/kg; $p < 0.03$), whereas at the highest dose, time until death remained at control levels (17.4 ± 4.0 min). The toxicity of IPPO alone was very low for the two lower doses (no deaths at 125 µg/kg; 1.7% deaths at 250 µg/kg), but was significant at the highest dose of 500 µg/kg (45% deaths; $p < 0.02$). Picrotoxin, which binds to the same site and has been used clinically to treat barbiturate toxicity, also reduced PB mortality in this model, but substantially decreased time until death in those animals that did die. Picrotoxin also caused a 90% mortality rate when given alone at a dose comparable to 250–500 µg/kg of IPPO. The effects of IPPO on reducing mortality seemed specific to barbiturates, since IPPO did not alter death rates from large doses of the anesthetic ketamine (which is not thought to interact at the chloride ionophore site).

   In an analogous study, mice were given 5 g/kg of ethanol intraperitoneally, followed by IPPO or vehicle, and the duration of the loss of the righting reflex (LRR) was determined. As seen in Figure 4-11, 500 µ/kg of IPPO greatly reduced the duration of the loss of the righting reflex from 84.1 ± 6.5 min to 39.3 ± 6.9 min ($p < 0.002$).

   These data suggest, then, that *in vitro* observations of PB binding at or near the dihydropicrotoxinin site may have some functional significance and that at least some aspect of the various toxic—but not hypnotic—qualities of PB may be mediated by this site. It seems possible that some pharmacological agent acting at the dihydropicrotoxinin site might be a clinically useful antidote for barbiturate or ethanol poisoning.

Relation of PB to BZ Recognition Site Function: Hypnotic, Anticonvulsant, and Anxiolytic Properties

   As mentioned earlier, PB may facilitate anion-dependent enhancement of BZ binding (Skolnick *et al.*, 1981c). This raises the possibility

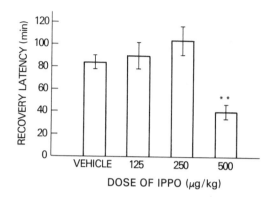

FIGURE 4-11. A 500 μg/kg dose of IPPO reduced the duration of loss of righting reflex induced by 5 g/kg ethanol in mice. **, $p < 0.002$. (From Mendelson *et al.*, 1985a. Reprinted by permission.)

that some pharmacological properties of PB are mediated by its indirect effect at the BZ recognition site. Mendelson *et al.* (unpublished) examined this issue by observing the effects of agents that bind at the BZ recognition site on various actions of PB. In a study of sleep induction, CGS 8216 and PB were given alone and in combination to rats. As expected, 10 mg/kg intraperitoneal PB decreased sleep latency from control values of 22.9 ± 3.1 min to 12.2 ± 9 min ($p < 0.003$) in a group of 16 rats; CGS 8216 (5 mg/kg) alone did not significantly affect sleep latency (27.3 ± 3.1 min). CGS 8216 pretreatment did not block the tendency of PB to shorten sleep latency (10.0 ± 1.6 min; $p < 0.0005$).

The possible role of the BZ recognition site in the anticonvulsant effect of PB was also examined. Because of the mild proconvulsant actions of CGS 8216 (File, Lister, and Nutt, 1982), β-CCT, which has no known proconvulsant properties, was used as a blocker. Pentylenetetrazole (PTZ), 80 mg/kg intraperitoneally, was found to induce seizures in 80% of mice tested. Treatment with 15 mg/kg of PB reduced seizures to 26% ($p < 0.01$). Pretreatment with 5 or 10 mg/kg of β-CCT did not reverse the anticonvulsant effects of PB, with seizures occurring in 28% and 35% of the mice, respectively.

In contrast to the hypnotic and anticonvulsant properties of PB, the "anxiolytic" properties measured by anticonflict activity in an animal model are sensitive to manipulation of the BZ recognition site. Mendelson *et al.* (1983b) examined the effects of CGS 8216 in this system. In a modification of the Vogel test (J. Vogel, Beer, and Clody, 1971), a water-deprived rat was placed in a situation in which it received a 0.55 mA shock for every cumulative 3 sec of licking a water tube. As can be seen in Fig. 4-12, treatment with diazepam produced significant ($p<0.01$) increases in shocks. A low dose of CGS 8216 actually reduced them slightly (a proconflict effect). Pretreatment with either dose of CGS 8216, however, prevented the anticonflict effect of PB (Fig. 4-13).

These data suggest that anxiolytic—but not hypnotic or anticonvulsant—properties of PB may have some functional link with the BZ recognition site. This suggestion is supported by studies showing that CGS 8216 antagonizes anticonflict effects of meprobamate, PB, and diazepam (Bernard et al., 1981). It should, however, be noted that Petersen et al. (1982) found that β-CCE, but not RO 15-1788 (another BZ recognition site blocker), antagonized the anticonflict effects of PB. The possibility should be explored that CGS 8216 and RO 15-1788 have slightly different spectrums of effects. Higher doses of CGS 8216, for instance, were found to have proconflict ("anxiogenic") effects in the Vogel model (J. Vogel et al., 1971), and high doses of RO 15-1788 may have some BZ antagonist (File et al., 1982) or agonist (Albertson, Bowyer, and Paule, 1982; Dantzer and Perio, 1982) properties, depending on the model used. Both CGS 8216 and RO 15-1788, however, seem relatively specific in their binding to the BZ recognition site.

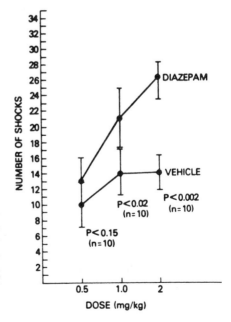

FIGURE 4-12. Effects of diazepam on conflict responding in rats. Each pair of points represents a separate study in which 10 rats received diazepam or vehicle in a randomized sequence with a 1-week interval between studies. Diazepam produced a dose-dependent increase in the number of shocks received. (From Mendelson et al., 1983b. Reprinted by permission.)

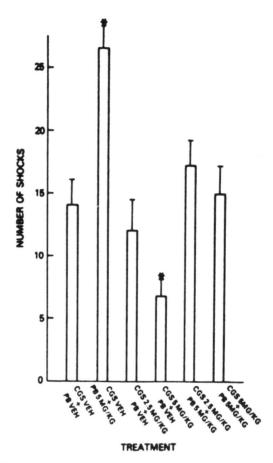

FIGURE 4-13. Effects of CGS 8216 and PB on conflict responding. Values are the mean±SEM of six independent groups of 10 rats each. *, $p<0.01$ compared to vehicle condition. Other significant contrasts include PB+CGS vehicle versus PB+CGS 2.5 mg/kg ($p<0.01$); PB VEH+CGS 2.5 mg/kg versus PB+CGS 2.5 mg/kg ($p<0.04$); and PB VEH+CGS 5 mg/kg versus PB+CGS 5 mg/kg ($p<0.01$). (From Mendelson *et al.*, 1982b. Reprinted by permission.)

    Another question as to the functional coupling of PB and the BZ recognition site blockers comes from the observation (B. A. Weissman, personal communication) that CGS 8216 in concentrations up to 500 nM does not affect [^{35}S]-*t*-butyl-bicyclophosphorothionate (TBPS) binding at the chloride ionophore site, where PB may bind. This preliminary observation raises the possibility that the blockade of PB actions by CGS 8216 may be the result of a pharmacological interaction rather than a molecular antagonism, or alternatively that PB binding to the dihydropicrotoxinin site has different qualities than those of TBPS.

In summary, CGS 8216 administration can prevent the anticonflict ("anxiolytic") effects of PB. This effect seems relatively specific to the anticonflict property, insofar as CGS 8216 does not block sleep induction and β-CCT does not prevent the anticonvulsant effects of PB.

HETEROGENEITY OF BZ RECEPTORS

As has been the case with other receptors, the years after the initial characterization have led to the subtyping of central nervous system BZ receptors. Work with a triazolopyridazine, CL 218,872, led to the concept that there are two biochemically distinct classes of BZ receptors. In this scheme, type 1 BZ receptors, which may mediate anxiolytic effects, have a high affinity for both BZs and triazolopyridazines (Kepner et al., 1979; Lippa, Meyerson, and Beer, 1982); type 2 receptors, which might mediate other BZ actions, have a high affinity for BZs and a low affinity for triazolopyridazines. Type 1 may be postsynaptic, whereas type 2 may be presynaptic. It was originally thought that CL 218,872, which may preferentially bind to type 1 receptors, is as potent as diazepam in anticonflict and anticonvulsant models, but that at anxiolytic doses, it does not produce ataxia or decrease motor activity (Lippa et al., 1979a,b). Lo, Trifiletti, and Snyder (1983) have divided receptors according to their ease of solubilization from membranes. An "insoluble" receptor ("SE") may correspond to type 1 receptors, whereas receptors more easily extracted by detergent ("DE") resemble type 2 receptors. Interestingly, calcium and other divalent cations may enhance [³H]flunitrazepam binding to the DE receptor, which suggests that it is associated with a calcium ionophore.

In order to determine whether the subdivision of BZ_1 and BZ_2 subtypes have some functional significance in terms of sleep, Mendelson et al. (1985c, in press, f) administered CL 218,872 alone and in combination with flurazepam to rats, and sleep studies were performed. Intraperitoneal CL 218,872 (2.5 and 5.0 mg/kg) increased total sleep but did not affect sleep latency. Intraperitoneal flurazepam (40 mg/kg) increased total sleep and decreased sleep latency. Pretreatment with CL 218,872 did not alter the flurazepam effects. To whatever degree CL 218,872 is specific for type 1 receptors, this result might suggest that their stimulation affects sleep maintenance, whereas type 2 receptors could conceivably be more involved in sleep induction.

A number of cautions should be considered in evaluating the possible roles of BZ receptor subtypes. It should be remembered that the preferential binding of CL 218,872 for type 1 receptors is only relative and that some degree of binding to type 2 may occur. Indeed, Braestrup et al. (1982) have suggested that the anxiolytic effects of CL

281,872 are dependent on type 2 binding. Other authors have shown that flunitrazepam and methyl-β-carboline-3-carboxylate bind significantly at both pre- and postsynaptic sites, with varying degrees in different brain regions (Tietz, Chiu, and Rosenberg, 1985). Thus assignment of pre- or postsynaptic localization to CL 218,872 binding, or any conclusions regarding the function of these sites, remains tentative. It is also not entirely clear that types 1 and 2 are distinct or whether they are biochemically identical but differ at the binding site as the result of conformational changes related to their association with other functional units (e.g., GABA receptor, chloride ionophore).

ISSUES FOR THE FUTURE

Many intriguing questions remain unanswered about BZ receptors. A convincing endogenous ligand for the BZ recognition site has yet to be found, and aside from GABA little is known about endogenous substances that might bind to other components of the BZ receptor complex. Another interesting possibility is that the study of receptors may lead to compounds that separate the traditional pharmacological properties of BZs, that is, their hypnotic, anxiolytic, muscle relaxant, and anticonvulsant effects. Interesting advances have been made in both of these areas in recent years.

Endogenous Compounds

As discussed in Chapter 2, the purines inosine and hypoxanthine have been considered as possible ligands for the BZ recognition site (Marangos et al., 1983). Their affinity is relatively greater than that of most compounds tested (IC_{50} of 10^{-3} M), but this still represents relatively weak binding. Although inosine is all the more intriguing because of its possible effects in anxiety-related behaviors (Crawley et al., 1981), the search continues for a compound that interacts significantly with the BZ receptor at lower concentrations.

There is some evidence that derivatives of certain endogenous steroids may bind with high affinity to the dihydropicrotoxinin site. At nanomolar to low micromolar concentrations the progesterone metabolite 3alpha-hydroxy-5alpha-dihydroprogesterone and the deoxycorticosterone derivative 3alpha,5alpha-tetrahydrodeoxycorticosterone (THDOC) have been reported to inhibit TBPS binding, increase flunitrazepam binding, and enhance $^{36}Cl^-$ uptake into brain vesicles (Majewska et al., 1986). Similarly, they may potentiate the inhibitory actions of GABA on cultured neurons. Some could conceivably affect

CNS excitability by such a mechanism, which might also explain the actions of steroidal anesthetics (Child *et al.*, 1971). Mendelson *et al.* (1986c) found that 10 mg/kg of intraperitoneal THDOC had potent hypnotic effects in rats (Fig. 4-14). This raises the possibility that THDOC or some other steroid might have some role in sleep–wake regulation.

Separation of Pharmacological Properties

Another intriguing possibility is that drugs can be developed to manifest a desired pharmacological effect selectively, rather than the several closely associated properties of traditional sedative–hypnotics or analeptics. Among the many preliminary indications that this is possible are observations with two groups of compounds: the β-carbolines and the quinoline derivatives PK 8165 and PK 9084. As discussed earlier, β-CCT clearly has awakening effects in animals but is not proconvulsant. Both PK 8165 and PK 9084 have been reported to have anxiolytic effects, but little anticonvulsant, sedative, or muscle relaxant properties (Lefur *et al.*, 1981). Such work suggests that the development of anxiolytics and hypnotics that are much more selective, with fewer undesirable effects, is indeed possible.

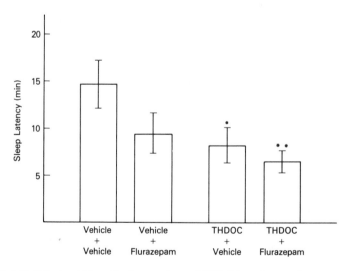

FIGURE 4-14. Effects of 10 mg/kg intraperitoneal THDOC and 20 mg/kg flurazepam on sleep latency in the rat. *, $p < 0.05$ compared to vehicle–vehicle; **, $p < 0.01$ compared to vehicle–vehicle.

SUMMARY

The discovery of high affinity, stereoselective binding sites for BZs was a major step in understanding the molecular mechanism by which these widely used sedative–hypnotics exert their pharmacological effects. It has become clear that the BZ receptor complex has functional significance in terms of the anxiolytic, anticonvulsant, and muscle relaxant properties. Until recently, its role in the sleep-inducing properties was unclear. This chapter has reviewed a series of studies indicating that the BZ receptor complex does indeed mediate the hypnotic effects of flurazepam. Nifedipine, which inhibits flux across potential-dependent calcium channels, inhibits BZ effects on $^{45}Ca^{2+}$ transport *in vitro* and blocks the hypnotic effects of flurazepam. BAY K 8644, which may enhance calcium flux, potentiates sleep induction by flurazepam. Such studies raise the possibility that the hypnotic—though not other—pharmacological actions of BZs may be mediated by alterations in calcium flux.

Pentobarbital and ethanol also affect chloride and calcium flux, although the significance of this in terms of their pharmacological effects is still being evaluated. Some of their actions—notably the toxicity of both compounds and anticonflict effects of PB—may be blocked by altering the chloride channel and the BZ recognition site function, respectively.

Benzodiazepine receptor complexes have been subdivided into type 1, which may be postsynaptic and to which barbiturates may bind, and type 2, which may be presynaptic. BZ binding to type 2 receptors may be sensitive to calcium concentrations. CL 218,872, which binds relatively selectively to type 1 receptors, has a potent sleep-maintaining effect. The molecular and functional significance of the subtyping of BZ receptors, however, requires more elucidation.

The search for a convincing endogenous ligand for the BZ receptor continues. Recently THDOC, a deoxycorticosterone derivative, has been found to have significant hypnotic activity in rats. Experience with some compounds that bind at the BZ receptor suggests that in the future, drugs may become available that are much more specific for individual desired effects.

CHAPTER 5

Neuroendocrinology and Sleep

It has become clear that anterior pituitary hormones are secreted in a pulsatile manner, and that their rhythms bear some relationship to sleep. The nature of this relationship varies with the hormone. Some appear to be associated with a specific EEG stage of sleep, others with the REM-non-REM cycle or the sleep-waking cycle. In some cases, the nature of the relationship varies with age. The association of secretion to sleep may be statistically significant yet account for only a portion of the variance of plasma levels of a hormone. Other influences that may act simultaneously on secretion include circadian mechanisms, the light–dark cycle, and the pulsatile secretion of other hormones.

Several types of studies need to be done in order to characterize the relationship of a hormone—or any physiological event—to sleep. These include:

1. Twenty-four–hour studies with repeated blood sampling to determine if a circadian and/or ultradian rhythm occurs. It seems clear that the frequency of sampling must not be substantially longer than the plasma half-life of the hormone studied. Experience with the gonadotropins emphasizes the need to perform such studies on subjects of all ages.

2. Studies of delayed sleep onset and a reversed sleep–waking cycle to determine if the secretion is related specifically to sleep or to the time of day or to both.

3. Studies of secretion under conditions of constant lighting and of secretion in blind subjects to determine if secretion is related to the light–dark cycle.

4. Studies of sleep deprivation and modified sleep–wake cycles (e.g., 3 hr, 33 hr) to determine if secretion is related to sleep and waking. A disadvantage here is that drastic changes in the sleep cycle length may distort percentages of various sleep stages.

5. Analyses relating hormone levels to specific sleep stages. A basic characterization may be made by determining what percentage of the variance in hormone levels is accounted for by the presence of a particular sleep stage.

6. Determination of whether the sleep-related secretion of a hormone is regulated by a second sleep-related system. There is, for example, some preliminary evidence that sleep-related secretion of testosterone may be influenced by sleep-related secretion of prolactin (PRL).

7. Pharmacological manipulation of sleep-related secretion to provide indirect data on the types of neural pathways that might regulate sleep-related secretion. Drug actions must be assessed in terms of the effects on sleep-related secretion as well as secretion during pharmacological provocative stimulation tests. As will be seen in the discussion of growth hormone, the same drug may have different effects on these two types of secretion.

8. Studies to determine what effects administration of the hormone has on the occurrence of the sleep stages. A similar approach is to study sleep in animals in which the endocrine gland under study has been removed, and in patients with diseases of over- and undersecretion. The drawback of the latter type of study is that there is always some question as to whether any abnormalities in sleep are due to modified hormone levels or to CNS lesions that may have produced the endocrine disease.

These types of studies are necessary for the most basic characterization of the relationship of secretion of a hormone to sleep. Before the results of these investigations are described, a brief review of the major endocrinological systems is in order.

BASIC CONCEPTS IN NEUROENDOCRINOLOGY

This discussion will center on the pituitary and pineal glands, which are anatomically contiguous with, and physiologically intimately involved with, the central nervous system. The pituitary gland is a small structure that rests in the sella turcica, a cavity in the sphenoid bone of the skull. It is attached by the pituitary stalk to the ventral surface of the diencephalon, just posterior to the optic chiasm. It is divided into the adenohypophysis (anterior pituitary), neurohypophysis (posterior pituitary), and intermediate lobe or zone. The anterior pituitary synthesizes and releases the following protein hormones: growth hormone (GH), adrenocorticotropic hormone (ACTH), beta-endorphin, prolactin (PRL), thyroid-stimulating hormone (TSH), luteinizing hormone (LH), and follicle-stimulating hormone (FSH). Although melanocyte-stimulating hormone (MSH) is well recognized in amphibians, in primates its chemical nature is uncertain and its existence controversial. The posterior pituitary secretes two hormones— vasopressin (or antidiuretic hormone) and oxytocin.

Some of these hormones may directly affect nonendocrine tissues, (GH and PRL) or may stimulate the release of hormones from endocrine glands elsewhere in the body (ACTH, TSH, LH, and FSH) (Fig. 5-1). There is also some evidence that GH, LH, and TSH may be formed in various parts of the nervous system, where they presumably have some neuromodulating role.

Anterior pituitary hormone secretion is thought to be regulated by two types of mechanisms. The first is open loop control, which refers to regulation of the anterior pituitary by stimulation from the central nervous system. This is mediated by releasing or inhibiting peptides that are carried from the hypothalamus to the pituitary by portal blood vessels. These include GH-releasing hormone, GH-inhibiting hormone (somatostatin), corticotropin-releasing hormone (CRH), prolactin-releasing hormone, prolactin-inhibiting hormone (PIH), thyrotropin-releasing hormone (TRH), and gonadotropin-releasing hormone (GnRH). Several of these substances may also act directly on the extra-hypothalamic nervous system as in the mediation of some stress responses by CRH. Neural pathways in the hypothalamus are thought to be mediated by the biogenic amines, particularly serotonin, norepinephrine, and dopamine. Epinephrine appears to play a more limited role. The amines are also thought to be involved in the pathways that regulate the sleep stages (see Chapter 2). A wide variety of peptide and amino acid neurotransmitters may also play modulatory roles. Later, it will be seen that many of the drugs that influence anterior pituitary hormone secretion (as well as the sleep stages) are thought to do so by stimulating or inhibiting these neural pathways. Other mechanisms of drug action might include direct effects on the pituitary.

The second type of control of anterior pituitary secretion is the closed loop mechanism, regulation by a negative feedback system sensitive to circulating hormone levels. When ACTH is released, for in-

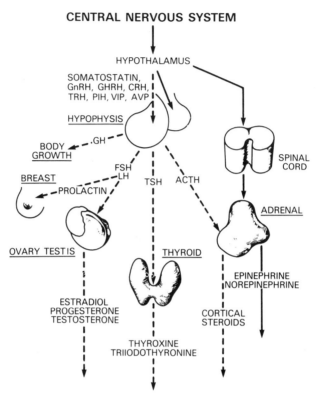

FIGURE 5-1. Schematic representation of pituitary function. (Modified from Morgan, 1973. Reprinted by permission.)

stance, there is a resultant rise in cortisol secretion by the adrenal cortex. The increased cortisol in turn affects the pituitary to reduce the secretion of ACTH; it may also affect the secretion of CRH. Negative feedback loops have been demonstrated for ACTH, LH, FSH, TSH, and GH; the closed loop mechanism for GH is mediated by somatomedin C, a peptide produced primarily in the liver under the influence of GH. These "long-loop" mechanisms are complemented by the effect of pituitary hormones on hypothalamic secretion and on their own production (short loop and ultrashort loop mechanisms, respectively). A rise in PRL, for example, increases hypothalamic dopamine turnover, and enhanced secretion of this potent RPL inhibitor tends to restore homeostatic equilibrium.

The intermediate lobe of the pituitary, which is well developed in lower species, is largely vestigial in man; it is represented by small cystic areas and nests of cells between the anterior and the posterior lobes. Its physiological importance lies in the fact that many of the pro-opiomelanocortin cells, which produce ACTH and endorphins, are found in this area (some are in the posterior lobe) and in the adjacent area of the anterior lobe.

The posterior pituitary gland, or neurohypophysis, is derived embryologically from nerve tissue. Peptidergic cells in the hypothalamus synthesize vasopressin and oxytocin and transport these hormones down their fibers to the neurohypophysis, where they are released into the blood. Vasopressin release is triggered by cells, sensitive to blood osmolality, located in the hypothalamus, and from cells sensitive to stretch, located in the right atrium of the heart and elsewhere. These latter cells send fibers to the brain via the vagal nerves. In addition, stimulation of the midbrain emetic center by dopaminergic stimuli releases large quantities of vasopressin. Oxytocin secretion is stimulated by suckling, and stimulation of the cervix and vagina.

The pineal gland is a small conical structure lying on the dorsum of the diencephalon, projecting backward over the tectum of the midbrain. In lower vertebrates it contains cells that are directly sensitive to light. In humans this is not the case, but the secretion of its hormone, melatonin, is influenced by the amount of lighting via neural pathways from the retina. The pineal gland is bathed in CSF, and it is not clear whether melatonin is released into the blood, the CSF, or both. As will be discussed later, melatonin is of particular interest because there is some evidence that it may be released by the pineal gland to directly influence other parts of the CNS.

The structure and actions of each hormone are summarized at the beginning of the appropriate section. Detailed discussions of these endocrine systems are provided by Daughaday (1985) and Reichlin (1985).

GROWTH HORMONE*

Secretion in Sleep and Waking

Since the 1960s, a growing body of evidence has linked GH secretion to sleep. This relationship has now been described in more detail than is available for any other anterior pituitary hormone. The nature of the hypothalamic control mechanisms of secretion and the relation of this phenomenon to psychiatric illness are less well understood.

*Portions of this section come from Mendelson (1982d). Reprinted by permission.

Growth hormone has a variety of known functions, including stimulation of growth of long bones, in which epiphyses have not closed, as well as endochondral bone and cartilage. It influences the growth of nearly all soft tissues and organs, although various tissues differ greatly in their sensitivity to its effects. Many of these actions may be mediated by the release from the liver and possibly the kidney of a group of peptides, the somatomedins. There has been particular interest in somatomedin C insulinlike growth factor I (Underwood, 1984). Growth hormone has also been found in the central nervous system (Pacold et al., 1978), and injections of GH into mice have been shown to enhance isolation-induced aggression (Matte, 1981). Such observations imply that GH has direct behavioral effects.

Growth hormone has been reported to modify carbohydrate, protein, and lipid metabolism; its secretion in turn is altered by changes in their blood levels (Brown and Reichlin, 1972). Decreases in plasma free fatty acids induced by nicotinic acid, for instance, result in increase blood GH (Irie et al., 1967), and the infusion of several amino acids, including arginine, is followed by increased GH secretion (Knopf et al., 1965). Of particular interest is the relation of GH to blood glucose levels. Hypoglycemia induced by insulin injection increases GH secretion (J. Roth et al., 1963; Brown and Reichlin, 1972). This action seems to be specifically related to hypoglycemia, rather than to other actions of insulin, since GH secretion is increased by hypoglycemia induced by, for example, infusion of 2-deoxy-D-glucose or the hypoglycemia seen with certain mesenchymal tumors with low levels of endogenous insulin (J. Roth et al., 1963). Oral glucose ingestion decreases GH, whereas fasting results in increased secretion (Glick et al., 1965).

Among the earliest observations on GH secretion at night is a report by Hunter, Friend, and Strong (1966), who took hourly measurements of GH concentrations by day, and up to three measurements at night in nine subjects. Growth hormone concentrations at night were found to be elevated, which was thought to be a response to the subjects not having eaten for some hours. Quabbe, Schilling, and Helge (1966), studying fasting human subjects, noted peak concentrations of GH several times throughout the night that were unrelated to blood glucose levels. Although there was no EEG monitoring, they suggested that the GH peaks were related to the "deeper" periods of sleep. The relation of a GH peak to sleep onset was carefully demonstrated by Takahashi, Kipnis, and Daughaday (1968). In seven out of eight human subjects a plasma GH peak (13–72 ng/ml) occurred during the first 90 min of sleep and lasted 1.5–3.5 hr (Figs. 5-2 and 5-3). If sleep onset was delayed, the GH peak also occurred later. If the subjects were awakened for 2 to 3 hr and then allowed to sleep, another GH peak appeared. Smaller peaks occurred throughout the night and seemed to be related to stages 3 and 4; 43% of the peaks were during these stages, even though they comprised only 15% of total sleep time. The GH secretion was not related to plasma levels of glucose, insulin, or cortisol.

Patterns of GH secretion over a 24-hr period vary greatly with age. In the first few weeks of life, plasma GH levels show no difference between sleep or waking, and no difference between "quiet" and "active" sleep (Shaywitz et al., 1971). After the third month, waking values drop considerably and are significantly less than levels during sleep (Vigneri and D'Agata, 1971). At about this time, "quiet" sleep, which is thought to be analogous to the adult slow-wave sleep, comes to dominate the infant's sleep cycle (Stern et al., 1969). Prepubertal children secrete GH during sleep but little during the waking state (Finkelstein et al., 1972; Illig et al., 1971). During adolescence, both sleep-related secretion and daytime secretion increase. In young adults sleep-related secretion is somewhat less than in adolescents; in the elderly sleep-related secretion is reduced (Carlson et al., 1972). It has been speculated that this decreased secretion in the elderly is related to their diminished slow-wave sleep (Rubin et al., 1974).

Initially, GH secretion seemed to be tied closely to sleep, since there was little evidence of any circadian influence. Sassin et al. (1969), for instance, found that a 12-hr reversal of the sleep–waking cycle was followed immediately by reversal of the pattern of GH secretion, which remained related to slow-wave sleep. More recent evidence suggests that there may also be some circadian aspects to the regulation of GH secretion. A study of jet lag, for instance, found that after subjects flew from Chicago to Brussels, GH tended to be secreted during the later part of the night (Golstein et al., 1983). Flights in either direction

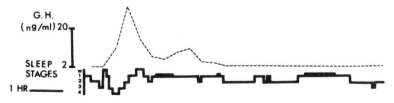

FIGURE 5-2. Sleep-related GH secretion in a normal young male, age 21, plotted in relation to sleep stages.

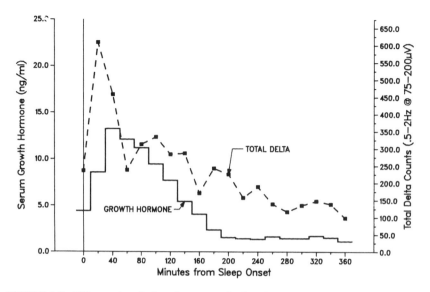

FIGURE 5-3. GH secretion during sleep may also be plotted with reference to total delta power in the EEG (see Chapter 9). (From Kupfer *et al.*, unpublished. Reprinted by permission.)

resulted in increased GH secretion, due primarily to increase in magnitude of peaks; a return to normal was more delayed (at least 11 days) after the westward flight. It has also been found that monkey anterior pituitary tissue *in vitro* releases GH and PRL periodically, approximately every 8 min (Stewart *et al.*, 1985). It has been reported that GH secretion may be greater during insulin tolerance tests conducted in the evening compared to the morning (Nathan *et al.*, 1979), although this was not found in an earlier study (Ichikawa *et al.*, 1972).

The nature of the relationship of GH secretion to slow-wave sleep also requires further description. As mentioned above, Takahaski *et al.* (1968) originally noted that a disproportionate amount of secretion occurred during slow-wave sleep. The problem, of course, is that there is normally a high percentage of slow-wave sleep in the first 2 hr of sleep, so that it seemed possible that the GH peak was related to sleep onset or to early sleep, and not to slow-wave sleep per se. There are several ways to resolve this issue. One approach is to examine GH peaks that occur late in sleep, when slow-wave sleep is relatively uncommon. Sassin *et al.* (1969) divided sleep late at night into slow-wave and non-slow-wave cycles. They found that the majority of peaks occurred in slow-wave cycles and that these were higher than those in cycles without slow-wave sleep. Using a similar principle, Karacan *et al.* (1975) examined 29 normal young men who slept for 2 hr in either the morning or the late afternoon. Their morning naps contained relatively more REM sleep and less slow-wave sleep than their afternoon naps. It was found that GH secretion was greater during sleep in the afternoon.

The association of GH secretion to slow-wave sleep has been further defined by a variety of studies. Pawel, Sassin, and Weitzman (1972) took plasma samples every 4 min during the first 90 min of sleep and found that delta activity (although not necessarily stage 3 using 30-sec epochs) always preceded GH release. Karacan *et al.* (1971) found that partial slow-wave sleep deprivation resulted in decreased GH secretion shortly after sleep onset. Generally, slow-wave sleep preceded GH secretion, but in some cases isolated peaks occurred. Conversely, periods of slow-wave sleep frequently were unaccompanied by episodes of GH secretion (Takahashi *et al.*, 1968). Flurazepam, which decreases slow-wave sleep, has been reported to have no effect on sleep-related GH secretion (Rubin *et al.*, 1973a). Conversely, ritanserin (see Chapter 2) may enhance slow-wave sleep without altering GH secretion during sleep (Clarenbach, Birmanns, and Jaursch-Hancke, personal communication). Medroxyprogesterone acetate and free fatty acid infusions can decrease GH secretion without influencing slow-wave sleep (Lucke and Glick, 1971b; Lipman *et al.*, 1972).

Weitzman *et al.* (1974) studied the relation of GH secretion to slow-wave sleep by manipulating the sleep-waking cycle. They allowed normal subjects to sleep for eight 1-hr periods during each 24-hr period. It was found that GH secretion was related to those periods in which more than 36 min of sleep occurred. There was no association between growth hormone secretion and duration of slow-wave sleep during these periods. The authors suggested that GH secretion is related to onset, but not duration, of slow-wave sleep. Such a premise might explain why Othmer *et al.* (1974a) found no relationship between total amounts of slow-wave sleep in the first 4 hr of sleep and amount of GH secretion or why GH secretion was normal in the flurazepam study (Rubin *et al.*, 1973a). Golstein *et al.* (1983), in the study of jet lag, found no correlation of total GH secretion during sleep with the amount of slow-wave sleep. Mendlewicz *et al.* (1985) reported that in depressed patients slow-wave sleep was reduced, but total amounts of GH remained normal. The timing of GH secretion, however, was altered.

It is also possible that GH secretion may be influenced by slow-wave sleep during periods of sleep prior to the one being studied. Othmer *et al.* (1974b), studying GH secretion during morning naps, reported that it was not related to the amount of slow-wave sleep during the nap or to the amount of GH secretion the previous night. It was found, however, that subjects who secreted the most GH during the morning naps were those who had had the least stage 3 sleep the previous night. It might be worthwhile to pursue the hypothesis that GH secretion is determined not only by the sleep stage present at the time of secretion, but also by the pattern of sleep stages over the previous 24-hr period.

The relationship, if any, between GH secretion and REM sleep is not clear. Studies of GH secretion during REM sleep deprivation have found either no change (Honda *et al.*, 1969) or increased (Daughaday, Othmer, and Kipnis, 1969) GH secretion. One tentative implication might be that REM sleep inhibits the secretion of GH-releasing factor (see Takahashi, 1974). In the jet lag study mentioned earlier (Golstein *et al.*, 1983), total amounts of GH secreted during sleep correlated negatively with the amount of REM sleep and were not significantly related to slow-wave sleep. A spike-by-spike analysis did show a significant relationship to the ratio of slow-wave minus REM (SW − REM) to slow-wave plus REM sleep (SW + REM). This ratio, which relates the amount of REM preceding the spike to the amount of slow-wave sleep during the spike, normally decreases from a value of $+1$ to -1 as the night progresses. These data were taken to suggest that there may be an inhibitory influence of REM sleep on GH secretion.

Although sleep stages may be related to the onset of specific peaks of GH secretion, there is some evidence that the total amount of GH secreted over 24 hr may be relatively constant in a given individual. In the Weitzman *et al.* (1974) study, total 24-hr GH secretion remained the same, although the pattern and times of sleep changed drastically. In an Arctic environment with extremes of daylight and darkness, sleep-related GH secretion stayed the same during all four seasons (Weitzman *et al.*, 1975). Golstein *et al.* (1983), however, did find greatly increased GH secretion as the result of transmeridian travel. In general, however, in the absence of such major manipulations of sleep, patterns of secretion differ greatly between subjects but may be relatively constant in any one person (Takahashi, 1974; Takahashi *et al.*, 1968). It has been suggested that traits with this combination of qualities are most suited for genetic studies, and the opportunity clearly seems to be here for such work.

The control of GH secretion may be examined by determining the effects of drugs on GH secretion in response to various standard stimuli or to sleep. Perhaps the most common provocative agents are insulin, arginine, L-DOPA, propranolol, clonidine, and GH-releasing hormone (Ho, Evans, and Thorner, 1985). Data comparing GH stimulation by these agents have been obtained in several studies (Lin and Tucci, 1974; Lucke, Hoeffken, and Morgner, 1974; Weldon et al., 1973). Sleep-related GH secretion seems to be as (or slightly more) consistent than secretion during pharmacological stimulation tests. Of the five subjects examined by Lucke et al. (1974), three had comparable values with all tests and one had a low response to arginine and L-DOPA but a normal response to sleep and insulin. Another subject had low values with sleep and subnormal responses to arginine and L-DOPA. Among the pharmacological stimuli, L-DOPA seemed to have the highest incidence of "false negatives." Analysis of the data of Underwood et al. (1971) shows that of 13 normal children who slept well, nine had good responses to both insulin and sleep; three had peak responses of less than 5 ng/ml to insulin but more than 5 ng/ml during sleep; and only one subject had less than 5 ng/ml during sleep but more than 5 ng/ml with insulin testing. Mace, Gotlin, and Beck (1972), drawing a single sample of blood 90 min after sleep onset, found that all of 46 normal children had levels of GH greater than 7 ng/ml; they compared this response with studies that reported comparable levels of GH in only 70–90% of subjects receiving insulin or arginine in provocative tests. A study by Lin and Tucci (1974), in which a sample was taken "1 to 2 hours after the apparent onset of nocturnal sleep" showed a relatively low percentage of GH peaks; such data point to the importance of serial blood sampling while monitoring sleep by EEG.

There is substantial evidence that neurotransmitter regulation of sleep-related GH secretion is very different from that of daytime insulin-stimulated GH secretion. Early indications that this might be the case came from studies of glucose infusions. Glucose will inhibit rising GH levels in resting awake subjects (Glick et al., 1965) as well as the response to exercise (Hunter et al., 1965) or arginine (Burday, Fine, and Schalch, 1968). In contrast, it does not inhibit sleep-related secretion (Parker and Rossman, 1971), at least until extremely high (>350 mg/100 ml) concentrations are reached (Lucke and Glick, 1971a). This section reviews the effects of pharmacological manipulation of neurotransmitters on insulin-induced GH secretion (chosen as an example of a daytime stimulation test) and sleep-related peaks in human normal volunteers. The studies that are described in detail in the text are summarized in Table 5-1. It will be seen that the relative roles of these transmitters (as inferred from the effects of pharmacological agents) are drastically altered in sleep.

TABLE 5-1. Effects of Substances on Sleep-Related GH Secretion in Humans

Drug	References	Effect on sleep-related secretion	Effect on insulin-stimulated secretion
Amylobarbital	Ogunremi et al., 1973	→[a]	—
Chlordiazepoxide	Takahashi et al., 1968		→
Chlorpromazine	Takahashi et al., 1968	→[b]	—
Clomiphene	Perlow et al., 1972	→	—
Diphenylhydantoin	Takahashi et al., 1968	↑	→
L-DOPA	Chihara et al., 1976c	↑	→
Free fatty acids	Lipman et al., 1972	→	→
Glucose	Lucke and Glick, 1971a	→ (>350 mg %)	—
Hydrocortisone	Krieger et al., 1972	↑	—
Imipramine	Takahashi et al., 1968	→	→
Isocarboxazid	Takahashi et al., 1968	↑	→
Medroxyprogesterone	Lucke and Glick, 1971b; Simon et al., 1967	→	→
Methscopolamine	Mendelson et al., 1978d	→	—
Methysergide	Mendelson et al., 1975b	←	—
Parachlorophenylalanine	Malarkey and Mendall, 1976	→[c]	—
Phenobarbital	Takahashi et al., 1968; Rosadini et al., 1983	↑ ; ↓	→
Phentolamine	Lucke and Glick, 1971a	↑	—
Pizotifen	Clarenbach et al., 1980	→	→
Prednisolone	Illig et al., 1971	→	—
Propanolol	Lucke and Glick, 1971a; Lewis et al., 1981	↑	←
Thyrotropin-releasing hormone	Chihara et al., 1977b	→	—
Tryptophan	Murri et al., 1973	↑[d]	—

[a] Increase reported during withdrawal.
[b] Dosage was 30 mg, substantially less than the amount with ITT by Sherman et al. (1971).
[c] Duchenne muscular dystrophy patients.
[d] Schizophrenic patients.

Effect of Alterations in Neurotransmitter Function on GH Secretion

Acetylcholine

There have been reports for some time that cholinomimetic agents may increase GH secretion. Cytidine diphosphate (CDP) choline and beta-methylchol: ie, which may enhance cholinergic acitity, increase GH levels in resting, awake depressed patients and in normal volunteers, respectively (Salvadorini *et al.*, 1975; Soulairac *et al.*, 1968). There is also evidence of cholinergic involvement in GH stimulation by arginine, glucagon, apomorphine, L-DOPA, clonidine, the enkephalin analogue FK 33-824, and exercise (Delitala *et al.*, 1982, 1983a,b; Casanueva *et al.*, 1984; Brillon, Nabil, and Jacobs, 1986). Mendelson *et al.* (1978d) compared the effects of methscopolamine bromide (a muscarinic cholinergic receptor blocker) on insulin-stimulated and sleep-related GH secretion. Methscopolamine (0.5 mg) was injected intramuscularly 30 min before bedtime in 8 normal male volunteers and 30 min before an insulin test in 12 volunteers, including 3 who had been in the sleep study. Methscopolamine had marginally inhibitory effects on insulin-induced GH secretion (Fig. 5-4). Peak concentrations, mean increments, and areas under the curve were not significantly affected ($p < 0.2$). An analysis of variance, however, did show a significant ($p < 0.01$) difference between drug and placebo values; as a percentage of area under the curves, this was approximately a 31% reduction. In contrast, sleep-related GH secretion was virtually abolished by methscopolamine (Fig. 5-5). The mean concentration, for instance, was reduced from 11.9 ± 3.11 ng/ml with placebo to 1.0 ± 0.2 ng/ml after methscopolamine ($p < 0.001$). Despite the virtual absence of GH secretion, no measured EEG sleep parameter (including slow-wave sleep) was altered. This suggests that muscarinic receptor blockade inhibits sleep-related GH secretion. [In passing, it should be noted that this may explain the report of Takahashi *et al.* (1968) that imipramine, which has anticholinergic properties, inhibits sleep-related GH secretion.]

There are few data on the possible role of nicotinic cholinergic receptors in GH secretion. Binding by alpha-bungarotoxin, which may be a marker of nicotinic receptors in the central nervous system (Morley, Kemp, and Salvaterra, 1979), occurs heavily in the mediobasal and basolateral hypothalamus (Silver and Billiar, 1976). More recently, such ligands as tritiated nicotine and acetylcholine have become available; their high-affinity binding sites, which have a different distribution than alpha-bungarotoxin, may represent the central counterpart of

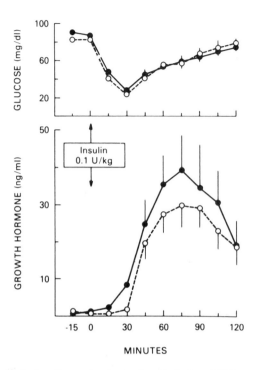

FIGURE 5-4. The effect of methscopolamine on insulin-induced GH secretion: concentrations of GH and glucose following administration of 0.1 unit/kg regular insulin; ●, control; ○, methscopolamine. (From Mendelson *et al.*, 1978d. Reprinted by permission.)

the ganglionic nicotinic cholinoceptor (Clarke, 1987). Mendelson *et al.* (1981c) gave 30-min intravenous infusions of 100 mg piperidine, a nicotinic receptor agonist, to seven volunteers, starting 15 min before an insulin test, and to eight volunteers, starting at sleep onset. During the insulin test, piperidine increased the area under the curve (3041 ± 78 ng·min·ml^{-1} on piperidine versus 2243 ± 214 ng·min·ml^{-1} on placebo; $p < 0.05$). The mean increase over baseline during the insulin test was also significantly enhanced (48.0 ± 5.3 ng/ml versus 36.83 ± 3.6 ng/ml; $p < 0.01$). Sleep-related secretion of GH was also increased by piperidine (Fig. 5-6). The mean GH concentration over the entire piperidine night was 6.1 ± 1.8 ng/ml compared to 4.2 ± 0.5 ng/ml on placebo ($p < 0.02$). When data for the first 2 hr of sleep were examined, this piperidine-induced increase was even more striking (15.2 ± 2.9 ng/ml versus 7.2 ± 1.2 ng/ml; $p < 0.01$). The EEG stages of sleep were unaffected. This suggests that nicotinic receptor stimulation enhances insulin-induced and sleep-related GH secretion.

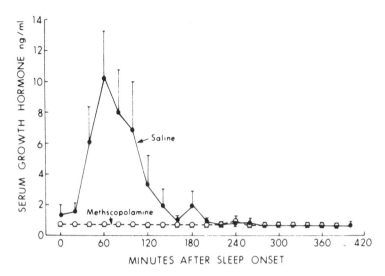

FIGURE 5-5. Effect of methscopolamine on GH concentrations during sleep. Normal volunteers were treated with (●) saline or (○) 0.5 mg of methscopolamine. (From Mendelson *et al.*, 1978d. Reprinted by permission.)

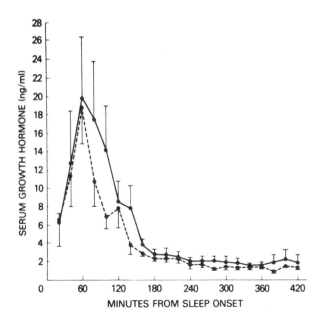

FIGURE 5-6. Sleep-related GH secretion in volunteers treated with 100 mg of piperidine (———) or saline (– – –). (From Mendelson *et al.*, 1981c. Reprinted by permission.)

Catecholamines

The involvement of monoamines in insulin-induced secretion was suggested by the observation that reserpine inhibits this form of GH secretion (Cavagnini and Peracchi, 1979). Blackard and Heidingsfelder (1968) found that insulin-induced GH secretion was inhibited by the α-adrenergic receptor blocker phentolamine and enhanced by the β-blocker propranolol. In contrast, phentolamine and propranolol have been reported to have no effect on sleep-related secretion (Lucke and Glick, 1971).

A role of dopamine in GH regulation may be inferred from several types of studies. L-DOPA (Boyd, Lobovitz, and Pfeiffer, 1970), the dopamine receptor agonist apomorphine (Lal *et al.*, 1973), and dopamine itself (Leebaw, Lee, and Woolf, 1978) all stimulate GH secretion when given alone to resting, awake subjects. Insulin-induced secretion has been reported to be diminished by chlorpromazine (Sherman *et al.*, 1971) and haloperidol (Kim *et al.*, 1971), possibly as a result of their dopamine receptor-blocking properties. On the other hand, prior stimulation of GH by dopamine blocks subsequent insulin-stimulated GH secretion (Leebaw *et al.*, 1978). Arginine stimulation, however, does not inhibit a later insulin-stimulated secretory episode (Woolf, Lantigua, and Lee, 1979). This suggests that insulin-induced GH secretion, which may be mediated in part by dopaminergic mechanisms, is inhibited after recent dopaminergic stimulation.

In contrast to insulin-stimulated secretion, sleep-related secretion of GH is not inhibited by chlorpromazine, at least in a somewhat smaller dose than that used in the previously described insulin study by Sherman *et al.* (Takahashi, Kipnis, and Daughaday, 1968). L-DOPA infusions, at a rate of 1 μg/min for several hours, have also been reported to have no effect on sleep-related GH secretion (Chihara *et al.*, 1976). A single patient with Tourette's disease was studied before and during chronic treatment with 5 mg of haloperidol (Fig. 5-7), again without effect (Caine, Mendelson, and Loriaux, 1979). Taken together, these data on dopamine and sleep-related secretion are somewhat less adequate than the data on the other neurotransmitters we will examine. It seems reasonable to tentatively conclude, however, that dopamine, which stimulates GH secretion in resting, awake subjects, may have a stimulatory role in insulin-inducing secretion of GH but little effect on sleep-related GH secretion.

Serotonin

There is reason to believe that serotonergic neurons enhance some forms of GH secretion. The serotonin precursor 5-hydroxytryptophan

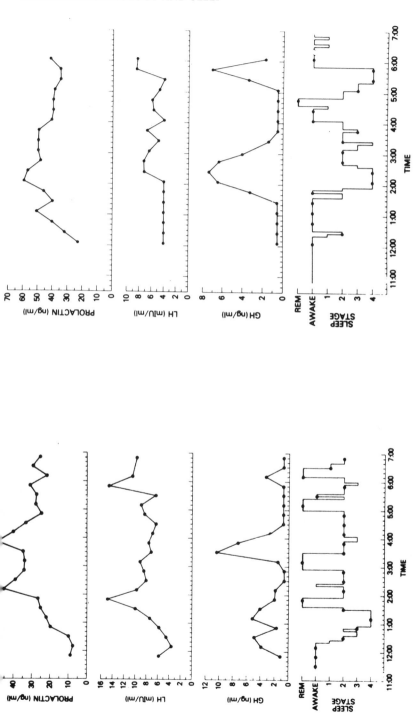

FIGURE 5-7. Prolactin, LH, and GH concentrations during sleep before (left) and after (right) 10 days of treatment with 5 mg/day of haloperidol in a patient with Tourette's disease. Student's *t*-test revealed an increase in PRL, a decrease in LH, and no change in GH. (From Caine, Mendelson, and Loriaux, 1979. Reprinted by permission.)

(5-HTP) increases GH concentrations in resting, awake subjects
(Yoshimura *et al.*, 1973), and agents with serotonin receptor blocking
properties, such as cyproheptadine, methysergide, and melatonin,
have been reported to inhibit insulin-induced GH secretion (Smythe
and Lazarus, 1974; Bivens, Lebovitz, and Feldman, 1973; Mendelson *et
al.*, 1975b). As with NE, the effects of some serotonergic agents on GH
may differ during insulin testing and sleep. Mendelson *et al.* (1975b)
gave the serotonin receptor blocker methysergide (2 mg orally) every 6
hr for 48 hr to 10 normal volunteers. In confirmation of previous work,
methysergide significantly ($p < 0.01$) decreased insulin-induced GH
secretion by 36% (Fig. 5-8). In contrast, serum concentrations during
nocturnal sleep were increased 46% by methysergide, compared to
placebo ($p < 0.001$; Fig. 5-9). Thus, a serotonin receptor blocker may inhibit GH secretion during a daytime insulin stimulation test but actually enhance secretion during nocturnal sleep. The more selective
serotonin type-2 receptor blocker ritanserin has been reported not to alter sleep-related GH secretion (Clarenbach, Birmanns, and Jaursch-
Hancke, personal communication); it is possible that this is the beginning of indications about functional significance of serotonin receptor
subtypes.

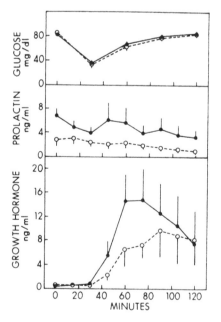

FIGURE 5-8. Glucose, PRL, and GH concentrations following administration of 0.1
unit/kg regular insulin in subjects pretreated with methysergide (–––) or placebo
(———). (From Mendelson *et al.*, 1975b. Reprinted by permission.)

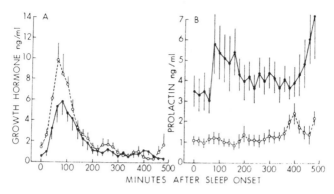

FIGURE 5-9. The effect of methysergide (————) or placebo (———) on sleep-related GH and PRL secretion. (From Mendelson *et al.*, 1975b. Reprinted by permission.)

Sedative–Hypnotics and GH Secretion

The role of hypnotics on GH secretion is not entirely clear. As mentioned earlier, flurazepam has been reported not to alter sleep-related GH secretion (Rubin *et al.*, 1973a). One laboratory has reported that diazepam may increase daytime secretion, an effect that may be reduced by the dopamine blocker pimozide, the GABA transaminase inhibitor sodium valproate, or naloxone (Koulu *et al.*, 1979, 1985). Other studies have found the stimulating effect of diazepam to be inconsistent (Levin, Sharp, and Carlson, 1984; D'Armiento *et al.*, 1984) or absent (Zaccario *et al.*, 1985). Phenobarbital has been reported to decrease both daytime and sleep-related levels of GH (Rosadini *et al.*, 1983).

Summary

The data presented here suggest that the systematic administration of agents that alter neurotransmitter function changes insulin-induced and sleep-related GH secretion, although any one agent may affect these two secretory processes differently. Phentolamine and propranolol inhibit and enhance insulin-induced secretion, respectively, but have no effect on sleep-related secretion. L-DOPA, apomorphine, and dopamine stimulate daytime secretion in resting, awake subjects. Chlorpromazine and haloperidol (which block dopamine receptors) inhibit insulin-induced secretion. L-DOPA, chlorpromazine, and haloperidol do not affect sleep-related secretion. Methysergide (a serotonin receptor blocker) inhibits insulin-induced secretion but actually enhances sleep-related GH secretion. Methscopolamine partially inhibits insulin-induced secretion and profoundly suppresses sleep-related secretion. Piperidine (a nicotinic receptor agonist) enhances both processes.

If one accepts that these pharmacological agents have relatively specific actions, the implications for neurotransmitter function might be summarized as follows: Some aspect of serotonergic receptor stimulation has facilitative effects on insulin-induced GH secretion but inhibits sleep-related secretion. Further work with receptor subtypes may show this to be more complex. α-Noradrenergic and dopaminergic pathways have facilitative effects on insulin-induced secretion and relatively little effect on sleep-related secretion. α-Noradrenergic pathways may have an inhibitory effect on insulin-induced secretion and little or no effect on sleep-related secretion. Muscarinic and nicotinic cholinergic mechanisms may facilitate both insulin-induced and sleep-related secretion. These concepts are represented schematically in Fig. 5-10. (This diagram should not be taken to imply the site of neurotransmitter action, but only the changes induced by them.) One way of viewing these findings is that the facilitative influence of the monoamines norepinephrine, dopamine, and serotonin on GH secretion is greatly diminished or even reversed during sleep. Cholinergic facilitation, however, is evident during sleep as well as in the day in response to several pharmacological stimuli. This may provide a possible foundation for models that can be tested using more basic neurophysiological techniques.

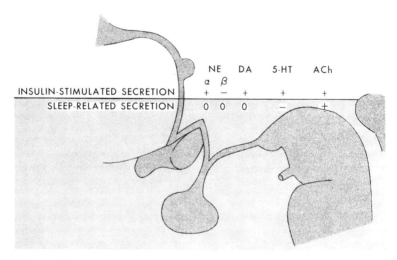

FIGURE 5-10. Schematic representation of neurotransmitter influence on insulin-induced and sleep-related GH secretion. (From Mendelson *et al.*, 1982d. Reprinted by permission.)

Before going on to possible mechanisms that might explain these findings, it is appropriate to mention that there are at least two findings that may not be consistent with the data summarized here. The first is that oral administration of 10 g of an acetylcholine precursor (choline chloride) did not change sleep-related GH secretion in a pilot study (Mendelson et al., unpublished data). Although this remains unresolved, the failure of oral choline to augment GH secretion may only mean that it did not enhance cholinergic transmission in relevant parts of the nervous system. Such a possibility is supported by the observation that choline infusions may not increase synthesis of acetylcholine in rats (Eckernas, Sahlstrom, and Aquilonius, 1977). The second issue is raised by a study (Chihara et al., 1976b) in which cyproheptadine, which is thought to have serotonergic blocking properties, decreased sleep-related GH secretion. It should be noted that, in prolactin studies, the effects of cyproheptadine differed from the effects of both methysergide and the serotonin antagonist metergoline (Crosignani et al., 1979). Cyproheptadine also has antihistaminic, dopamine-blocking, and anticholinergic properties (Stone et al., 1961; van Riezen, 1972). Insofar as the methscopolamine data suggest that anticholinergic drugs inhibit sleep-related GH secretion, perhaps this property of cyproheptadine is responsible for the reduced GH secretion reported by Chihara et al. (1976b).

Locus of Drug Effect

The only data presented here that help define the locus of effect come from the methscopolamine study. Insofar as quaternary ammonium derivatives are largely unable to cross the blood–brain barrier (Domino and Corssen, 1967; Innes and Nickerson, 1970), it seems likely that methscopolamine acts in the areas of the median eminence or the pituitary, which are less well protected by the barrier. The site of action of the other pharmacological agents is unknown. Mueller, Nistico, and Scapagnini (1977) have outlined possible paths that include indirect connections from distant parts of the brain, direct axodendritic or axosomatic contact of cells employing these neurotransmitters with the cells that secrete inhibiting or releasing factors, the presence of cell elements that contain both monoamines and inhibiting or releasing factors, and other possibilities. Elegant studies by Martin (1974) have shown that GH secretion in the rat may be elicited by electrical stimulation of a number of areas, including the hippocampus and the locus ceruleus. Insofar as the latter, which contains primarily noradrenergic cells, is thought to play an important role in the regulation of sleep and waking (Chapter 2), this may be one connection by which monoaminergic areas related to sleep are associated with sleep-related GH secretion.

Somatostatin

Another possibility is that somatostatin plays a role in the nocturnal rise of GH. It has been reported that somatostatin administration will block the sleep-related peak of GH (Parker et al., 1974b; Lucke, Hoffken, and Muhlen, 1976; Cabranes et al., 1984). However, there may be little change in plasma somatostatin concentrations during sleep, and no negative correlations with the sleep-related peak of GH (Saito et al., 1983). Assays for somatostatin are still being improved, and there is also some uncertainty about the relation of circulating peripheral coi.centrations of somatostatin to amounts secreted by the hypothalamus (Chihara, Arimara, and Schally, 1979; Tsuda et al., 1981). It seems too early, then, to draw conclusions about the role of somatostatin in sleep-related GH secretion.

Secretion of GH in Psychiatric Patients

One might well ask what bearing these findings have on psychiatric illness. Perhaps the most obvious association comes from reports that GH responsiveness to insulin is decreased in adult (Mueller, Heninger, and McDonald, 1969; Sachar et al., 1973b; Gruen et al., 1975; Amsterdam, Schweizer, and Winokur, 1987) and childhood (Puig-Antich et al., 1984a) depression and remains lower after recovery (Gruen et al., 1975; Puig-Antich et al., 1984c). Decreased responsiveness of GH secretion to L-amphetamine (Langer et al., 1976) and 5-HTP (Takahashi et al., 1974) in depressed patients has been reported. Sleep-related GH secretion in depression has not been fully characterized. Schilkrut et al. (1975) studied five patients with unipolar and one patient with bipolar depression and found a normal GH peak associated with sleep onset in only one. Three others (including the bipolar patient) had GH peaks substantially later at night, and two (aged 51 and 59) had no peaks. (As will be discussed later, sleep-related GH secretion in normal persons over 50 is decreased, so the relevance of this finding to depression per se is not clear.) Mendlewicz et al. (1985) found that depressed patients had elevated 24-hr GH secretion as the result of enhanced release during the day. The total GH secretion during sleep was normal, although unipolar, but not bipolar, patients tended not to have a secretory GH episode in early sleep. In contrast, patients with both endogenous and nonendogenous childhood depression have been reported to have elevated sleep-related GH secretion (Puig-Antich et al., 1984b). This observation, coupled with the failure to find short REM latencies in childhood depression (Chapter 9), seems to suggest that depression in childhood may be very different from depression in adulthood.

There is some evidence that sleep-related GH secretion is disturbed in alcoholics. Othmer *et al.* (1972) found, in eight alcoholics, abnormally small amounts of both slow-wave sleep and GH. Secretion of GH occurred seemingly at random throughout the night, with no obvious relation to slow-wave sleep. When the patients drank, there was an increase in slow-wave sleep, but not GH, in the first 2 hr of sleep.

Sleep-related GH secretion in schizophrenics has been examined in two studies. Vigneri *et al.* (1974) found that three chronic schizophrenics had normal daytime GH responses to insulin but that GH levels throughout the night were relatively constant, with no relationship to sleep onset or any sleep stage. A single acute schizophrenic patient had a normal response to insulin and had one nocturnal peak in relation to sleep onset and one peak late at night, which was seemingly unrelated to slow-wave sleep. Murri *et al.* (1973) reported no consistent rises during sleep in four chronic schizophrenic patients.

There are, then, reports of abnormalities of sleep-related GH secretion in schizophrenia, alcoholism, and adult depression, all of which are characterized by a decrease in slow-wave sleep. Since the pharmacological reduction of slow-wave sleep does not necessarily inhibit GH secretion (Rubin *et al.*, 1973a), it sems likely that this alone does not explain the altered GH secretion under these pathological conditions. Depression (Coppen, 1967; Schildkraut, 1974), schizophrenia (Woolley and Shaw, 1954a,b), and alcoholism (Zarcone and Hoddes, 1975) have all been postulated to be associated with abnormalities of biogenic amine metabolism, which might be related to changes in GH secretion. Whether these endocrine changes are an inherent part of the pathological process or a consequence of some more basic abnormality, or bear some other relationship, is unknown.

Secretion of GH in Disease

Several studies have compared sleep-related secretion and pharmacological provocative tests in children with short stature (Eastman and Lazarus, 1973; Mace *et al.*, 1972; Underwood *et al.*, 1971; Illig *et al.*, 1971). Generally, children with constitutional short stature or with histories of prolonged corticosteroid treatment for asthma, who have good GH responses to insulin tests, also have comparable sleep-related GH peaks. Secretion in patients with short stature related to hypopituitarism that is idiopathic or the result of space-occupying CNS lesions is usually decreased during both tests. On the other hand, there are cases in which insulin provocative tests give ambiguous results

(Underwood *et al.*, 1971). Tanner *et al.* (1971), for instance, described a patient whose growth rate following treatment with GH clearly indicated a GH deficiency, but whose secretion was normal during an insulin tolerance test. One might speculate that sleep-related GH secretion in such a patient would be decreased. There are, in fact, some documented cases of this phenomenon. Eastman and Lazarus (1973) described an abnormally short patient with a history of surgery for craniopharyngioma who had a normal response to arginine (20.4 ng/ml), a significant but blunted response to insulin (7.4 ng/ml), and a poor response to sleep (4.0 ng/ml). Similarly, Howse *et al.* (1974) described two children with clinical GH deficiency who had normal responses to insulin but low sleep-related GH secretion. Another example of dissociation of these two GH responses involved a patient in whom an adrenal adenoma had been excised (Krieger and Glick, 1974). Insulin-induced GH secretion, which had been decreased before surgery, returned to normal in four months; sleep-related GH secretion, however, remained abnormally low until eight months after surgery. It seems possible, then, as Eastman and Lazarus (1973) and Tanner *et al.* (1971) speculated, that some patients may respond normally to pharmacological stimuli and yet may be unable to produce normal amounts of GH regularly.

Spiliotis *et al.* (1984) described children with neurosecretory dysfunction who have decreased growth velocity and normal responses to daytime pharmacological stimulation tests, but a low 24-hr total secretion of GH. Cumulative, sleep-related GH secretion in these children has been reported to be as little as one-half that of controls; like the controls, however, they tended to have their first peak during slow-wave sleep as well as peaks in other stages. This suggests that there is a spectrum of degree of GH dysfunction, running from classically GH-deficient patients to those with neurosecretory dysfunction, to normal. There are also children of short stature with normal amounts of immunoreactive GH, for whom the possibility of a biologically inactive GH has been raised (Underwood, 1984). Sleep data are not yet available for this group.

Children with disturbed home environments may develop a reversible GH deficiency in "psychosocial dwarfism." They may grow at unusually slow rates at home and show subnormal GH responses to insulin, yet return to normal when removed from their usual environments and placed in the hospital (Krieger and Mellinger, 1971). Subjective sleep reports have related periods of slow growth to disturbed sleep, and periods of more rapid growth to normal sleep (Wolff and Money, 1973). Stage 4 sleep has been found to be decreased in these patients (Guilhaume, Benoit, and Richardet, 1981; Guilhaume *et al.*,

1982) and to return to normal after hospitalization and social intervention. In contrast, slow-wave sleep has been reported to be increased in GH-deficient dwarfs (Vogel *et al.*, 1972).

Studies of the sleep-related secretion of GH in acromegalics have generally found high, fluctuating levels throughout sleep, with no peak associated with sleep onset or slow-wave sleep (Carlson *et al.*, 1972; Sassin, Hellmand, and Weitzman, 1972b; Cryer and Daughaday, 1969). The latter study reported slightly lower levels during sleep than waking. Sassin *et al.* (1972b), who plotted values as percentages of 24-hr secretion, found highest concentrations from midnight to 10:00 AM. Values often rose before sleep onset and were briefly high after the end of sleep. A single patient, however, clearly had a peak associated with sleep onset. They speculated that the adenoma present in this disease is not completely autonomous and that a loss of hypothalamic control may be involved in the pathogenesis of acromegaly. Chihara *et al.* (1977) found no difference between daytime and nighttime GH levels in seven acromegalic patients. 2-Bromo-alpha-ergocriptine significantly reduced 24-hr secretion in six cases, following which levels during sleep were higher than those during waking.

Growth hormone secretion has also been examined during sleep apnea (Chapter 6) and narcolepsy (Chapter 7). Clark, Schmidt, and Malarkey (1979a) found that 57% of a group of 28 patients with one or both disorders had diminished sleep-related secretion, and 81 and 44% failed to respond fully to L-DOPA and arginine.

Sleep-related GH secretion and percentage slow-wave sleep are decreased in treated (remission five months to two years) and untreated patients with Cushing's disease, as well as in some patients with "eucorticoid" hypothalamic tumors (Krieger and Glick, 1974). On the other hand, nocturnal GH secretion that was decreased in a patient with an adrenal adenoma returned to normal eight months after corrective surgery. These data have been taken to imply a neural dysfunction in Cushing's disease, as well as some direct effect of excess cortisol on GH secretion. Administration of hydrocortisone for one night (Krieger *et al.*, 1972) and prednisone for two weeks (Stiel, Island, and Liddle, 1970) or two years (Krieger and Glick, 1974) did not modify sleep-related GH secretion in these patients. It seems likely that studies involving multiple doses, infusions at different times of the day, and infusions of different duration will be needed to characterize the relationship of corticosteroids to GH secretion.

Because of the relation of GH secretion to slow-wave sleep and reports of increased slow-wave sleep in patients with hyperthyroidism, GH secretion in this illness is of interest. Dunleavy *et al.* (1974) reported that in two adult patients, nocturnal GH secretion was higher than might be expected, and that it decreased along with total slow-wave sleep after treatment with carbimazole.

Aging and GH

Growth hormone secretion is altered in the elderly. Carlson et al. (1972) reported that in four of six normal volunteers over 50 years old there were no sleep-related peaks. This may parallel the decline in 24-hr GH secretion (Finkelstein et al., 1972) and in insulin-induced secretion (Laron, Doron, and Amikam, 1970) in the elderly, although there may be relatively little effect of age on stimulation by arginine (Dudl et al., 1973). There is a growing literature on altered neurotransmitter function in the elderly, including observations of decreased choline acetyltransferase and tyrosine hydroxylase in the caudate in the normal human elderly (McGeer and McGeer, 1976), and cholinergic receptor loss with aging in animals (Freund et al., 1980). Cholinergic dysfunction has been speculated to be related to cognitive deficits in senile dementia (Davis and Yamamura, 1978). Given the reports of decreased sleep-related GH secretion in the elderly, and the evidence of a facilitative cholinergic effect on this form of secretion, one wonders whether sleep-related GH might be used experimentally to measure central cholinergic function.

Effects of GH Administration

Acute GH Administration and Sleep

The focus of the discussion so far has been on how sleep-related neural mechanisms participate in the regulation of GH secretion. The converse of this—that GH may have a role in the regulation of sleep—will now be examined. This may be approached by assessing the effects of GH administration on sleep. Several animal studies have suggested that this might be fruitful. It has been reported, for instance, that, in rats, labeled GH rapidly enters the brain after intraperitoneal injection (Stern et al., 1975a) and that within 15 min of injection, brain concentrations of norepinephrine and serotonin significantly decrease (Stern et al., 1975b). In rats (Drucker-Colin et al., 1975) and in cats (Stern et al., 1975c), there is some evidence that GH administration increases REM sleep; and in mice, it may influence memory (Hoddes, 1979).

Mendelson et al. (1981b) performed sleep studies on 18 young adult normal volunteers who had been injected intramuscularly with 2 ($n = 8$)

or 5 ($n = 10$) units of GH or saline in random sequence. In addition, 15 subjects (all but two of whom had participated in sleep studies) received injections of GH at 8:00 AM and then underwent a battery of psychological tests involving serial learning of word lists, a mood and behavior scale, and 100-mm line scales of sleepiness, energy, and anxiety. The 2-unit dose had no effect on sleep, and neither dose altered the various psychological measures. Administration of 5 units of GH, however, decreased slow-wave sleep from 86.0 ± 6.8 min on placebo to 69.7 ± 5.7 min after GH ($p < 0.01$). In addition, REM sleep time rose from 97.6 ± 6.5 min on placebo to 109.9 ± 6.0 min after GH ($p < 0.05$). Total sleep time and sleep latency were unaffected.

In order to determine blood concentrations, two subjects who had previously been in the study were given GH, and blood samples were drawn every 20 min throughout the night. The peak concentrations were 64.5 and 56.4 ng/ml (Fig. 5-11A,B), in contrast to peak concentrations in untreated normal volunteers from the same laboratory, which were in the 6–10 ng/ml range (Mendelson et al., 1975b, 1978d).

The acute administration of human GH to normal volunteers, then, results in decreased slow-wave sleep and increased REM sleep. Plasma concentrations of GH were higher than those normally found but much lower than those sometimes observed in acromegaly (Carlson et al., 1972; Cryer and Daughaday, 1969). The finding that GH administration enhances REM sleep confirms similar findings in animals (Stern et al., 1975c; Drucker-Colin et al., 1975). The decreased slow-wave sleep raises the possibility that GH may play a role in the regulation of slow-wave sleep by a negative feedback mechanism. Further support for this view comes from reports of decreased slow-wave sleep in acromegalics (Carlson et al., 1972) and increased slow-wave sleep in GH-deficient dwarfs (Vogel et al., 1972). This would not, however, fit the finding of a further increase in slow-wave sleep after GH administration to three dwarfs in the latter study or with the unchanged slow-wave sleep when GH was decreased by methscopolamine in the study presented earlier.

The GH-induced increase in REM sleep is evocative of a study reporting that 24-hr REM deprivation resulted in increased GH secretion (Othmer, Daughaday, and Guze, 1969). It has also been observed, by such authors as Stern et al. (1975d), that there is an ontogenic relation between GH secretion and REM sleep (e.g., infants have high amounts of both and the elderly low amounts of both). Up to 80% of the sleep of neonates is composed of REM sleep, which drops to roughly 30% after 6 months or so (Williams, Karacan, and Hursch, 1974). Similarly, the waking mean GH level in neonates is very high, in the area of 20

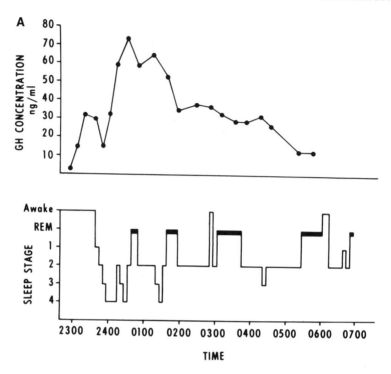

FIGURE 5-11. Plasma GH concentration in two volunteers who received 5 units of GH intramuscularly 15 min before going to bed. (A) A 24-year-old male; (B) a 22-year-old male. (From Mendelson *et al.*, 1981b. Reprinted by permission.)

ng/ml, dropping to roughly 6 ng/ml after 6 months (Vigneri and d'Agata, 1971). Thus the data reported here, the REM deprivation data, and ontogenic observations leave open the possibility that GH may be involved in sleep stage regulation, perhaps by inhibiting slow-wave sleep or (more likely) by somehow preparing the central nervous system for REM sleep.

The study of acute GH administration could be interpreted as suggesting that GH may play a role in the regulation of sleep in the nervous system. One is reminded of studies showing that insulin concentrations and insulin receptors in the central nervous system vary independently of peripheral insulin levels (Havrankova, Roth, and Brownstein, 1979) and that estradiol-concentrating cells (Pfaff and Keiner, 1973) and estrogen receptors (Maclusky *et al.*, 1976) are found widely throughout the central nervous system. Although these studies do not clearly demonstrate that GH, insulin, or estrogens have functional roles in neural regulation, they are at least compatible with this

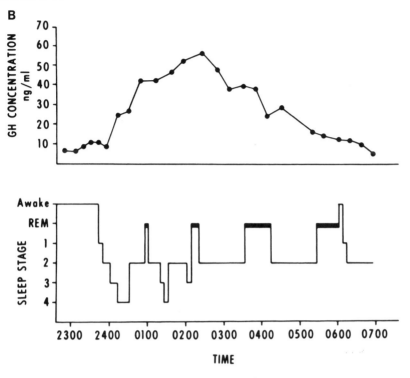

FIGURE 5-11. (*Continued*)

concept. This leaves open the possibility, for future work, that hormones traditionally thought to act only as peripheral target organs may also affect the central nervous system.

Repeated GH Administration Effects on GH Secretion

It has been known for some time that GH administration may result in decreased endogenous GH secretion in the rat (Mueller and Pecile, 1966) and decreased daytime insulin-induced GH secretion in humans (Abrams, Grumbach, and Kaplan, 1971). In order to determine whether such a negative feedback mechanism operates for sleep-related secretion, Mendelson, Jacobs, and Gillin (1983c) gave 2 units of GH every 12 hr for a total of five injections and then measured sleep-related GH in six volunteers. The final injection was given 6 hr before the beginning of the sleep period, so that (in contrast to the acute study) little or no exogenous GH would be circulating, although the activity of somatomedins (or other substances mediating feedback) might be stimulated. Little effect on sleep stages was observed, but GH secretion was profoundly suppressed. As can be seen in Figure 5-12, this effect was most evident during the first 2 hr of sleep, when the mean GH concentration after saline injections was 10.2 ± 2.3 ng/ml compared to 3.8 ± 0.40 ng/ml after hormone administration. Thus, pretreatment with GH appears to inhibit sleep-related GH secretion in a manner analogous to that reported for daytime insulin-induced secretion.

THE PITUITARY–ADRENAL AXIS

It has been known for some time that cortisol, which is secreted in response to adrenocorticotropic hormone (ACTH) from the pituitary, has a circadian cycle. Blood cortisol concentrations are lowest in the early hours of sleep (1:00–3:00 AM) and highest from 4:00–8:00 AM (Hellman et al., 1970a; Weitzman et al., 1971). Hellman et al. (1970a) found that cortisol is secreted in multiple discrete episodes, the total time of which may be 6.25 hr out of 24 hr; the rest of the time, the adrenals may be quiescent. Over one-half of the 24-hr secretion occurs during sleep.

As radioimmunoassays for ACTH became available, it became clear that, as expected, ACTH levels are lowest in the few hours before and just after sleep onset, increase after 3 to 5 hr of sleep, and peak shortly

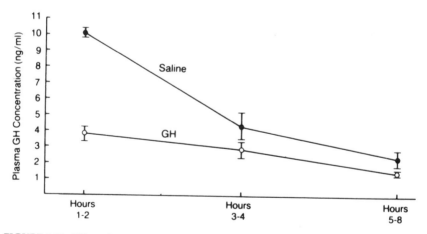

FIGURE 5-12. Effect of pretreatment with parenteral GH (2 units every 12 hr for a total of five injections) on subsequent sleep-related GH secretion. (From Mendelson, 1982b. Reprinted by permission.)

after awakening (Liddle, 1974; Gallagher et al., 1973; Berson and Yalow, 1968). Individual episodes of ACTH secretion are, in general, closely related to episodes of cortisol secretion, which tend to occur about 10 min later (Gallagher et al., 1973). It is evident, however, that some ACTH peaks are not followed by cortisol peaks and, conversely, that some elevations of cortisol are not preceded by ACTH peaks (Desir et al., 1980).

Adrenocorticotropic hormone secretion is thought to be primarily affected by circadian processes and by various physiological stresses, presumably by way of CNS mechanisms (an open loop system) and by closed loop negative feedback from glucocorticoid levels (Daughaday, 1985). The episodic nature of the secretion, the acute response to various stresses, and the disruption of ACTH secretion following deaferenation (sectioning of neural pathways) of the medial ventral hypothalamus (Halasz, 1969) emphasize the importance of neural regulation. This is accomplished by way of a corticotropin-releasing factor (CRH) from the hypothalamus. Release of CRH may be stimulated by cholinergic or serotonergic neurons and inhibited by noradrenergic neurons. The beta blocker propranolol may elevate circulating cortisol levels in humans (Lewis et al., 1981b).

One interesting feature of the closed system of negative feedback from circulating corticosteroids is that its importance relative to the central nervous system may vary cyclically during the day. Ceresa et al. (1969) found that although maximum intravenous doses of dexamethasone could decrease urinary 17-hydroxycorticosteroid levels at any time, submaximal doses could only effect such decreases from 4:00 to 8:00 AM. Adrenal sensitivity to ACTH may not change over the 24-hr day (McDonald et al., 1969).

In recent years, it has become more evident that, in addition to peripheral actions, glucocorticoids have a number of effects on the CNS. These include inhibition of growth, regulation of myelination, promotion of serotonergic development, suppression of high-affinity GABA transport in the hippocampus, and enhancement of vasoactive intestinal peptide concentrations in the hippocampus (McEwen, 1985). Thus, glucocorticoids may interact with neuropeptides and neurotransmitters, separately and together. They may also play a role in regulating the permeability of the blood–brain barrier (Long and Holaday, 1985).

Relation to the Sleep–Waking Cycle

The daily rhythm of corticosteroid secretion appears to involve both circadian rhythmic and sleep-related effects (Parker et al., 1981).

The relationship to sleep appears to be less close than is the case for GH. A urinary 17-hydroxycorticosteroid diurnal rhythm was found to persist despite 205 hr of sleep deprivation (Poland *et al.*, 1972). It also continues in human subjects kept under constant lighting conditions for 21 days (Krieger, Kreuezer, and Rizzo, 1969). Altering the sleep–waking cycle for one day by greatly lengthening or shortening sleep time has no effect on the diurnal plasma cortisol cycle; after chronic changes to 19- or 33-hr sleep–waking cycles, or reversal of the 24-hr cycle by 180°, the cortisol cycle adjusts to the new sleep–wake pattern in one to two weeks (Weitzman *et al.*, 1968a; Orth, Island, and Liddle, 1967; Parker *et al.*, 1981). During the period of realignment after 180° reversal, both the circadian and sleep-related aspects of secretion may be more apparent (Parker *et al.*, 1981). In a study of jet lag after flights between Brussels and Chicago, cortisol and ACTH rhythms did not return to normal patterns for about 11 days (Desir *et al.*, 1980). Adaptation of ACTH and cortisol rhythms was faster after eastward than westward flight. Since psychological and sleep difficulties are greater after eastward flights (see Chapter 10), there seems to be little relationship between this particular endocrine disturbance and the sleep difficulties of jet lag.

The effects of sleep on cortisol secretion can also be seen when volunteers are put on 3-hr days (1 hr of sleep followed by 2 hr of waking). In this situation, the circadian rhythm of cortisol persists but superimposed on it is an ultradian rhythm in which plasma cortisol is lowest during sleep periods and highest in the first hour after waking (Weitzman *et al.*, 1974). The importance of influences other than the light–dark cycle is emphasized by the observation that blind persons may have some irregularity in corticosteroid rhythm but continue to show diurnal secretion with a high point at the end of sleep (Bodenheimer, Winter, and Faiman, 1973; Krieger and Rizzo, 1971). When sighted humans live in the dark but continue to have 24 hr-periodic social cues, the corticosteroid rhythmicity is essentially normal (Aschoff *et al.*, 1971).

The relation of cortisol to a specific sleep stage is complicated by its loose association with the sleep–waking cycle and by its half-life of about 68 min (Hellman *et al.*, 1970a), which is relatively long compared to the various EEG events that are measured. It is possible that studies relating ACTH to sleep stage will be more helpful, since it has a half-life of only about 10 min (Liddle, 1974). Mandell and Mandell (1969) reported that all 14 episodes of REM in four normal subjects were associated with elevated urinary 17-hydroxycorticosteroids. Perhaps one of the most careful studies of plasma cortisol levels and sleep stages was provided by Hellman *et al.* (1970a). In one subject, they found that all three peaks of plasma cortisol occurring in sleep were in juxtaposition to REM episodes, as were four out of five in a second subject. Rubin, Kales, and Clark (1969), monitoring sleep stages and urinary 17-hydroxycorticosteroids in subjects given glutethimide, found that secretion was related more closely to phasic events (eye movement density) than to percentage REM sleep. Since glucocorticoids tend to increase hepatic gluconeogenesis, it has been suggested that the function of increased glucocorticoid secretion during REM sleep is to prepare nutrients for use by the brain (Mandell and Mandell, 1969).

REM sleep and cortisol secretion can, however, clearly be dissociated, as in 12-hr sleep–waking cycle reversal studies (Weitzman *et al.*, 1968a) in which, for several days, there were multiple episodes of REM sleep during the day with little cortisol secretion. During the study of 3-hr sleep–waking cycles described above (Weitzman *et al.*, 1974), the total 24-hr plasma cortisol secretion was unchanged, although the total amount of REM sleep was reduced by almost half. The relation of cortisol secretion to REM sleep is, then, clearly not well defined.

Another adrenal steroid, aldosterone, may be secreted in relation to REM sleep (Rubin *et al.*, 1975b). Because aldosterone is an important regulator of renal function, it is discussed in the section of this chapter dealing with antidiuretic hormone. It should be noted here, however, that ACTH is a minor determinant of aldosterone secretion, in addition to the renin–angiotensin and volume controls that exert major control.

Sleep-Related Cortisol Secretion in Disease

The circadian rhythm of cortisol secretion remains intact in a variety of disease states. Cortisol secretion in Cushing's syndrome has been studied by Hellman *et al.* (1970b) and Krieger and Gewirtz (1974). In the former study, a patient with idiopathic Cushing's syndrome with adrenal hyperplasia had episodic secretion, with retention of a diurnal rhythm the low point of which occurred early in sleep. Secretion was remarkably normal, except for the larger amounts of cortisol secreted. The authors suggested that if cortisol secretion were found to be constant in patients with autonomous adrenal tumors, then serial sampling of cortisol might help in distinguishing idiopathic Cushing's from neoplasms. Krieger and Gewirtz (1974) measured ACTH and cortisol secretion in a tumor patient, although sampling was done only every 3 hr. There was in fact a loss of the circadian pattern. In addition, there was a loss of the ACTH, cortisol, or GH response to hypoglycemia or vasopressin administration. These endocrine responses to hypoglycemia and vasopressin returned three and one-half months after surgical removal of the tumor. In contrast, the circadian rhythm of ACTH did not return until seven months after surgery. The authors suggested that these differing time-courses for recovery imply the existence of separate mechanisms governing responses to pharmacological provocation and circadian rhythmicity. (It will be recalled that the issue of multiple CNS control mechanisms has also been raised regarding GH.) As in idiopathic Cushing's syndrome, there is also evidence that plasma ACTH retains its diurnal rhythm in cortisol-deficient patients with Addison's disease (Graber et al., 1965).

Gallagher (1971) and Perlow et al. (1971) have described cortisol patterns in narcolepsy. The patient in the former study had a history of cataplectic attacks, but all sleep episodes documented by EEG were slow-wave sleep. In the latter study, three patients, all of whom had secondary symptoms of narcolepsy, had daytime sleep attacks of REM sleep and nocturnal sleep-onset REM. In both cases, the 24-hr cortisol secretory patterns were normal. Gallagher (1971) also reported on a patient with parkinsonism, whose cortisol secretory patterns remained normal, including decreased cortisol secretion early in sleep. Treatment with L-DOPA, which ameliorated the motor symptoms of parkinsonism, did not change the pattern of cortisol secretion. The implication is that in this patient L-DOPA in amounts sufficient to affect striatal dopaminergic function may not affect hypothalamic pathways controlling CRH secretion.

A variety of studies have been performed on cortisol secretion in depression (Fullerton et al., 1968a,b; Doig et al., 1966; McClure, 1966; Bridges and Jones, 1966). The general direction of the findings is an incease in the degree of diurnal variation of plasma cortisol, with either the 6:00 AM "high" point or the mean cortisol value higher than controls. These findings should be taken in the context of sleep stage disturbances (which often include multiple wakenings and decreased slow-wave and total sleep time), which are discussed in Chapter 9. There is some tendency to change toward normal upon recovery, although some studies (Bridges and Jones, 1966) found absolute levels to be lower in recovered patients than in controls. Doig et al. (1966) noted that in seven of ten depressed patients, the highest peak occurred at 3:00 AM, but on recovery moved to the more normal 6:00 AM. Similarly, the nadir of serum cortisol levels has been reported to occur 3 hr earlier in depressed patients than in controls (Fullerton et al., 1968a,b). As will be seen in Chapter 9, such findings have been interpreted by some authors as evidence of a circadian phase advance in depression.

McClure (1965), citing studies in which ACTH treatments were associated with wakefulness, suggested that the increased plasma cortisol in depressed patients might be responsible for their early morning awakenings.

The topics of steroid secretion and sleep also come together in depression research because of the interest in the dexamethasone suppression test (DST). Along with a decreased TSH response to TRH and the short REM latency, the DST is a possible biological marker of depression. There is little relationship between patients with positive DST tests (in whom dexamethasone fails to suppress cortisol secretion) and those with short REM latencies (Rush *et al.*, 1982). It has also been suggested that nonsuppression of dexamethasone predicts a beneficial response to sleep deprivation treatment (Nasrallah and Coryell, 1982). One added complication of interpreting DST data is that sleep deprivation procedures may induce nonsuppression of dexamethasone in normal subjects (Klein and Seibold, 1985).

Effects of Cortisol and ACTH on Sleep

We have mentioned earlier that corticosteroids may have a variety of effects on the CNS, such as altering nerve conduction velocity (Henken *et al.*, 1968) and thresholds for smell (Henkin and Bartter, 1966) and hearing (Henken and Daly, 1968). Corticosteroids may alter metabolism of the monoamines (Maas and Mednieks, 1971; Grelak *et al.*, 1970; Green and Curzon, 1968), which in turn are involved in the regulation of sleep stages (Chapter 2). A corticosterone derivative that binds to the chloride ionophore site of the benzodiazepine receptor complex has been reported to have hypnotic properties in rats (Mendelson *et al.*, 1986c; see Chapter 4). Thus, there was some basis for the expectation that subjects receiving exogenous corticosteriods and patients with excessive endogenous adrenal activity might have disturbed sleep stage regulation.

Krieger and Gewirtz (1974), whose study of Cushing's syndrome is mentioned above, found that their patients had virtually no slow-wave sleep, a reduction in REM periods, and an increase in stage 1 sleep. This pattern did not return to normal until 16 months after surgical removal of the adenoma. These observations with slow-wave sleep agree with data by Gillin *et al.* (1974a) on patients with adrenal insufficiency. In the baseline period, during which patients were receiving replacement therapy, slow-wave sleep was slightly higher than that of normal controls. When replacement therapy was discontinued, slow-wave sleep increased markedly. Similarly, when cortisol secretion was decreased in normal subjects following administration of metyrapone (SU 4885), there was an increase in slow-wave sleep.

Gillin *et al.* (1972a) observed that single oral doses of 60 mg prednisone given to normal volunteers decreased REM sleep time and increased REM sleep latency, with no change in slow-wave sleep. These may only be acute responses, since there is some evidence that asthmatic patients who chronically receive prednisone have sleep patterns similar to those not receiving it (Kales *et al.*, 1968). Dexamethasone (1 mg) has also been given to depressed patients but apparently has had little effect on sleep except for lowering REM activity (Feinberg *et al.*, 1984).

It is clear that circulating corticosteroids are not needed for REM sleep to occur. Jouvet (1965b), for example, reported that complete removal of the hypothalamus and hypophysis in the pontine cat is still compatible with the appearance of REM sleep. Although circulating steroids would have left the body in a few hours, REM sleep continued to appear (although in declining amounts) until death on the sixth or seventh day. Injections of ACTH and posterior pituitary extracts restore REM sleep periodicity in these animals. Thus, although REM sleep can clearly occur in the absence of corticosteroids, it is possible that corticosteroid secretion may have some modulating effect on its appearance.

Other evidence of a possible modulating role of corticosteroids on the maintenance of sleep cycles comes from the work of Johnson and Sawyer (1971). They put rats on a 1-hr light–dark cycle and found that although REM sleep began to appear in a 1-hr ultradian rhythm, the basic circadian rhythm persisted. Most of the total 24-hr REM sleep still occurred in what had formerly been the daylight hours. Following adrenalectomy, however, the circadian rhythm of REM sleep disappeared. Administration of cortisol in the late afternoon established a new circadian rhythm, which was out of phase with the original one. They speculated that cortisol may be released by stress ur exposure to drugs, resulting in REM sleep, which, in turn, might encourage biochemical repair of the central nervous system (Oswald, 1970). Since REM sleep in humans is decreased by pharmacological doses of prednisone (Gillin *et al.*, 1972a) or ACTH (Gillin *et al.*, 1974b) and in patients with adrenal adenomas (Krieger and Gewirtz, 1974), the observation in this study of increased REM sleep after cortisol administration, as well as the hypotheses derived from the observation, must await confirmatory studies. Interpretation of this study is also made more difficult by the authors' use of cortisol, which in the rat is not a major glucocorticoid. (Corticosterone plays the more important role in rats.)

Gillin *et al.* (1974b) found that infusions of ACTH begun at 8:00 AM or 3:00 PM, but not at 11:30 PM, decreased REM sleep. Since this effect was more marked in normal volunteers than in patients with Addison's disease, the implication was that changes in sleep induced by ACTH may be mediated by adrenocortical steroid secretion. The REM suppressive effect seemed to require 4 hr of infusion and to persist for at least 12 hr. Thus, the effects on REM sleep last some time after the ACTH and adrenocortical steroid levels had probably returned to normal. Slow-wave sleep also decreased after infusions of ACTH at 8:00 AM.

In rats, $ACTH_{1-24}$ has been reported to shorten chlordiazepoxide-induced enhancement of "sleeping time" as measured by loss of the righting reflex (Vellucci, 1984). It is known that ACTH and some of its analogues have no effect on the binding of benzodiazepines to their receptors (Braestrup and Squires, 1978; also see Chapter 4). Whether this interaction of ACTH and chlordiazepoxide is a nonspecific result of activation due to ACTH or some more specific interaction is unknown.

PROLACTIN

Prolactin, a single-chain polypeptide, participates in the initiation and maintenance of lactation and has some metabolic effects similar to GH in animals; it may also be related to such behaviors as nesting in birds (Daughaday, 1985). Both catecholamines and serotonin may play a role in central nervous system regulation of PRL. The beta agonist isoproterenol may increase (Imura and Kato, 1974) and the beta blocker acebutolol (Lewis *et al.*, 1981) may decrease PRL plasma concentrations. Agents which deplete amines by synthesis inhibition (alpha-methyldopa) or by release (reserpine) increase PRL concentrations (Lancranjan *et al.*, 1979). Drugs with dopamine receptor blocking properties, such as phenothiazines, butyrophenones, and procainamide derivatives (e.g., metoclopramide), will also increase PRL secretion (McCallum *et al.*, 1976; Lal *et al.*, 1976). Such observations are consistent with the view that the dominant physiological inhibitory factor is dopamine (Shaar and Clemens, 1974), although other transmitters such as GABA may also have an inhibitory effect (Neill, 1980). The results of studies on the serotonergic system are less clear. Although Coppola (1971) and Talwalker, Ratner, and Meites (1963) were unable to find a role for indoleamines in PRL release, Kamberi, Mical, and Porter (1971b) demonstrated that intraventricular administration of serotonin and intraperitoneal injection of 5-HTP increased plasma PRL in rats. Similarly, such ergot derivatives as ergocornine, ergonovine, and LSD inhibit PRL release in several species (Meites and Clemens, 1972). There is some evidence that this is the result of effects on the anterior pituitary and on hypothalamic release of prolactin inhibiting hormone (Meites, 1973). MacIndoe and Turkington (1973) observed that intravenous L-tryptophan increased serum PRL in humans and that this effect was decreased by pretreatment with methysergide. There is no known long loop hormonal negative feedback in the control of PRL secretion (Turkington, 1972).

Sassin *et al.* (1972a) demonstrated that plasma PRL concentrations have a diurnal rhythm. There is an initial rise 60–90 min after sleep onset, with subsequent peaks resulting in maximal levels at 5:00–7:00 AM. During the hour after awakening concentrations begin to drop, reaching a nadir from about 10:00 AM to noon. Van Cauter *et al.* (1981) described a bimodal rhythm, with a mean nocturnal peak at about 4:23 AM, a nadir at about 11:30 AM, and a second but smaller peak at about 5:03 PM.

Studies in which the hours of sleep were shifted over the 24-hr day demonstrated an immediate shift of PRL to the new hours of sleep (Sassin *et al.*, 1973; Parker *et al.*, 1981). In this sense, PRL secretion is more like GH than ACTH, which, as described earlier, seems to be under relatively greater control by circadian mechanisms in addition to some relationship to sleep. For PRL, sleep appears to have a dominant effect which is stimulatory, and any endogenous circadian rhythmicity is probably low amplitude and easily obscured (Parker *et al.*, 1981).

In nonpregnant women, PRL secretion appears to be the same (Sassin *et al.*, 1972a) or slightly higher (Nokin *et al.*, 1972) than that in men, and both sexes have a similar diurnal rhythm. However, PRL concentrations increase during pregnancy. Although a study in which blood samples were drawn every 4 hr suggested that the circadian rhythm of PRL is not present in pregnancy (Nokin *et al.*, 1972), a study with sampling every 20 min found this rhythm to be intact (Boyar *et al.*, 1975).

Unlike GH, PRL secretion does not seem to be related to a specific sleep stage. Sassin *et al.* (1972a) found no gross relationship, although a detailed analysis was not undertaken. Parker, Rossman, and Vanderlaan (1974a) reported that although secretory peaks did not occur with specific stages, PRL concentrations decreased during REM sleep and increased during subsequent non-REM sleep. This study, however, involved 58 recordings performed on 14 subjects. Since there are large differences between individuals, the repeated use of some subjects (up to 11 times) may have influenced the results. Sultan *et al.* (1980)

reported peaks during REM sleep in pubertal boys. Mendelson *et al.* (1975b) and Van Cauter *et al.* (1982), however, were unable to relate PRL secretion to the REM–non-REM cycle. In monkeys, PRL concentrations have been reported to be higher after slow-wave sleep onset than after REM sleep onset, but the appropriate cross correlations were not significant (Quabbe *et al.*, 1982).

Relation of PRL to Other Hormones

Thyrotropin-releasing hormone (TRH) is a potent stimulator of PRL secretion; there is some suggestion of a circadian aspect to this effect, since PRL responses may be greater in the evening than in the morning (Nathan *et al.*, 1982; Caroff and Winokur, 1984). An association of PRL secretion to sleep, and possibly indirectly to oxytocin secretion, has been postulated by Voloschin and Tramezzani (1984). They found that, in lactating rats, suckling by pups induced PRL release, but lactation occurred only after the mothers showed evidence of EEG-defined sleep. They suggested that PRL release induced sleep, which is necessary for the subsequent release of oxytocin needed for lactation.

The initial rise of PRL after sleep onset often coincides with the rise of GH, but peak values may occur some 40 min after the GH peak (Sassin *et al.*, 1972a). Thus, although there is some temporal relationship in initial sleep-related PRL secretion, there are often cases when PRL is released with no changes in GH. This is particularly true late in sleep, when overall values of PRL are increasing, but GH release is less frequent (Sassis *et al.*, 1973). Rubin *et al.* (1975a) reported a positive correlation between PRL and testosterone levels.

Drugs and Sleep-Related PRL Secretion

Several studies have been done on the effects of drugs on acute daytime PRL secretion. These include observations that phenothiazines, tricyclic antidepressants, reserpine, and methyldopa increase (Turkington, 1972) and L-DOPA decreases (Kleinberg, Noel, and Frantz, 1971) daytime secretion in humans. In contrast, there are few data on the effect of drugs on sleep-related PRL secretion as ascertained by multiple frequent samplings. Bixler *et al.* (1977) reported that thioridazine increased the total nightly secretion of PRL in two subjects; the interpretation of what mechanisms are involved is hampered by the multiple neurochemical effects of phenothiazines, which include adrenolytic and anticholinergic effects. Mendelson *et al.* (1975b) reported that the serotonin receptor blocker methysergide greatly decreased sleep-related PRL secretion. An implication might be that serotonergic pathways may stimulate sleep-related PRL secretion.

Sleep-Related PRL Secretion in Disease

It has been reported that men with primary testicular failure and elevated gonadotropin levels have increased PRL concentrations in response to TRH or metoclopramide, although basal levels may be normal (Spitz et al., 1981). However, PRL secretion in these patients during sleep may be normal (Spitz et al., 1982). In a report of two men with gynecomastia but normal daytime PRL levels, it was found that at sleep onset there was a transient increase followed by a decline throughout the night (Buckman et al., 1980). These studies suggest that, as with GH, it is important not to generalize from responsiveness in daytime pharmacological tests to what may be happening during nocturnal sleep.

FOLLICLE-STIMULATING HORMONE AND LUTEINIZING HORMONE

Follicle-stimulating hormone (FSH) and luteinizing hormone (LH) are glycoproteins, somewhat similar in structure to TSH and human chorionic gonadotropin. FSH is related to follicular development and spermatogenesis in the testis; LH is synergistic with FSH in stimulating maturation of the follicle, is involved in ovulation, estrogen secretion, and maintenance of the corpus luteum of the ovary as well as the production of androgens by Leydig cells of the testis (Daughaday, 1985; Ross, 1985). Both LH and FSH are released from the pituitary upon stimulation by luteinizing hormcne-releasing hormone (LHRH) from the preoptico-hypothalamus, which is carried to the pituitary by the portal vessels. LHRH release is sensitive to feedback from circulating gonadal steroids, which may be mediated by changes in alpha adrenergic receptors both in the hypothalamus and in the midbrain (Chappel, 1985). Since many elevations of FSH do not correspond to LHRH pulse frequency, some authors have speculated that there is also a specific FSH releasing hormone (Coutifaris and Chappel, 1983).

Relation of LH and FSH Secretion to Sleep

The relation of gonadotropins to sleep is in many ways a study of the ontogeny of endocrine function. Prepubertal children of both sexes and adult men show no consistent relationship between LH secretion and the sleep-waking cycle (Rubin *et al.*, 1975a; Boyar *et al.*, 1972a,b, 1974; Rubin *et al.*, 1973a; De Lacerda *et al.*, 1973). In contrast, LH levels increase in pubertal boys and girls during sleep (Boyar *et al.*, 1972a, 1974; Kapen *et al.*, 1974; Fevre *et al.*, 1978). After experimentally delayed sleep onset in pubertal subjects, LH secretion was also delayed and maintained its relation to sleep. In sleep reversal studies, LH secretion also shifted to maintain a relation to daytime sleep, but there was still some cyclic increase during waking time at night (Boyar *et al.*, 1974; Kapen *et al.*, 1974). It has been speculated that increases in LH, which may reach levels two to four times higher than during waking, may be responsible for Leydig cell stimulation and increasing chorionic gonadotropin responsiveness that occur during puberty. Sleep-related increases in LH and FSH have also been found in girls with precocious puberty (Matthews *et al.*, 1982; Beck and Stubbe, 1984).

As described above, LH secretion seems not to be related to the overall period of sleep in adult men. In adult women, LH and FSH increase in the morning compared to the evening (Alford *et al.*, 1973a). Kapen *et al.* (1973) reported decreased LH levels during the first few hours of sleep. In contrast, Naftolin *et al.* (1973) found no relationship of LH or FSH to sleep in adult women. There is, of course, in women a monthly cycle of "basal" LH levels, probably the result of variations in the magnitude of ultradian secretory pulses, which is reflected in waking (Yen *et al.*, 1972) and sleep (Naftolin *et al.*, 1973) studies.

It is not clear whether FSH has a diurnal rhythm in adults. Bodenheimer *et al.* (1973) reported a cycle with its high point at 8:00 AM in a study in which plasma was sampled every few hours in normal and blind men. Studies with sampling every 20 or 30 min in men and women failed to show a circadian or an ultradian rhythm (Rubin *et al.*, 1972, 1973a; Naftolin, 1973).

Boyar *et al.* (1972a), studying the increases in LH secretion during sleep in puberty, reported that LH plasma levels varied in an ultradian manner, with cycles of 75–100 min. They noted that this is approximately the periodicity of the non-REM–REM cycle (see Chapter 1) and pointed out that increases in LH usually began in non-REM sleep, whereas decreases tended to occur in close proximity to REM sleep episodes. Several studies of LH and FSH in adults that found no relation to the sleep–waking cycle also found no association with specific sleep stages (Naftolin *et al.*, 1973; Alford *et al.*, 1973a; Kapen *et al.*, 1973; Boyar *et al.*, 1972b). A study of adult men by Rubin *et al.* (1973a), however, found that although there was no circadian rhythm of LH or FSH, there was a small but significant association of increases in LH with REM sleep. This is consistent with the observation by Clemens *et al.* (1972) of increases in LH during REM sleep in rats. Schiavi *et al.*

(1984) found no relation to a specific sleep stage, but mean values during sleep were higher than during nocturnal waking.

Relation of Testosterone Secretion to Sleep

As with LH, testosterone increases during sleep in pubertal subjects (Judd *et al.*, 1974; Boyar *et al.*, 1974). The latter study included a delayed sleep onset experiment in one subject in whom testosterone remained related to sleep, and a sleep–waking reversal subject, in which testosterone continued to be related to sleep in a more intimate manner than was the case with LH. Evans *et al.* (1971a) also noted that testosterone secretion stayed in phase with sleep during sleep–waking reversal in one subject.

It is not clear whether this relation of testosterone to sleep holds true in adults. Most studies have reported a diurnal rhythm in which plasma levels are highest late in sleep, when a fluctuating pattern may be superimposed (Rubin *et al.*, 1975a; Schiavi *et al.*, 1974; DeLacerda *et al.*, 1973; Piro *et al.*, 1973; Rose *et al.*, 1972; Evans *et al.*, 1971a,b). Other studies found no diurnal pattern (Boyar *et al.*, 1974; Alford *et al.*, 1973a). The adult studies have also been varied in terms of the relation of testosterone to individual sleep stages. Evans *et al.* (1971a,b), using a largely impressionistic approach, noted increases in testosterone either during or just before REM sleep. Roffwarg *et al.* (1974) found that there was some evidence of peaks around the non-REM–REM junction and that testosterone levels tended to rise just before this. They noted, however, that these trends accounted for only a small part of the total variance and suggested that any relation to REM sleep may be a relatively weak, time-linked association. In a later study, Roffwarg *et al.* (1982) found no difference in mean concentrations during REM and non-REM sleep but described a pattern of higher concentrations 10–30 min before REM onset. Schiavi *et al.* (1974) did not find a relation to REM sleep but did observe that testosterone levels were lowest during slow-wave sleep. They pointed out that this could be coincidental, since the diurnal rhythm of testosterone was such that testosterone was lower early in sleep, when slow-wave sleep is most heavily concentrated. A later study found mean concentrations higher during REM than during other sleep stages or wakefulness (Schiavi *et al.*, 1984).

Gonadotropin and testosterone secretion have been examined during the sleep of men with erectile dysfunction. In contrast to controls, testosterone concentrations in REM sleep were no higher than in other sleep stages (Schiavi *et al.*, 1984). There was no difference between patients and controls in frequency and amount of peak hormonal increases in LH and testosterone (Schiavi *et al.*, 1984).

The control of nocturnal episodic testosterone secretion during puberty seems to be related to LH secretion (Boyar et al., 1974). As
described above, however, some of the data in adults could be interpreted as showing a sleep-related diurnal rhythm of testosterone but
not of LH. Thus, one might have to look at other mechanisms in addition to LH secretion for the control of a diurnal rhythm of testosterone.
Rubin et al. (1975a) found some positive relations of PRL and testosterone levels and suggested that PRL might play a role in regulation of
nocturnal testosterone secretion. The later observation that suppression of PRL secretion by methysergide did not alter nocturnal testosterone secretion (Jacobs et al., 1978) makes this seem less likely. The
secretion of testosterone, as well as of LH and FSH, has been reported
to be unchanged in blind men (Bodenheimer et al., 1973), suggesting
that the light–dark cycle does not play a role in the regulation of these
hormones. Although there are some conflicting data, it may well be
that this is also the case with cortisol and GH release (Weitzmann et al.,
1972).

Effects of Sex Hormones on Sleep

One indirect indication of the relation of sex hormones to sleep is
the examination of sleep during the menstrual cycle. Ho (1972) studied
three women at three time points: premenstrually, when progesterone
and estrogen levels were high; during menses, when both levels were
low; and early in the cycle, when progesterone levels were low and estrogen levels were rising. The only parameter that varied significantly
was slow-wave sleep, which decreased premenstrually. Similar results
at a corresponding time of the cycle were found for three women taking oral contraceptives. Other measures, including amounts of REM
sleep, did not vary. Kapen et al. (1972) examined four women on days
5–28 of the cycle. Their findings were generally negative, except for a
single subject who had a large increase in REM sleep time on the 18th
day of the cycle, when there was a marked increase in LH. Parry et al.
(personal communication) studied eight normal women weekly
throughout the menstrual cycle and found few changes. Intermittent
waking time was slightly higher and stage 3 sleep was lower (in a manner reminiscent of the Ho study) during the fourth week. Overall,
though, the general impression from these studies is that the menstrual cycle changes the sleep architecture only minimally.
    There have been many animal studies on the effects of sex hor-
mones on sleep. Colvin, Whitmoyer, and Sawyer (1969) reported
decreased REM sleep following estrogen administration. Branchey,
Branchey, and Nadler (1971b) reported decreased REM when estrogen

was given to ovariectomized female rats; they also found that both REM and non-REM sleep decreased when progesterone was also given. This effect did not occur in males (Branchey, Branchey, and Nadler, 1971a). An interesting sexual dimorphism was observed; males castrated since birth had the same response as ovariectomized females, but there was no effect on the sleep of males castrated in adulthood (Branchey, Branchey, and Nadler, 1973). Sawyer (1969) summarized a series of studies from his laboratory, elaborating on the observation that coitus in female rabbits stimulated slow-wave sleep, followed by "hippocampal overactivity."

It is possible that testosterone plays a role in reported sex differences in response to the hypnotic effect of barbiturates (Kato, Chiesara, and Frontino, 1962; Dundee, 1954). The effect of exogenous testosterone on barbiturate sensitivity may vary with length of pretreatment with testosterone. This may reflect an effect on induction of enzymes for barbiturate metabolism, as well as a true synergistic effect (Gessner and Gessner, 1973).

Sleep-Related FSH and LH Secretion in Disease

Nocturnal secretory patterns have been studied in various disease states. Cerone *et al.* (1975) found no unusual pattern in the episodic release of LH and FSH in an uncontrolled study of chronic schizophrenics. In contrast, the nocturnal secretion of LH and FSH is reduced in patients with anorexia nervosa (Kalucy *et al.*, 1975). Patients with the Chiari–Frommel syndrome, which involves postpartum amenorrhea and galactorrhea, may have unusually low nocturnal LH secretion (Kapen *et al.*, 1975). Children with idiopathic precocious puberty and congenital adrenal hyperplasia with precocious puberty are reported to have the episodic LH release and sleep-related increases seen in normal adolescents (Boyar *et al.*, 1973). This observation seems analogous to the finding of intact cyclic secretion of cortisol in idiopathic Cushing's syndrome with adrenal hyperplasia, described previously.

THYROID-STIMULATING HORMONE

Thyroid-stimulating hormone (TSH) is a glycoprotein that stimulates the growth and vascularity of the thyroid gland, increasing iodotyrosine and iodothyronine formation and triiodothyronine (T_3) release. Secretion of TSH is controlled by negative feedback from circulating levels of thyroid hormones and by thyrotropin-releasing hormone (TRH) from the hypothalamus (Ingbar, 1985). A noradrenergic system may be involved in the release of TRH (Reichlin, 1974). In addition to its effect on TSH, TRH also stimulates prolactin secretion (Reichlin, 1974).

Although some studies have failed to show diurnal variation in TSH release (Hershman and Pittman, 1971; Webster, Guansing, and Paice, 1972), a large body of evidence suggests that a diurnal rhythm is in fact present (Weeke, 1973; Patel, Alford, and Burger, 1972; Alford et al., 1973b; Vahaelst et al., 1972, 1973; Nicoloff, Fisher, and Appleman, 1970; Azukizawa et al., 1976; Weeke and Gundersen, 1978). Although the time of increases and maximum values vary in each study, the tendency is to report increases in TSH sometime before sleep onset (8:00–11:00 PM). Peak values may occur anywhere from 10:00 PM–3:00 AM (Alford et al., 1973b) to 4:00 AM–6:00 AM (Vanhaelst et al., 1972). In the elderly, the 24-hr mean concentration remains the same, but the amplitude of the circadian fluctuation and the peak nighttime levels decline (Barreca et al., 1985). This sleep-related peak may be absent in patients with central hypothyroidism (Caron et al., 1986). There seems to be general agreement that the circadian fluctuation of TSH is decreased in depression. Although some studies found an absence of nighttime secretion only in unipolar patients (Goldstein et al., 1980), others reported it also in bipolar illness (Kjellman et al., 1984; Weeke and Weeke, 1978). It is not clear whether the circadian pattern returns to normal upon remission (Kjellman et al., 1984) or remains altered after recovery (Kijne et al., 1982). The TSH response to TRH administration is also reduced in some endogenously depressed patients. There seems to be little relationship of this possible biological marker to the presence of a short REM latency (see Chapter 9) or dexamethasone nonsuppression in individual patients (e.g., Rush et al., 1982, 1983; Kupfer, Jarrett, and Frank, 1984). It has been reported that a significant increase in maximal TSH secretion following TRH may be predictive of a favorable outcome after total sleep deprivation treatment for depression (Kvists and Kirkegaard, 1980).

In addition to a diurnal rhythm, TSH, like GH, ACTH, and PRL, is released episodically with an ultradian rhythm of 1–3 hr (Alford et al., 1973b; Vanhaelst et al., 1972, 1983; Weeke, 1973; Patel et al., 1972).

The regulatory mechanism of the diurnal rhythm of TSH is not well understood. Administration of maintenance doses of hydrocortisone given to patients with Addison's disease and pharmacological doses of glucocorticoids to normal subjects suppresses TSH secretion (Patel et al., 1974; Nicoloff, Fisher, and Appleman, 1970). This has led these authors to speculate that rhythmic glucocorticoid secretion may play a role in the physiological control of TSH release. Similarly, infusion of 1 mg of somatostatin has been found to suppress nighttime levels of TSH, raising the possibility of its role in TSH regulation (Klaff *et al.*, 1982). Indirect evidence for this includes the observation that the TSH response to TRH is less in REM sleep than in slow-wave sleep, during which somatostatin secretion is thought to be lower (Peters *et al.*, 1981). In rats, *in vivo* anti-somatostatin antiserum elevates TSH levels, which suggests a tonic physiological inhibitory role. Plasma somatostatin concentrations in humans, however, seem to have little relationship to TSH during the night, which makes this seem less likely (Saito *et al.*, 1983).

TSH Secretion and Sleep

Relatively few data are available on the relationship of TSH to sleep stages. Alford *et al.* (1973b) found, in four normal adults, that TSH concentrations correlated positively with wakefulness and slow-wave sleep and negatively with non-slow-wave sleep and REM sleep. Noting the large difference between subjects, these authors postulated that there was no temporal relationship between TSH levels and specific sleep stages. Johns *et al.* (1975) measured the free thyroxin index (FTI) from plasma samples taken from normal subjects just before sleeping, after awakening, and in the middle of the day. The index just before sleep varied directly with the amount of subsequent delta sleep and inversely with the amount of REM sleep. The authors suggested that thyroid function is indirectly related to sleep and is possibly mediated by effects of the general metabolic rate on biogenic amine metabolism.

There is also a growing body of evidence that sleep may inhibit TSH secretion. During studies of acute sleep–waking reversal, the normal nighttime rise in TSH is greatly increased when subjects are kept awake (Parker, Pekary, and Hershman, 1976; Parker *et al.*, 1981).

Sleep in Hyperthyroidism and Hypothyroidism

The relation of thyroid function to delta sleep observed by Johns *et al.* (1975) and Alford *et al.* (1973b) is consistent with the findings of Dunleavy *et al.* (1974) that patients with hyperthyroidism have increased delta sleep and decreased REM sleep. Conversely, delta sleep has been reported to decrease in hypothyroid adults (Kales *et al.*, 1967a). After treatment, the delta sleep returned to normal. Studies of hypothyroid infants (Schulte and Parmelee, 1970; Schultz *et al.*, 1968) found decreased sleep spindles, a finding thought to represent a lack of normal maturation of the central nervous system.

Central Nervous System Actions of TRH

It seems likely that TRH itself may also have a direct effect on the central nervous system. Breese *et al.* (1974) and Prange *et al.* (1974) showed that in mice TRH reduced the sleeping time and hypothermic effects produced by ethanol and pentobarbital. Since these effects were not produced by T_3, it is likely that they were produced by TRH. There is also some evidence that TRH may be useful in the treatment of depression (Prange *et al.*, 1972; Kastin *et al.*, 1972; Whybrow and Prange, 1981). Injections of 2 mg of TRH have been reported to have no effect on REM percentage (Nakazawa *et al.*, 1979).

ANTIDIURETIC HORMONE AND RENIN

Antidiuretic hormone (ADH) is a pentapeptide ring closed by an S–S bridge, with a tripeptide side chain. It is secreted from the posterior pituitary gland in response to changes in blood osmolality and volume. The main peripheral action of ADH is to increase the permeability of tubule cells in the collecting ducts of the kidney to water and urea, resulting in increased retention of water and more concentrated urine. Antidiuretic hormone, as well as vasoactive intestinal peptide (VIP), is also found in the suprachiasmatic nucleus (see Chapter 10), which raises the possibility that it may be involved in the regulation of circadian rhythmic processes (Stopa *et al.*, 1984).

Another hormone important in kidney function regulation is aldosterone, a steroid secreted by the adrenal gland, which increases the reabsorption of sodium, and hence water, by the kidneys. Its secretion is thought to be related to changes in renal blood perfusion resulting from variations in blood pressure and blood volume. Decreased perfusion results in release of the substance renin from the kidney, which converts a circulating substrate to angiotensin. This, in turn, stimulates the release of aldosterone. The ultimate effect of aldosterone is thought to be an isosmotic decrease in volume, whereas ADH also decreases the volume but results in a more concentrated urine.

Urine output decreases at night, during which time perhaps one-third of the 24-hr volume is excreted (Brod, 1973). This probably results from the action of a complex group of factors including decreased glomerular filtration and increased reabsorption of water (Brod, 1973), a circadian rhythm of renin release (Leaf and Liddle, 1974), and other factors. In addition, there is some evidence suggesting sleep-related ultradian changes in urine volume and osmolality.

ADH and Renin Secretion during Sleep

Mandell *et al.* (1966) and Mandell and Mandell (1969) reported that urine volume decreased and osmolarity increased in association with REM sleep in seven urological patients. They speculated that this was the result of periodic secretion of ADH from the posterior pituitary during REM sleep. Bailey, Jenner, and Wheeler (1971) similarly found that urinary sodium, potassium, and chloride increased during REM sleep. In the former study, urinary 17-hydroxycorticosteroid secretion increased during REM sleep; in the latter, no relationship to sleep states was found. Neither study, however, provided formal statistical analyses. With the development of a radioimmunoassay for ADH, it became possible to do direct blood determinations, rather than to gather data indirectly by determining urine osmolalities. Rubin *et al.* (1975), employing such an assay, found that ADH, like the anterior pituitary hormones, is secreted in a pulsatile manner. There was, however, no relationship to specific sleep states. Interestingly, aldosterone was found to increase during REM sleep.

There is no evident circadian pattern of plasma renin activity, but an ultradian rhythm with a period of about 100 min has been described (Brandenberger *et al.*, 1985). Levels may begin to peak at the transition from REM to stage 2, with highest levels in slow-wave sleep.

Effects of ADH on Sleep

Faure (1962) demonstrated that injections of large amounts of ADH resulted in increased REM sleep in rabbits. Similarly, Jouvet (1965b) found that hyperosmolarity induced by water deprivation or hypertonic saline infusion—which presumably stimulates ADH release—increased the duration and the frequency of REM sleep episodes. Conversely, hypoosmolarity of the blood, induced by the ingestion of large volumes of water and by small amounts of exogenous ADH, reduced REM sleep. There may be, as Mandell and Mandell (1969) suggested, a relationship between neural mechanisms controlling ADH release and those that regulate REM sleep. Whether this represents a normal physiological system or whether it is only seen under unphysiological laboratory conditions is not clear.

MELATONIN

All the hormones discussed in this chapter have been products of the pituitary gland or one of its target organs. Another area of interest in the study of neuroendocrinology and sleep is the role of melatonin, which is released from the pineal gland.

Melatonin (5-methoxy-N-acetyltryptamine) is a serotonin derivative synthesized mainly in the pineal gland in mammals. It causes contraction of skin melanophores in fish and frogs, and in rats it decreases the concentrations of LH (Fraschini, Collu, and Martini, 1971). This seems to fit well with data from early-morning blood samples from human subjects, which suggest that melatonin levels are lowest at the time of ovulation and highest during menstruation (Wetterberg et al., 1976). This implies that low melatonin levels may be a permissive factor for ovulation. Conversely, high concentrations of melatonin may be involved in the early-morning rise of PRL (Ronnekiev, Krulich, and McCann, 1973). Administration of melatonin to humans has been reported to decrease GH secretion during insulin tolerance testing (Smythe and Lazarus, 1974).

The rate-limiting step in the synthesis of melatonin is its acetylation, which is catalyzed by serotonin N-acetyltransferase. In the rat, the activity of this enzyme and pineal concentrations of melatonin itself have a circadian rhythm, with levels highest at night; the precursor serotonin has a reciprocal rhythm, with the highest level occurring midday (Axelrod, 1974). Two human studies of melatonin in urine suggest a similar pattern (Lynch et al., 1975; Pelham et al., 1973).

In the rat, the circadian rhythm of melatonin synthesis is maintained by discharges of the noradrenergic sympathetic fibers that innervate the pineal gland and stimulate receptors (for a general review see Erlich and Apuzzo, 1985). The basic rhythm appears to rely on a mechanism located in or near the suprachiasmatic nucleus of the hypothalamus, which receives input from the eyes via the retino-hypothalamic tract (see Chapter 10). Exposure to light decreases sympathetic discharge, resulting in low levels of serotonin N-acetyltransferase activity (Axelrod, 1974). In a rat study, enzyme activity increased 1 hr after the onset of darkness, at 6:00 PM (Deguchi and Axelrod, 1972). This effect was prevented by keeping the lights on after that time. Darkness during the daytime, however, did not increase activity. The implication is that both darkness and nighttime are necessary for melatonin synthesis by the pineal gland. In human subjects, during the nocturnal sleep period, plasma melatonin is highest during spontaneous awakenings and lowest in REM sleep (Birkeland, 1982). It has been speculated that during brief awakenings, melatonin might have a physiological role in inducing sleep. During 64 hr of continuous wakefulness, in humans, high plasma levels of melatonin were associated with decrements of performance and increased subjective sleepiness (Akerstedt, Gillberg, and Wetterberg, 1982). In passing, it should also be mentioned that benzodiazepines may suppress nocturnal melatonin secretion in human subjects (Kabuto, Namura, and Saitoh, 1986).

Effects of Melatonin on Sleep

Two studies of administration of melatonin to humans during the day have reported that it has sleep-inducing effects (Cramer *et al.*, 1974; Anton-Tay, Diaz, and Fernandez-Guardiola, 1971). Cramer *et al.* (1974) found that melatonin given at night shortened sleep latency but did not change the total duration of any sleep stage. Administration of 2 mg orally at 5:00 PM for four weeks has been reported to increase a sense of fatigue but did not alter subjective reports of sleep (Adrendt *et al.*, 1984). Such a dose might be expected to raise plasma concentrations to 10–100 times the typical maximum nighttime secretion (Arendt *et al.*, 1985). James and Mendelson (1987) gave 1 and 5 mg orally to 10 normal volunteers at night and found no changes in sleep latency or total sleep. The only significant effect was an increase in REM latency at the higher dose. Similarly, Mendelson *et al.* (1987b) found virtually no effect from the same doses in chronic insomniacs. It seems unlikely, then, that melatonin will be a useful sedative for clinical use.

Direct application of melatonin to the preoptic region of the hypothalamus in cats may induce sleep (Marczynski *et al.*, 1964), whereas intraventricular administration may enhance non-REM sleep but suppress REM sleep (Goldstein and Pavel, 1981). Daytime intraperitoneal administration of 10 mg/kg to rats has been reported to decrease sleep latency and increase non-REM and REM sleep (Holmes and Sugden, 1982). Mendelson *et al.* (1980) gave 833 μg/kg of melatonin intraperitoneally to rats during the morning in the light and at night in the dark. In the morning, it decreased non-REM sleep; at night it did not have this effect. Propranolol, which might be expected to reduce *N*-acetyltransferase activity, did not alter non-REM sleep when given in the morning, but increased it at night. It also decreased REM sleep both at night and in the morning.

One interpretation of the observation that daytime administration of melatonin induces wakefulness in rats and sleepiness in humans might be that, in both cases, it induced the typical nighttime behavior of the particular species. In an analogous process, melatonin given to hamsters and other animals that breed when days are long had an antigonadal effect, but it stimulated gonadal activity in sheep and other animals that breed when days are short (Lincoln, 1983). Thus, in terms of effects on wakefulness and fertility, melatonin secretion provides information on lighting conditions; each species uses that information in ways that fit its own needs.

SUMMARY

The anterior pituitary hormones ACTH, GH, PRL, TSH, LH, FSH, and the endorphins are secreted in a pulsatile manner, in response to several influences including the sleep–wake and non-REM–REM cycles and circadian rhythmic processes. Some hormones (GH, PRL) are relatively more influenced by the sleep–wake cycle, others (ACTH) are affected more by circadian mechanisms. Several, including GH, LH, TSH, ACTH, and PRL, may have fairly evident ultradian rhythmicity as well. The ultimate pattern of secretion results from the combined effects of these factors, whose relative strength may change across the course of a lifetime (e.g., LH). A major aspect of anterior pituitary hormone regulation is achieved by open loop control mechanisms mediated by releasing or inhibiting factors from the hypothalamus. Some of these (e.g., GH-releasing factor, somatostatin, TRH), may also act directly on the central nervous system. Corticotropin-releasing hormone, for instance, may play a key role in mediating a variety of stress responses as well as controlling the secretion of ACTH. In addition, the anterior pituitary hormones are also under the control of a closed loop negative feedback system. Hypothalamic pathways in the open loop system may be mediated by the neurotransmitters norepinephrine, dopamine, serotonin and acetylcholine, which have also been implicated in control mechanisms of sleep. A number of peptide neurotransmitters are also involved. In the case of GH, it is possible that the neural mechanisms that control sleep-related secretion may differ from those regulating secretion in response to provocative tests by pharmacological agents. For LH and cortisol, the relation to sleep persists even in the presence of some diseases of oversecretion. Growth hormone, ACTH, and possibly TSH and melatonin, are influenced by sleep, and in turn may themselves affect sleep. It may turn out, then, that one major aspect of sleep regulation is this two-way interaction between neural mechanisms of sleep and endocrine activity.

PART II

Pathology of Sleep

INTRODUCTION

In Part I, we showed how anatomical, pharmacological, and endocrinological studies provide some basic understanding of normal sleep.
Several themes emerged, the most important being that there is a
unique physiology and pharmacology of sleep. For example, some
drugs may have very different effects on endocrine systems when
given when the patient is awake rather than asleep (Chapter 5). In
Part II, we will see that there are also unique pathologies of sleep. Various disorders that appear during sleep may be undetectable during the
waking state. In the sleep apnea syndromes, for instance, a person will
repeatedly have epidsodes of greatly decreased respiration, even
though the most careful pulmonary examination is often normal during
the day (Chapter 6). Patients generally do not realize that they have
these disorders, although they are only too aware of some of the
consequences—the uncomfortable experience of insomnia or of daytime sleepiness. Thus, poor sleep or excessive sleepiness are not disorders per se, but rather are symptoms of underlying pathological
conditions. These range from clearly disordered physiology (e.g., sleep
apnea) to psychiatric illnesses (e.g., depression) to difficulties currently
best described in psychological terms (e.g., persistent psychophysiological insomnia). We will now describe the major disorders of sleep,
and the available treatments. One theme seen throughout is that many
can be best understood as aberrations in the known physiology of
sleep. As we will see in Chapter 7, for instance, many of the symptoms

181

of narcolepsy can be viewed as the inappropriate appearance of components of REM sleep. Similarly, the particularly severe apneas that appear during REM sleep (Chapter 6) make more sense when one is aware of the irregularity of respiration that normally occurs in that state. Let us turn, then, to the known pathologies of sleep.

Sleep-Related Breathing Disorders

INTRODUCTION

The sleep apnea syndromes comprise the single most common diagnosis in contemporary sleep disorder centers. Although there has been a resurgence of interest in this area in recent years, reports have been in the literature since the last half of the nineteenth century (Lavie, 1984). After individual cases of what might now be considered sleep apnea were described by Broadbent (1877), Caton (1889), and Morrison (1889), the first account viewing this as a specific sleep disorder was written by Silas Weir Mitchell in 1890. He described patients in whom breathing was normal only in the waking state, during which voluntary efforts supplement automatic mechanisms. During sleep, when voluntary control diminished, the disordered automatic activity was not adequate, and respiratory failure would occur. As a consequence, the patient would awaken with a sense of suffocation. Accounts also appeared linking upper airway obstruction with somnolence and sleep disturbance (Lamacq, 1897; Wells, 1898). In 1889 Christopher Heath, commenting on the presentation of Caton's patient, pointed out the resemblance to Joe, a character in Charles Dickens' *Pickwick Papers* (1837). After later references by Bramwell (1909) and Osler, and a detailed modern description by Burwell *et al.* (1956), the Pickwickian syndrome of obesity and hypersomnolence became part of our medical heritage. In 1966, Gastaut, Tassinari, and Duron related the daytime somnolence of Pickwickian patients to primarily obstructive apneas that occurred during sleep. Subsequently we have come to distinguish sleep apnea from the obesity–hypoventilation syndrome which may result from apneas, a primary defect in alveolar ventilation, or both (Millman, 1986). The literature has flourished, with approximately 100 papers a year on sleep-related respiratory disorders published in the early 1980s.

SNORING

Although the relation of snoring to sleep apnea syndrome is not entirely clear, a widely accepted view is that the two represent the mild and severe extremes on a continuum of airway disruption during sleep. Lugaresi, Coccagna, and Cirignotta (1978) found that in mild snoring alveolar ventilation as well as pulmonary and systemic circulation do not change significantly. In louder and more continuous snoring, however, there are some significant changes; thus, heavy snorers may have increased pulmonary and systemic arterial blood pressure and increased arterial partial pressures of CO_2 compared to normal subjects, although these pressures are lower than they are in obstructive sleep apnea patients. The authors also described cases in which patients with the Pickwickian syndrome lost weight, resulting in decreased apneas but increased snoring. This suggests that snoring may be a way-station on the road to the sleep apnea syndrome.

A study of over 5000 citizens in the tiny republic of San Marino found that 24.1% of men and 13.8% of women reported snoring regularly (Lugaresi et al., 1982), and this incidence increased with age. Systemic hypertension and cardiac disease were found to be higher among persons who snored. The relationship of snoring to hypertension was seen in nonobese as well as obese persons.

Although the medical consequences of snoring are not as severe as those associated with sleep apnea syndromes per se, the social consequences are very real. In many households, it disrupts the harmony of the marital bed and can affect intimate relationships. An extreme case of ill effects of snoring comes from the history of the Western desperado John Wesley Hardin, who is said to have shot a man to stop his snoring in an adjacent hotel room (Sifakis, 1982).

INCIDENCE OF SLEEP APNEA SYNDROMES

Since data on snoring can presumably be reliably obtained by history, there is more demographic information available on snoring than on sleep apnea syndromes. Among patients who have been studied at a sleep disorder center (and hence are clearly not representative of the general population) sleep apnea syndromes were found in 43.2% of those who complained of excessive sleepiness and in 6.2% of those who complained of insomnia (Coleman et al., 1982; Fig. 6-1). Approximately 1% of presumably healthy industrial workers in Israel were found to be affected (Lavie, 1983). In a study of 100 persons of both sexes and with a wide age distribution, who had no subjective difficulty with their sleep, none had the clinical condition of sleep apnea syndrome, which is defined as 30 apneas or more a night (Bixler et al., 1982a). Twelve percent, however, had between 3 and 29 apneic events. In another study of 30 men and 19 women, all of whom were asymptomatic, 20 men were found to have a cumulative total of 264 episodes of oxygen desaturation or abnormal breathing (Block et al., 1979). None of the women experienced oxygen desaturation, although three had a total of nine apneic episodes. Obesity and increasing age correlated with these respiratory disturbances in the men. Carskadon, Van den Hoed, and Dement (1980) studied 24 subjects over 65 who had no complaints about their sleep. During sleep, nine had between 70 and 216 apneas or hypopneas, which were primarily central in nature. Reynolds et al. (1985) found the incidence of sleep apnea (defined as five or more disordered breathing events an hour) to be 4.3% among 23 healthy elderly controls. It was much more frequent in depressed (17.6%) and demented (42.9%) patients. The relationship of sleep apnea syndrome to depression and dementia is actively being explored. As we will see later, significant numbers of apnea patients have many of the symptoms of depression and exhibit cognitive deficits.

Bliwise et al. (1984) performed a longitudinal study on 10 middle-aged and 15 elderly persons selected for having few or no sleep-related respiratory disturbances. Among the middle-aged subjects who were followed up after approximately 8.1 yr, there was an increase in the respiratory disturbance index (RDI) (number of apneas and hypopneas an hour) (Guilleminault, Van den Hoed, and Mitler, 1978) in the group as a whole, with four having pathological values of five or more. The mean RDI for the elderly, with a mean follow-up time of 2.8 yr, also rose, largely because of a major increase in one individual. This suggests a progressive process in these individuals; as the authors pointed out, however, it is also not clear how long it might take for the pathological consequences of the respiratory disturbance to appear.

There are some indications that laboratory studies of sleep apnea may underestimate its prevalence if recordings are performed for only one night. Bliwise, Carey, and Dement (1983), who also reported a correlation between respiratory disturbance and age in healthy elderly subjects, found a marked increase in RDI across two nights. Using an index of five as an arbitrary lower limit for the clinical condition, 11 subjects met this criteria on night 1, whereas 22 did so on night 2. The difference could not be accounted for by the change in the amount of REM sleep across the two nights. There was no further increase in respiratory disturbance across nights 2 and 3 in those subjects in whom a third night was recorded. The implication is that prevalence studies that involve two nights of recording would reveal a higher rate in the population.

REGULATION OF RESPIRATION IN SLEEP

Before considering the clinical manifestations of sleep apnea syndromes, it might be well to review the regulation of breathing during sleep. During sleep, both the mechanics of respiration and the degree of drive in response to blood gases clearly change. In terms of the mechanics, there is a decrease in general muscle tone in non-REM sleep, which tends to spare the diaphragm, and a further decrease in REM sleep. Additionally in REM sleep, there is relatively less respiratory involvement of the intercostals and relatively more involvement of the diaphragm. Hence, Tusiewicz *et al.* (1977) reported that in human subjects the rib cage contributed 44% to tidal volume in waking and non-REM sleep, but during REM sleep, its contribution decreased to 19%. During waking, one function of intercostal activity is to stiffen the

Disorders of Excessive Sleepiness (DOES)				
Diagnosis*	N	% DOES	Range/Center, %	% Total
Sleep apnea syndromes	857	43.2	23.9-81.2	22.0
Narcolepsy	496	25.0	7.7-32.2	12.7
Idiopathic CNS hypersomnia	175	8.8	0.0-26.9	4.5
No hypersomnia abnormality	106	5.4	0.0-16.4	2.8
Other hypersomnia	99	5.0	1.9-7.9	2.5
Psychiatric disorders	73	3.7	0.0-25.3	1.9
Sleep-related myoclonus and RLS	70	3.5	0.0-13.7	1.8
Medical, toxic, and environmental	53	2.7	0.0-5.1	1.4
Drug and alcohol dependency	30	1.5	0.0-4.4	0.8
Psychophysiological	22	1.1	0.0-4.3	0.6
Total	1,983	99.9	. . .	51.0

FIGURE 6-1. Diagnoses of patients complaining of excessive daytime sleepiness in a 5000-patient multicenter study. (From Coleman *et al.*, 1982. Reprinted by permission.)

rib cage; while the intercostals are hypotonic during sleep, the negative intrapleural pressure induced by diaphragmatic contraction can cause an inward movement of the rib cage during inspiration.

A second aspect of the mechanics of respiration involves the muscles of the upper airway, as described by Orr (1984). The activity of the genioglossus muscle, for example, is enhanced during inspiration, presumably stabilizing the tongue to keep the airway open (Sauerland and Harper, 1976). However, tonic activity of the genioglossus drastically declines during REM sleep. Other pharyngeal musculature, such as the medial pterygoid and tensor palati, have decreased activity in non-REM, which decreases further in REM sleep (Sauerland, Orr, and Hairston, 1981). A similar process may occur in the laryngeal musculature (Berger, 1961). The timing of the pharyngeal constrictors vis-à-vis the respiratory cycle is less clear (Sherry and Megirian, 1975; Sauerland et al., 1981; Hill, Guilleminault, and Simmons, 1978). Strohl et al. (1980) have demonstrated that some upper airway muscles have bursts of activity immediately before inspiration. There is, then, an elaborate system of precisely timed alterations in upper airway muscle tone during the respiratory cycle. Given the intricate nature of this process, it is possible that pathological changes in tone or timing of muscle activity could lead to functional obstruction.

In the waking state, respiration is under both metabolic and behavioral control. Metabolic control is thought to be centered in the medulla, which contains tissue sensitive to CO_2, and also oxygen sensors in the carotid bodies. Behavioral control includes voluntary alterations in respiration for speaking and swallowing. As one goes to sleep, behavioral control diminishes and automatic regulation becomes more important. During waking, a number of diseases can alter arterial oxygen and CO_2 content, but few disorders alter the respiratory rate. (Exceptions are severe central nervous system disorders associated with a poor prognosis.) In sleep, however, many changes occur in the respiratory rate. At sleep onset, the minute volume falls, often with a small increase in the arterial CO_2, and a declining oxygen content. In the transition between sleep stages, there are often brief (about 10 sec) pauses in respiration, a phenomenon that may be particularly common in children and the elderly.

Sleep also alters responsiveness to hypoxia and hypercapnea (for reviews, see Phillipson, 1977, 1978; Cherniak, 1981; Guilleumault, 1982). During non-REM sleep in humans, the ventilatory response to CO_2 declines, as manifested by a shift of the curve to the right, and a diminished slope (Cherniak, 1981). On average, there may be relatively little change in response to hypoxia, although in some individuals it may decrease or even increase (Cherniak, 1981). Santiago, Scardella, and Edelman (1984) noted that in goats there was a decreased respiratory responsiveness to hypoxia during non-REM and REM in the eucapnic state, but that this difference disappeared under conditions of hypocapnea. This suggests that differences in P_{CO_2} might help explain differing results among studies. In dogs, there is a further decrease in response to both stimuli in REM, but the response to hypoxia is reduced less than to hypercapnea (Phillipson et al., 1978). It is not clear if there is a further decrease in phasic REM sleep (during which eye movements and other phasic processes occur; see Chapter 1) as opposed to tonic REM sleep. Sullivan et al. (1979) reported that in dogs the response to CO_2 in tonic REM is similar to that in non-REM, although it is further decreased in phasic REM. Netick, Dugger, and Symmons (1984), however, saw no such change in phasic REM in cats and suggested that these differences may be species-specific. In humans, the respiratory response to hypercapnea may depend on gender. Berthon-Jones and Sullivan (1984) found that in men there was a progressive decrease in respiratory response from waking to non-REM to REM. In women the response was about the same in all three states, and was roughly comparable to the level of response during non-REM in men.

Thus far, we have described the alterations in respiration that follow changes in blood gases. Another reaction to hypoxia and hypercapnea is arousal. As Guilleminault (1982) pointed out, an arousal need not refer to a return to full consciousness, but rather to a brief excitation of the reticular activating system resulting in a changed level of functioning of the autonomic nervous system. An apneic period, for instance, may be ended by a brief arousal followed by resumption of respiration. In terms of the EEG this is often reflected in the appearance of K complexes or a brief burst of alpha activity. The arousal response to hypoxia is presumably mediated by the carotid bodies. In dogs, arousal from sleep has been reported to occur when oxygen saturation dropped to 83% in non-REM sleep and 70% in REM sleep (Bowes, 1984). When the carotid bodies were denervated, there was no arousal even when saturations of 60% (non-REM) and 50% (REM) had been reached. One report indicated that, in male humans arousal occurred from approximately equal degrees of hypercapnea in stage 2 and REM sleep, whereas higher levels were required for stage 3 and stage 4 sleep (Berthon-Jones and Sullivan, 1984). In females, there was little difference across stages. This is again somewhat at variance with the animal literature, which reports less sensitivity during REM, so this will need further clarification. The arousal response also depends on the quality of sleep. There is evidence in animals that fragmentation of prior sleep will raise the subsequent arousal threshold to hypercapnia and hypoxia (Phillipson *et al.*, 1980; Bowes, 1984). One might speculate, then, that a snowball effect may occur in the sleep apnea syndromes, such that arousals due to previous apneas may lead to progressive difficulty having arousals in response to subsequent ones.

Another respiratory change in sleep involves nasal ε r resistance. The overall supralaryngeal resistance has been reported to rise during sleep (Hudgel and Robertson, 1984). This may not be due to an increase in total nasal resistance, which may not change with sleep, but rather may possibly reflect an increase in pharyngeal resistance. There is, however, a cyclical change in resistance between the two sides of the nose that is not dependent on gravity (Hudgel and Robertson, 1984). One significance of this observation is that if one side of the nose is blocked (e.g. by a deviated septum or the sequelae of a fracture), then periodically throughout the night, there will be a near-total occlusion as resistance rises on the "good" side.

Respiration during sleep can also be affected by medications and by illness. As discussed later, a number of drugs, including some hypnotics and alcohol, may have little effect on respiration during waking but will suppress respiration during sleep. Similarly, a variety of illnesses, including chronic obstructive pulmonary disease (COPD) and spinal or rib cage conditions that limit chest wall movement, may have relatively greater effects on ventilation during sleep (and particularly in the irregular respiration of REM sleep). Altitude may also affect respiration during sleep, with higher altitudes possibly enhancing sleep apneas.

METHODS OF RECORDING AND MEASURING
SLEEP-RELATED RESPIRATION

In addition to the standard measures of sleep, polygraphic recordings for sleep apnea require several additional channels (see Chapter 1; Bornstein, 1982; Fig. 1-1). Thermistors or thermocouple transducers are used to track air flow from both the nose and the mouth. Both are important, since there is often a shift between the two from waking to sleeping. In general, during the awake state, air resistance is lower in the mouth than the nose; when the individual is asleep and recumbent, the reverse is usually the case. Movements of the chest wall and abdomen are detected by a variety of techniques, including use of mercury-filled strain gauges, pressure-sensitive pneumatic devices, or instruments that record alterations in inductance. In addition to measuring the presence or absence of movement, which is necessary to distinguish between the central and obstructive types of disordered breathing events (DBEs), information about the phase relationship between the chest and abdomen is obtained. As will be discussed later, this is important in characterizing obstructive events. The energetic diaphragmatic exertions during obstructive events cause the abdomen and chest to move out of phase with each other, as can be seen in the tracing (Fig. 6-2). Finally, arterial oxygen saturation must be measured. This is usually obtained with an oximeter, a noninvasive instrument that indirectly determines oxygen saturation as a function of the light absorption of blood in the earlobe or fingertip. Currently available instruments require 20 or 30 sec to determine this, and hence, oxygen saturation curves printed out on the polygraphic record tend to lag 20 or 30 sec behind the data for the other channels. A less widely used approach involves a skin oximeter, which reports data in terms of partial pressures of oxygen. The EKG is monitored to observe the respiration-related changes in heart rate and to detect any possible arrhythmias. As will be described later, the heart rate generally declines during an obstructive event and often accelerates immediately afterward. Heart rate may also be studied without polysomnographic monitoring by use of a Holter monitor, which can provide 24-hr data. These may be displayed as computer-generated printouts of the R-R interval and may give indirect evidence of disordered breathing events (Bornstein, 1982). Esophageal balloons may be used to determine if there is enhanced negative intraesophageal pressure during inspiration, which would be taken as evidence of upper airway obstruction.

Several measures of disordered breathing events are commonly used. Generally, DBEs may be considered to be comprised of *apneas* and *hypopneas*. In a general sense, apneas refer to virtually complete cessation of air flow as measured by the thermistor channels, while hypopneas refer to decreased flow. Defined in more technical terms (Bornstein, 1982), apneas refer to events in which the amplitude of the thermistor tracing falls to less than 50% of basal values. During an obstructive apnea, the strain gauges continue to move at the respiratory frequency but increase in amplitude by at least 20% compared to baseline. Often the movements of the two strain gauges fall out of phase, resulting in "paradoxical" movement, and oxygen saturation falls. The event often terminates in a brief arousal, characterized by K complexes or brief bursts of alpha waves, and body movements. In contrast, central apneas are characterized by cessation of air flow measured in the thermistor channels, accompanied by cessation of respiratory effort on the strain gauge channels (Fig. 6-3). In practice many disordered breathing events are

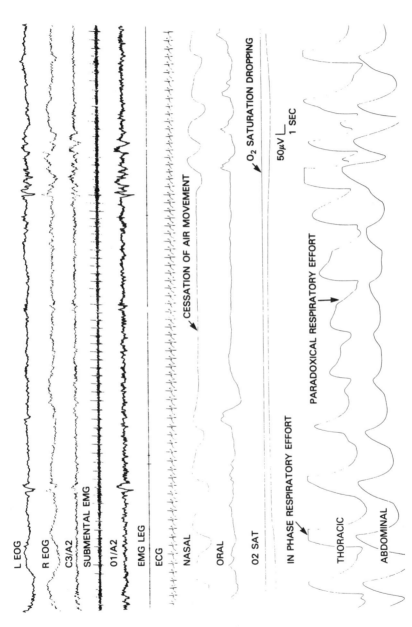

FIGURE 6-2. Polysomnogram of an obstructive apnea.

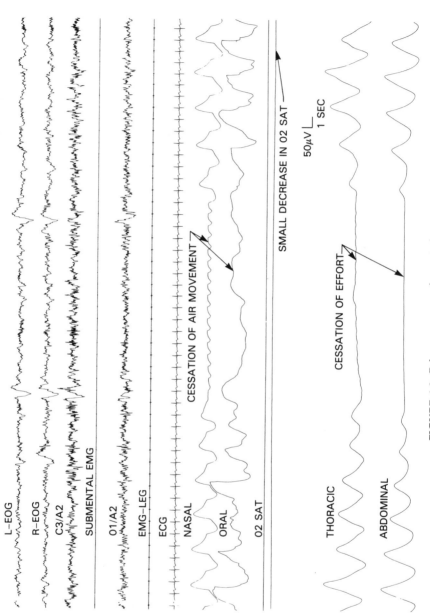

FIGURE 6-3. Polysomnogram of a central apnea.

mixed types in which typically a brief period of central apnea with no respiratory effort is followed by an obstructive period during which respiratory effort takes place. Hypopneas may be defined as decreases in air flow on the thermistor channels to one-third of baseline, accompanied by a decrease in arterial oxygen saturation and decreased respiratory effort. The definition of sleep apnea syndrome is usually considered to be the presence of at least 30 apneas of at least 10-sec duration. As mentioned earlier, it is often expressed as the apnea and hypopnea index (respiratory disturbance index):

$$RDI = \frac{\text{No. of apneas and hypopneas}}{\text{Total sleep time (min)}} \times 60$$

Again, reflecting the observation that occasional respiratory irregularities may occur in many asymptomatic persons, an index value is not considered abnormal until it is above five.

CLINICAL SYNDROMES

Sleep-related respiratory disturbances are often divided into sleep apnea and hypoventilation syndromes. Sleep apnea syndromes are, in turn, divided into obstructive and central types.

Obstructive Sleep Apnea

Clinical Features

These patients often present with a complaint of excessive daytime sleepiness. General clinical characteristics have been described by a number of authors, including Guilleminault, Van den Hoed, and Mitler (1978) and Waldhorn (1985). Classically, a patient may be observed snoring; there is then an absence of sound as the airway becomes obstructed, usually at the end of an expiration (Martin *et al.*, 1980). During this time the diaphragm and accessory muscles of respiration continue to function in an attempt to move air past the obstruction. As the arterial oxygen saturation falls, a bradycardia (or arrhythmia) occur. Suddenly, the patient "breaks through" with a brief arousal on the EEG, often making a loud inspiratory gasping sound, and respiration resumes. There may be a brief tachycardia at this point. Often the patient is entirely unaware of these events, and presents only with the complaint of sleepiness during the day and a vague sense of having slept poorly. The cause of daytime sleepiness is not clear, although there is some correlation with the degree of nocturnal oxygen desaturation (Orr, Imes, and Martin, 1979). A patient may describe awakening during the night with a sensation of choking or awakening in the morning with a headache or nausea. Guilleminault, Van den Hoed, and Mitler (1978), in a case series of 50 patients, point to a number of other related symptoms. These include difficulty in concentration and focusing attention, which occurred in all 39 patients who complained of sleepiness, as well as in two who did not. The symptoms often seemed worse in the morning. Of these patients, 48% appeared to have personality changes, which were often manifested as anxiety or depression, 16% had actually sought psychiatric help, and 42% reported impotence. Other symptomatology included nocturnal enuresis (30%), sleepwalking or falling out of bed (54%), hypnagogic hallucinations (44%), automatic behavior (58%), and systemic hypertension (52%). The depressive symptoms seen in apneic patients have been emphasized by Reynolds et al. (1984b), who found that 40% of 25 patients with primarily mixed apneas met the Research Diagnostic Criteria for affective disorder or alcohol abuse. Cognitive deficits appear on formal neuropsychological testing (Bell and Govindan, 1986; Berry et al., 1986; Norman, Levin, and Cohn, 1986). The latter group, for instance, found that patients with sleep apnea had particular difficulty with learning word pairs, verbal memory, visual–motor tracking skills, and changing cognitive set. Patients with sleep-related respiratory disorders may also tend to display somatic concerns and dysphoric mood (Fiss, Lavie, and Hasselbrock, 1983). Another study has emphasized hypochondriacal and hysterical personality characteristics (Beutler et al., 1981).

Examination of the patient's oropharynx often reveals a number of characteristic findings. These may include an elongated uvula, as well as a narrow opening of the nasopharynx and velopharyngeal port.

The daytime sleepiness of the obstructive sleep apnea patient has been well documented in multiple sleep latency test (MSLT) studies (see Chapter 7). Walsh, Smitson, and Kramer (1982), who examined a severely ill group (mean apneic episodes per hour was 59.0), found that the mean sleep latency on MSLT was similar to that for narcoleptics. It should also be noted that eight of the 14 patients had at least one REM-onset sleep episode (four had one episode, three had two, and one had three). These REM-onset sleep episodes presumably reflect REM deprivation resulting from frequent awakenings at night. This serves to remind us that REM onset episodes are not confined to narcolepsy.

Age

Patients with obstructive sleep apnea syndrome tend to be middle-aged and male. In the Guilleminault, Van den Hoed, and Mitler (1978) series, the mean age was 45.5 years (range 28–62), and 90% were men. The sleep apnea syndrome may also occur in children, in whom anatomical problems such as enlarged tonsils and adenoids, choanal atresia, or nasal septum deviation may occur (Mark and Brooks, 1984). Clinical features associated with obstructive sleep apnea in children include difficulty breathing during sleep, a history of apneas observed by parents, snoring, restless sleep, chronic rhinorrhea and mouth breathing when awake (Brouilette *et al.*, 1984). This author's impression is that behavioral or school performance changes are often major features of this disorder in children.

Complications

Patients often develop pulmonary hypertension with resultant cor pulmonale. The former may be the long-term consequence of the normal hypoxic reflex, by which the pulmonary vasculature constricts in response to hypoxia. The stress placed on the heart during episodes of hypoxemia in sleep was demonstrated by Shepard *et al.* (1984) in COPD patients. They found that the demand for coronary blood flow during these episodes was transiently as great as during maximal exercise. Systemic hypertension may occur in many of these patients apparently as the result of increased sympathetic tone (Fletcher *et al.*, 1987). The origin of decreased libido and impotence in obstructive sleep apnea syndrome is unclear. Fletcher and Martin (1982), studying a somewhat different population—20 men with COPD—found subjective measures of sexual dysfunction to be very common in the group as a whole, but objective measures of loss of nocturnal penile tumesence (NPT) in six patients. Upon oral glucose testing, occult diabetes mellitus was found in four, of whom two were among the patients with NPT deficits. Otherwise, there was little evidence of endocrine disturbance; only one patient was found to be androgen deficient. Subjective measures of sexual dysfunction correlated significantly with pulmonary impairment as well as age. Coming from the other direction, Schmidt and Wise (1981) studied 15 patients with secondary impotence, seven of whom had abnormal NPT. The latter subjects had significantly more episodes of apneas and hypoventilation compared to the patients with normal NPT. Foreman *et al.* (1986) found sleep apnea syndrome in 17% of 30 patients complaining of impotence, with both normal and abnormal NPT. At this time it is not clear whether the apnea and the impotence have a common etiology or whether the impotence sometimes results from the chronic hypoxemia (Timms, 1982).

Associated Conditions

Obstructive sleep apnea may be brought out or worsened by a variety of illnesses that compromise the upper airway. These include congenital micrognathia, hypothyroidism, acromegaly (Cadieux *et al.*, 1982), lymphoma (Zorick *et al.*, 1977), and other disorders. Allergic rhinitis may produce frequent hypopneic events associated with "microarousals" (Lavie *et al.*, 1981). The common theme among these disorders is a reduction in the functional size of the upper airway.

Neurological Components of Obstructive Sleep Apnea?

Although anatomical considerations are obviously very important in understanding the obstructive apnea process, it is well to bear in mind the possible neurological aspects of this disorder. There is evidence that in the period immediately preceding obstructive apneas, airway resistance increases while ventilation decreases. During this period, the swings in gastric pressure (a measure of diaphragmatic activity and abdominal muscle tone) decline. One interpretation of this progressive suppression of respiratory musculature is that there are central aspects to "obstructive" sleep apnea, and this may help explain the existence of mixed apneas (Martin *et al.*, 1980). Onal, Lopata, and O'Connor (1982) found that diaphragmatic and genioglossal activity increased and decreased cyclically during sleep and that obstructive apneas occurred at the nadir of these cycles (Fig. 6-4). Cerniak *et al.* (1980) proposed that if the neural drive to upper airway musculative were disproportionate to that to the diaphragm and accessory respiratory muscles, obstructive apneas might appear. A similar process has been invoked to explain the rare cases in which medroxyprogesterone exacerbates sleep apnea (Strohl *et al.*, 1981). Given the complex interactions of the upper airway musculature and the diaphragm, it seems likely that a centrally induced disturbance of these relationships might be manifest as an apparently obstructive apnea. There may also be a reflex inhibition of respiration as the result of activation of supraglottic mucosal receptors during passive oropharyngeal airway closure (Issa and Sullivan, 1986). Conceivably, then, airway closure could be manifested as an apparently central apnea. These observations imply that both obstructive and central sleep apneas might be different manifestations of one underlying disorder.

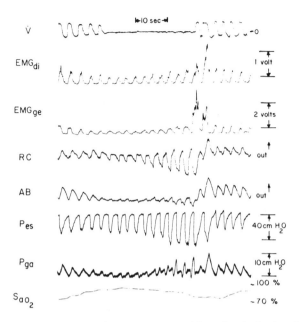

FIGURE 6-4. A representative obstructive apnea. Note that both the diaphragm and genioglossus electromyograms (EMGs) (EMG$_{di}$ and EMG$_{ge}$) gradually decreased as oxygen saturation (SaO$_2$) increased; the muscular activity reached the nadir of the cycle when SaO$_2$ was highest. After upper airway occlusion onset, both EMGs increased with decreasing SaO$_2$. Genioglossal activity during the first unoccluded breath is out of proportion to that of the diaphragm. Paradoxical thoracoabdominal motion, phasic expiratory increases in gastric pressure (P$_{ga}$), and an increase in baseline gastric pressure are seen during the course of the apnea. Note that the esophageal pressure (P$_{es}$) during the occlusive phase is relatively higher than that during the unoccluded phase, despite the decreased diaphragmatic EMG. (From Onal, Lopata, and O'Connor, 1982. Reprinted by permission.)

Central Sleep Apnea

Clinical Features

In central sleep apnea, a patient is observed to have normal air flow, which then ceases in conjunction with an absence of movement of the respiratory musculature. Once again, arterial oxygen saturation falls. An arousal will occur, accompanied by resumption of breathing. As in the obstructive sleep apnea syndrome, the patient is often unaware of these events. Snoring may be present but tends to be milder and less common than in obstructive sleep apnea. In addition to insomnia, roughly 30% of patients complain of not feeling rested in the morning, and approximately 20% describe daytime tiredness. In

general they go to sleep quickly but awaken during the night, sometimes feeling that they cannot breathe.

In general, patients with central sleep apnea tend to be somewhat
older than those with obstructive sleep apnea. In the Guilleminault,
Van den Hoed, and Mitler (1978) series, the mean age was 57 (range
27–79), and all were male. These patients often had normal body
weights and tended to score higher on the depression scale of the
MMPI. Central apneas may also appear in elderly persons without
sleep complaints. In a study of 24 asymptomatic elderly subjects, nine
(five women and four men) were found to have predominantly central
respiratory disturbances (Carskadon et al., 1980). Central sleep apnea
may, of course, occur in infants and may be involved in the apnea of
prematurity and in the sudden infant death syndrome. It may also appear in other adult conditions, including narcolepsy. In passing, it
should be mentioned that central sleep apneas have also been observed
in rodents (Mendelson et al., 1987d).

Complications

The medical complications of central sleep apnea are not so clear as
those in obstructive sleep apnea. Aside from the discomfort of insomnia and fatigue, some patients complain of loss of libido or impotence.
Whether this is related to repeated hypoxia or some other cause is not
known. Daytime sleepiness may indeed be a consequence of central
sleep apnea. In the Carskadon et al. (1980) study, the subjects who
had central apneas were significantly more sleepy during daytime
MSLT testing than were subjects with normal respiration during sleep.
Another concern is that an apneic episode could lead to full respiratory
arrest or trigger an arrhythmia in a susceptible individual. As will be
discussed later, there is some evidence that such respiratory suppressant drugs as hypnotics or anxiolytics may enhance disordered breathing in these patients.

Mixed Apneas

Many disordered breathing events are of mixed type. Typically, the
event appears as a central apnea, with no diaphragmatic activity, followed by an obstructive period with vigorous respiratory effort. Clinically, symptoms are usually a mixture of those in obstructive and
central types. The existence of mixed apneas is instructive in that it
suggests possible common etiological factors for both forms of the apnea syndromes. We mentioned earlier the study of Martin et al. (1980),
which showed a progressive decrease in respiratory effort prior to the

onset of an apnea, possibly suggesting a neurological component to this process. Onal *et al.* (1982) found that during the sleep of apnea patients the amplitude of respiration periodically increased and decreased, in a manner similar to Cheyne–Stokes breathing. Hypopneas and obstructive apneas occurred at the nadirs of these cycles, and mixed apneas began as episodes of no inspiratory activity, at that time. One interpretation of these findings is that obstructive apneas and mixed apneas, in particular, may be extreme cases of a periodic cycle of amplitude of respiration during sleep.

Hypoventilation Syndromes

Patients with a variety of medical conditions affecting respiration may have an augmentation of these difficulties during sleep. These illnesses might be peripheral (e.g., COPD) or central (e.g., Ondine's curse). A common situation is for a COPD patient to be barely compensated, with a marginal oxygen saturation when awake; during sleep, however, episodes of desaturation occur (Flick and Block, 1977; Wynne *et al.*, 1978a). These presumably result from the decreased respiration of non-REM, or the irregular respiration of REM sleep. Anecdotally, such a situation is often found in patients who have had COPD for many years and are now being evaluated for a relatively recent onset of sleepiness or difficulty concentrating. One's retrospective impression is that perhaps they retained relatively good oxygen saturation even in sleep and that the additional symptomatology occurred when they were no longer compensated during sleep. Thoracoskeletal deformities and myotonic dystrophy (Coccagna, Martinelli, and Lugaresi, 1982) may be other disorders that produce hypoventilation syndromes, as are such neurological disorders as poliomyelitis, spinal cord lesions, and encephalitis.

The congenital central alveolar hypoventilation syndrome (Ondine's curse) is manifest as severe episodes of hypoventilation during sleep (Coccagna *et al.*, 1984). There may be CO_2 retention and, eventually, cor pulmonale may develop. Ventilatory capacity is often normal, but responses to hypoxemia and hypercapnea are minimal. It is not clear whether this involves a defect of central chemoreceptors or a problem in the integration of chemoreceptor information (Guilleminault *et al.*, 1982). Ondine's curse may occur without apparent cause or it may follow encephalitis, a cerebrovascular accident, or trauma. Treatment by diaphragm pacing will be described later.

The Pickwickian syndrome (obesity-related hypoventilation syndrome) includes daytime somnolence, obesity, and often hypercapnea, without intrinsic lung disease (Burwell *et al.*, 1956). In these patients, the massive obesity may result in restrictive pulmonary dysfunction. The central aspects of the respiratory dysregulation have been emphasized by Lugaresi, Coccagna, and Ceroni (1968a). As we will see later, some patients who undergo surgery for Pickwickian syndrome and sleep apnea may continue to have hypercapnea because of a primary ventilation dysfunction (Rapoport et al., 1986).

TREATMENT

A variety of treatments have been proposed for obstructive sleep apnea, but relatively few are available for the central disorder. For obstructive apnea, these range from relatively benign interventions, such as weight loss, to major procedures such as chronic tracheostomy.

Obstructive Sleep Apnea

Protriptyline

In the early 1970s, individual case reports indicated that sleep apnea improved with tricyclic antidepressants (Kumashiro et al., 1971; Schwartz and Rochemaure, 1973). Insofar as most tricyclics are clinically sedating, interest turned to protriptyline which has little, if any, sedative qualities at moderate doses. In a study of 14 predominantly obstructive and mixed apnea patients with an average of more than 60 apneas a night, seven were managed successfully with 2.5–25 mg of protriptyline alone (Clark et al., 1979b). Both apnea time as a percentage of total sleep and mean duration of apneas decreased. Smith et al. (1983) gave protriptyline to 12 obstructive apnea patients with 50 to 108 DBEs per hour. In 10 of the 12 patients, there was an improvement in the subjective assessment of sleepiness and a small but significant increase in daytime wakefulness, as assessed by the MSLT.

It is not yet clear whether protriptyline is beneficial in both non-REM and REM sleep. In the Smith et al. (1983) study, there was no change in the frequency of DBEs, although the percentage of DBE time (apnea and hypopnea time) comprised of apneas dropped considerably from $60.4 \pm 27.2\%$ to $35.5 \pm 26.7\%$. The maximum fall in oxygen saturation also decreased. In REM sleep, there was no change in the frequency or composition of DBEs. Since the drug decreased the amount of REM sleep, however, it could be argued that there was less opportunity for the more severe events in REM sleep to occur. This view is supported by observations in five obstructive apnea patients, in whom protriptyline reduced REM apnea time as a fraction of total sleep but not as a fraction of total REM sleep time (Brownell *et al.*, 1982). On the other hand, a study of nine sleep apnea patients indicated that protriptyline decreased both the number of DBEs and the degree of desaturation in both non-REM and REM sleep (Fletcher *et al.*, 1984). Clark *et al.* (1979b) described several patients with predominantly non-REM events who improved, which does not support the argument that benefits are primarily the result of drug-induced suppression of REM sleep. Changes in upper airway function also seem unlikely. In the Smith *et al.* (1983) study, four of the 12 patients had abnormal pulmonary function tests; three of them developed better values while they were taking the drug, but a number of patients with normal pulmonary function tests also improved. Weight loss also did not seem a likely explanation. Although the group as a whole did lose weight, there were significant improvements in oxygen saturation and daytime somnolence in those patients whose weights did not change.

Side effects of tricyclic antidepressants that need to be considered include alterations in cardiac conduction and, possibly, myocardial contractility. This is of concern, insofar as sleep apnea patients may already be particularly susceptible to arrhythmias. Such anticholinergic symptoms as urinary hesitancy, dry mouth, and blurred vision may appear. Many male patients experience difficulty with erections.

Medroxyprogesterone Acetate

Progesterone, which may act as a respiratory stimulant, has been known to reduce Pa_{CO_2} in patients with the obesity–hypoventilation syndrome (Sutton *et al.*, 1975; Skatrud, Dempsey, and Kaiser, 1978; Skatrud, Dempsey, and Iber, 1981). Postmenopausal women have a much higher incidence of disordered breathing in sleep compared to premenopausal women, which perhaps implies that endogenous progesterone may have stimulating effects on respiration (Block, Wynne, and Boysen, 1980). Ross (1982) has suggested that alterations in endogenous progesterone in infants may contribute to the sudden infant death syndrome.

Orr, Imes, and Martin (1979) gave 60 mg of medroxyprogesterone acetate a day to seven obstructive sleep apnea patients, of whom five had congestive heart failure. For the group, as a whole, the incidence or the duration of apneas did not change significantly. The patients did, however, have a reduction in heart failure, and they reported less daytime somnolence. They were found to have increased daytime Pa_{O_2}, which may have been secondary to diuresis and an improvement in their cardiac status. Strohl *et al.* (1981) gave 60–120 mg of medroxy-progesterone a day to nine obstructive apnea patients. As a group there was no reduction in number of duration of apneas after six weeks of treatment. Four patients, however, had reduced daytime sleepiness and number of apneas during sleep. One patient had a marked increase in apneas. The only pretreatment difference that could be detected between responders and nonresponders was that the resting Pa_{O_2} during wakefulness was lower in the responders. A study of 21 postmenopausal women, of whom six had significant sleep-disordered breathing, found that medroxyprogesterone (30 mg/day for a month) had little effect on respiration (Block *et al.*, 1981). The only change noted was a reduction in the maximum duration of apneas. Dolly and Block (1983) examined the effects of 60 mg/day of medroxyprogesterone given for one month to 20 COPD patients. During the daytime, arterial Pa_{O_2} increased and Pa_{CO_2} decreased. During sleep, however, there was no change in the number of DBEs or in the episodes of desaturation or minimal desaturation, although percentage of sleep during which oxygen saturation was less than 90% declined nonsignificantly.

In summary, progesterone therapy has had limited benefits. The mechanism of action is unclear. As Strohl *et al.* (1981) pointed out, stimulation of such upper airway muscles as the genioglossus, as well as the diaphragm and intercostals, may occur. If the latter two are disproportionately stimulated, the increased negative pressure might actually enhance the obstruction. Conversely, the drug might preferentially stimulate the respiratory cycling of the upper airway musculature. Another interesting theory is that progesterone, which is known to have thermogenic properties, enhances respiration nonspecifically, as a consequence of raising the temperature. The benefits of progesterone also need to be weighed against its possible side effects, including alopecia and decreased libido. In the Strohl *et al.* (1981) study, these presented difficulties in one patient each.

Other Pharmacological Approaches

As mentioned earlier, anticholinergic side effects will sometimes limit the use of protriptyline. Nomifensine, a newer antidepressant with relatively little anticholinergic activity, was given to five obstructive sleep apnea patients by George, West, and Kryger (1986). Daytime somnolence was reduced. Although there was no change in the number of apneas and hypopneas per hour, the percentage of sleep during which oxygen saturation was less than 80% declined. Nomifensine has subsequently been taken off the market because of reports of hemolytic anemia, so it seems unlikely to be studied further.

L-Tryptophan, in an average dose of 2500 mg, has been reported to help obstructive but not central apnea patients (Schmidt, 1983). Benefits were greater in patients whose apneas were primarily in non-REM sleep and in those with fewer than 70 apneas and hypopneas per hour.

Low Flow Oxygen

Another approach to treating sleep apnea is the administration during sleep of low flow oxygen (usually 2–10 liters/min). Results have been mixed. Motta and Guilleminault (1978) described an acute study of four patients (three obstructive, one central) in whom they measured four consecutive apneas each in non-REM and REM sleep, with and without oxygen administration. In the non-REM sleep episodes, the duration of apneas increased in all four patients, reaching statistical significance in three. In the three in whom blood gases were followed, there was an increase in P_{CO_2} and acidosis with oxygen administration. During REM sleep, oxygen administration was associated with increased duration of apneas, which reached statistical significance in two patients. In two patients in whom blood gases were obtained, there were once again increases in P_{CO_2} and acidosis compared to the studies on room air. The mean increase in duration of apneas was greater in REM sleep (52 ± 5 sec) compared to non-REM sleep (19 ± 5 sec).

Martin et al. (1982) studied acute daytime sleep in eight primarily obstructive sleep apnea patients and found that, as a group, oxygen administration decreased the number of apneas and the apnea time as a percentage of sleep time. Five patients then used oxygen at home for 39–90 days. Three had a decrease in percentage apnea time of over 60%. One patient had an increase in apnea time, and one had minimal improvement; both of these results reflect the earlier observations of the acute study. In another daytime sleep study, the effects of room air and oxygen were compared in 11 COPD patients (Kearley et al., 1980). Oxygen therapy was associated with reduced number of episodes of desaturation per hour and time spent in desaturation, with no change in the number or duration of DBEs. Fletcher and Levin (1984) studied the effects of an eight-week course of low flow oxygen on COPD patients with daytime hypoxemia and episodes of desaturation during REM sleep. In the six patients who completed the study, the mean sleeping pulmonary arterial pressure declined; in four of these patients, the total pulmonary resistance was lower and the cardiac output was higher.

Low flow oxygen administration, then, has had mixed results, and in one case, the unhappy consequence of prolonging the duration of apneas has been raised. One question that still needs to be answered is whether oxygen administration differentially affects episodes in non-REM and REM sleep, insofar as the respiratory regulatory mechanisms may differ. More positively, Martin *et al.* (1982) and others have suggested that episodes of oxygen desaturation during sleep might themselves have a central ventilatory effect that, in turn, increases the number of apneas. If this is so, then one might expect that low flow oxygen, by minimizing the desaturation, would help prevent this snowball effect.

Continuous Positive Air Pressure

The use of continuous positive air pressure (CPAP), applied by a mask at pressures of about 5–15 cm H_2O (Figs. 6-5, 6-7), has been described in case reports and patient groups (Sullivan *et al.*, 1981; Garay, Turino, and Goldring, 1981; Sullivan *et al.*, 1984; Rapoport *et al.*, 1982; Sullivan, Berthon-Jones, and Issa, 1983; Rapoport, Garay, and Goldring, 1983; Berry and Block, 1984; Sanders, Moore, and Eveslage,

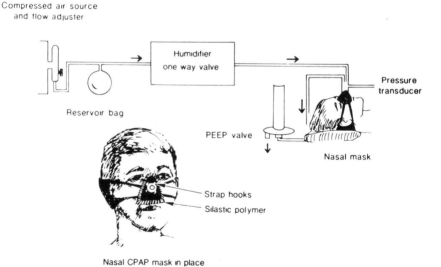

FIGURE 6-5. Nasal CPAP apparatus and the nasal mask. (From Berry and Block, 1984. Reprinted by permission.)

1983; Issa and Sullivan, 1984; McEvoy and Thornton, 1984; Rajagopal *et al.*, 1986). With one exception (Wagner, Pollak, and Weitzman, 1983), these reports have been relatively favorable, both in terms of use acutely in the hospital and at home. Representative of this work is the study of McEvoy and Thornton (1984), which is particularly interesting because there were no selection criteria for patients. In an acute study of 12 of 13 consecutively diagnosed patients with obstructive sleep apnea, each nighttime recording was divided into a control and a CPAP portion. The CPAP was found to decrease the apnea rate as well as to improve arterial oxygen saturation (Fig. 6-6). In three patients with lung disease and elevated Pa_{CO_2}, the hypoxemia persisted, however. Eleven patients used CPAP at home for 1–18 months. All reported less daytime sleepiness. At follow-up, there was a decrease in apnea rate (per hour), although there was no change in the total number of apneas and hypopneas per hour or in oxygen saturation.

Initial short-term studies on CPAP have been promising. Further work documenting changes in daytime functioning, as well as assessment of acceptability to the patient, will continue to characterize its utility.

The relative contraindications for CPAP include presence of fixed lesions of the upper airway, significant COPD, bullous emphysema, and significant congestive heart failure. In general, the negative aspects of use of CPAP include the inconvenience, the sound produced by the apparatus, and nasal stuffiness. In the McEvoy and Thornton (1984) study, only one patient discontinued treatment because of discomfort. In another case series, 87% of the patients tolerated CPAP in the laboratory, but only 75% actually began a trial at home. Long-term compliance was also of some concern; after 18 months, only 40% were still using home CPAP (Schweitzer *et al.*, 1987).

The mechanism by which CPAP produces benefits remains to be elucidated. Among the possibilities are (1) reduced airway resistance because airway collapse is prevented during sleep; (2) reduced resistance as the result of the dilation of the airway beyond its dimensions in the waking state; and (3) stimulation of mechanoreceptors leading to an increase in airway tone (Rapoport, Garay, and Goldring, 1983).

Uvulopalatopharyngoplasty (UPPP)

Following observations by Ikematsu (1964) that many persons who snore have narrow pharyngeal dimensions which could be corrected surgically, Fujita, Conway, and Zorick (1981) demonstrated the useful-

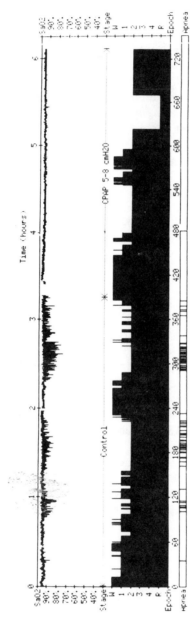

FIGURE 6-6. Typical sleep record of an obstructive sleep apnea syndrome patient treated with CPAP. Upper part of panel depicts oxyhemoglobin saturation (SaO2) measured by an ear oximeter, below which is the sleep state. Below this is a record of apneas; each vertical line represents an apneic event. Nasal CPAP (second part of study) resulted in an obvious improvement in SaO2, decrease in apnea frequency, and less disruption of sleep, compared with the control period. (From McEvoy and Thornton, 1984. Reprinted by permission.)

ness of the UPPP in some sleep apnea patients. Fundamentally, the procedure involves removal of redundant tissue from the lateral pharynx, uvula, and palate (Fig. 6-8). Typical of the case series that have emerged from the subsequent use of this procedure is that of Simmons, Guilleminault, and Silvestri (1983). Of 20 obstructive sleep apnea patients, nine were considered to have completely successful results (defined as oxygen desaturation to no more than 85% of normal or an improvement of 50%). Twelve reported virtually complete disappearance of snoring and daytime sleepiness; an additional five had no more snoring, but retained some subjective sleepiness. A detailed statistical analysis of polysomnograms was done on 14 patients. Although the number of arterial desaturations that fell below 80% was significantly reduced, both the number of apneas per hour and the degree of lowest desaturation were not altered. In a series of 13 surgical patients, Schoen *et al.* (1984) found that 77% had at least a 50% improvement in apnea index. Oxygen desaturation improved by approxi-

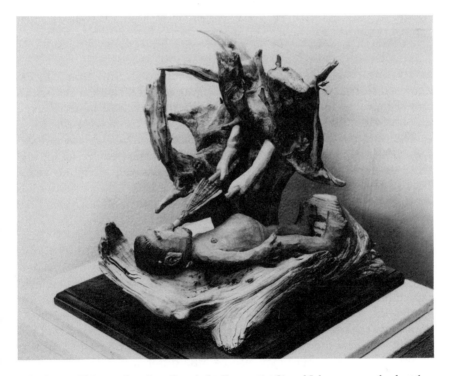

FIGURE 6-7. This woodcarving, *Genesis*, by Texas artist Sigurd Johnson may also be taken to express some aspects of CPAP treatment. (Reproduced by permission of Mr. Johnson.)

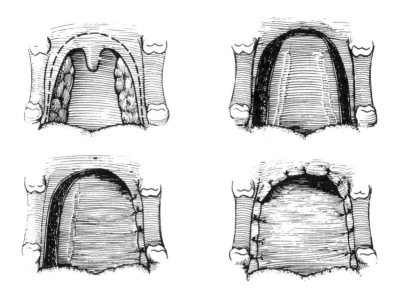

FIGURE 6-8. Procedure for UPPP. (From Simmons, Guileminault, and Silvestri, 1983. Reprinted by permission.)

mately one-third, overall. Reimao *et al.* (1986) found that UPPPs decreased apnea indices in all ten patients studied, with a return to normal levels in five. Before surgery, nine patients had minimal oxygen saturations of less than 80%; afterward, only three were this low.

The duration of benefits of UPPP is still under investigation. Zorick *et al.* (1984b) found that 33 patients who were helped by UPPP six weeks postoperatively tended to continue to do well after one year. Thorpy, Sher, and Spielman (1984a,b) followed four patients, two of whom deteriorated to a preoperative degree of apnea after a year. The two who did well had also lost the most weight.

In summary, the UPPP is a highly successful procedure for the complaint of snoring, and at present benefits perhaps 50 to 70% of sleep apnea patients. In assessing these results, one needs to consider both the polysomnographic data and the patients' impression, which may differ. Criteria for patient selection are uncertain. It is also not clear at this time whether the appearance of a "crowded pharynx" should favor surgery. Simmons *et al.* (1983), for instance, could find no relation between the appearance of the palate and pharynx and the success of surgery. There may also be little difference in the degree of severity of the syndrome and the outcome of surgery (Katsantonis *et al.*, 1985). The same study found no relationship between the surgically induced increase in cross-sectional area of the oropharynx and clinical outcome. Gereau *et al.* (1986) reported that a positive Muller maneuver (closure of the upper airway at the level of the soft palate) preoperatively will select patients with more likelihood to benefit from UPPP. In their series of 46 cases, 85% had a reduction in apneas per hour of at least 50%. One interesting possibility for the future is that opening pressures determined by a preoperative CPAP procedure might predict UPPP outcome. Another promising approach may be fluoroscopic examination during sleep, or somnofluoroscopy (Katsantonis *et al.*, 1985). Contraindications are also unclear, although many surgeons feel that extreme obesity is among them.

The UPPP may have a number of untoward effects such as nasal regurgitation of liquids and altered speech. A certain number of patients also require at least a temporary tracheostomy at the same time. This occurred in 20% (Simmons *et al.*, 1983), 61% (Gereau *et al.*, 1986), and 77% (Katsantonis *et al.*, 1985) in various case series. In practice, a patient often keeps the tracheostomy for a few weeks; a polysomnogram is then performed with it closed and a decision regarding its removal is made. Other procedures are also being examined. These include mandibular osteotomy and sectioning of the hyoid bone (Kaya, 1984).

Tracheostomy

Tracheostomy is in some sense the definitive, albeit very major, procedure for obstructive sleep apnea. In a long-term follow-up of 50 patients treated with tracheostomy, 45 considered themselves to be 100% improved in terms of daytime sleepiness and fatigue (Guilleminault *et al.*, 1981). At a follow-up recording with the tracheostomy tube open, all patients had apnea indexes under five, compared to values over 65 before surgery. When the tube was occluded, the apneas recurred in all patients in whom this was done. Among eight patients in whom hemodynamic studies were done, the mean pulmonary and femoral arterial pressures decreased.

There are a number of difficulties which can occur in the postsurgical period after a UPPP. Local infections occurred in 42% of the patients during the first six months in the Guilleminault *et al.* (1981) series. Inaccurately fitted tubes may cause dyspnea when the head is turned. Depressive symptoms are frequent, and counseling, as well as visits with similarly treated patients, may be indicated. Paradoxically, the increased wakefulness itself may be a problem. Patients often may have settled into low-key jobs as well as family relationships in which they are relatively inactive. Sometimes both professional and personal difficulties have developed because of the appearance of new energy and wakefulness in these unhappy but stable situations.

Although results of tracheostomy are usually very favorable, some authors have commented that not all postsurgery apnea patients become eucapneic (Garay et al., 1983). Rapoport et al. (1986) described eight patients with the Pickwickian syndrome and sleep apnea, of whom seven underwent surgery, and one CPAP treatment. Hypersomnolence and snoring were greatly diminished in all these patients. Four patients returned to eucapnea, whereas four remained hypercapneic. It is possible that the latter four patients, who might have been the true "Pickwickians," suffered not only from sleep apnea but also from a primary dysfunction that resulted in hypoventilation whether they were awake or asleep.

Central Sleep Apnea

Pharmacological Approaches

The section on treatment of central sleep apnea in any current article is likely to be rather short, since there are relatively few treatments available. Empirically, these patients are often given protriptyline although there are relatively little systematic data on their use in this situation. There is some tentative evidence that the carbonic anhydrase inhibitor acetazolamide may be of benefit. In an uncontrolled study of six central apnea patients, one week of acetazolamide (250 mg qid) decreased apnea-associated awakenings, and the apnea index dropped from 6.0 to 0.9/hr (White et al., 1982). There was some improvement in oxygen saturation and the subjective impression of daytime wakefulness. Results after one year, however, were mixed. Acetazolamide has not been found to protect elderly subjects whose apneas had been made worse by flurazepam (Guilleminault et al., 1984).

Diaphragm Pacing

Diaphragm pacing has been effectively used in some central apnea patients, although at present it is available at relatively few medical centers. The phrenic nerve is electrically stimulated along its descending path in the lower neck. Usually only one side at a time is stimulated, so that respiration is induced by a maximal contraction of the hemidiaphragm. Glenn, Phelps, and Gersten (1978) described their experience with this treatment for 29 patients with central alveolar hypoventilation (Ondine's curse). Treatment lasted 8 to 12 hr/day, for an average of 36 months. During this period, there were seven deaths: five the result of the primary illness, one the result of pacemaker failure, and one related to sedation. Sleep studies carried out in 27 of the patients found that 15 also had obstructive components as well, and most of these required tracheostomy. A registry of central alveolar hypoventilation patients indicates that some have been maintained for 10 years by diaphragm pacing (Hambrecht, 1980).

There is some possibility that occasionally the relatively rapid rise of negative pressures from a maximal contraction of the hemidiaphragm may collapse the pharyngeal musculature, to produce obstruction. In one case report, a patient placed on diaphragm pacing developed both paradoxical rib cage movements and upper airway obstruction during sleep (Hyland et al., 1981). A tracheostomy corrected the obstruction, but the paradoxical rib cage movement persisted. The obstruction was presumably the result of the diaphragmatic contraction being out of phase with the normal reflex that tends to maintain patency of the upper airway during inspiration; this emhasizes the importance of the coordination of these diverse muscle groups. It has also been suggested that the upper airway obstruction and paradoxical rib cage movement sometimes seen during diaphragm pacing may be related to afferent stimulation of the phrenic nerve (Trenchard and Meanock, 1982). In this particular study, pacing may have induced obstruction in three patients. Studies of the effects of pacing on nerve and diaphragm tissue continue to be performed (Kim et al., 1983), and the process appears to be relatively benign from that point of view. Experience with quadraplegics suggests that continuous low-frequency stimulation of both hemidiaphragms may be effective and that strength and endurance of diaphragm muscle may even improve (Glenn et al., 1984). Another intriguing possibility is that "closed loop" systems may be developed in which information on Pa_{O_2} or Pa_{CO_2} would be fed back to the system regulating the stimulator (Hambrecht, 1980).

Continuous Positive Air Pressure

Continuous positive air pressure has traditionally been regarded as a treatment for obstructive sleep apnea syndrome. In view of the possibility that both central and obstructive apneas might have common origins, Issa and Sullivan (1986) gave CPAP to eight predominantly central apnea patients, with substantial benefit. On the other hand, no improvement with CPAP was noted by Schweitzer et al. (1987) in five patients with mixed or antral apneas. Clearly, further studies are needed to elucidate this issue.

Adjunctive Treatment and Precautions

In addition to the treatments we have just reviewed, a number of other maneuvers may be of limited additional benefit.

Weight Loss

The upper airway is, of course, subject to changes in radius secondary to fat deposits. Since the area of a circle is proportional to the square of the radius, a relatively small change in radius has a disproportionally large effect on the cross-sectional area through which air may flow. Anecdotal reports of improvement with weight loss (Remmers, de Groot, and Sauaerland, 1976; Coccagna *et al.*, 1972) suggested that this might indeed be a useful practice. Guilleminault *et al.* (1978) examined the effects of weight loss on primary obstructive apnea patients and found differing benefits, depending on when the apneas tended to occur. Patients with intermittent apneas in both non-REM and REM sleep lost 20 to 45 kg and reduced both the apnea index (from 32 to 14) and their subjective sleepiness. Those whose apneas tended to occur in REM sleep lost over 30 kg, with no subjective improvement. The effects of weight loss were also examined in 50 patients who had received chronic tracheostomies for obstructive sleep apnea (Guilleminault *et al.*, 1981). Although a mean weight loss of 15 kg (range, 4–100 kg) occurred, it was not possible to close any tracheostomy. Harman, Wynne, and Block (1981) examined the effects of weight loss on four morbidly obese men, approximately two years after obesity bypass surgery. The mean weights before surgery and at follow-up were 213 and 123 kg, respectively. The number of apnea and hypopneas per hour before surgery was 78; it had declined to 1.4 at follow-up. In the two patients who were symptomatic (snoring, somnolence, elevated daytime Pa_{CO_2}), there was a dramatic improvement in minimal oxygen saturation. In summary, weight loss may benefit some patients, and indeed should be recommended. It is, however, often not sufficient by itself and should be considered an adjunctive treatment.

Sleep Position

Common experience suggests that snoring is greatest when a person sleeps on his or her back. There is some evidence that this holds true for obstructive apneas as well. Issa and Sullivan (1984) have shown that in apnea patients less negative inspiratory pressure is required to collapse the airway in the supine, as compared to the lateral, position. Cartright (1984) demonstrated a decline in the rate of DBEs during those times of the night when obstructive apnea patients slept on their sides compared to their backs; some actually entered the normal range at this time. Patients who were more obese had relatively little difference in rate of DBEs in the two positions. Chaudhary et al. (1986) similarly found marked improvement in apnea indices in four obstructive sleep apnea patients while they were sleeping on their sides. It may be of benefit, then, to encourage patients to sleep on their sides.

Avoid Drugs Which Are Respiratory Suppressants

A very important aspect of preventive care in these patients is to avoid drugs which are respiratory suppressants. These include many anxiolytics, hypnotics, and major analgesics. It has been observed that some hypnotics increase snoring (Lugaresi, Coccagna, and Cirignotta, 1978). Many of the older hypnotics, such as barbiturates, suppress respiration. The possible effects of long-acting benzodiazepines on sleep-related respiration have only been reported recently and will be reviewed here in more detail.

Benzodiazepines. There is no shortage of data documenting respiratory suppression by long-acting benzodiazepines in pulmonary patients in the waking state. Geddes, Rudolf, and Saunders (1976), for example, reported that flurazepam (15 mg) reduced ventilatory response to CO_2 in both normal subjects and chronic bronchitis patients. Nitrazepam (10 mg) may increase Pa_{CO_2} and decrease the respiratory response to CO_2 in chronic bronchitis patients (Rudolf et al., 1978). Model and Berry (1974) found that chlordiazepoxide (10 mg tid) increased mixed venous CO_2 tension and decreased 1-sec, forced expiratory volume in six out of seven chronic bronchitis patients. Model (1973) also described two COPD patients in whom 10 mg of nitrazepam induced CO_2 retention.

The effects of benzodiazepines on respiration during sleep have been examined in several studies (Table 6-1). Mendelson et al. (1981) have described a 38-year-old chronic insomniac who had 7 to 18 apneas a night under baseline conditions. When given 30 mg of flurazepam, he had 22 and 100 apneas on the first and second drug nights, respectively, and developed daytime sleepiness (Fig. 3-2). Upon drug withdrawal, the number of apneas returned to baseline levels. Two studies of asymptomatic adults indicated that 30 mg of flurazepam suppresses

TABLE 6-1. Effects of Benzodiazepines on Sleep-Related Respiration

References	Subjects (N)	Drug (dose)	Duration (nights)	Results
Mendelson et al., 1981	Insomniac with 7–18 apneas (1)	Flurazepam (30 mg)	2	Increase in DBEs (22–100); onset of sleepiness
Dolly and Block, 1982	Asymptomatic adults (20)	Flurazepam (30 mg)	1	Increase in DBEs, total duration of apnea, and degree of desaturation
Cummiskey et al., 1983	COPD patients (5)	Flurazepam (15 mg)	7	No significant change during sleep
Hedemark and Kronenberg, 1983	Normal adults (8)	Flurazepam (30 mg)	1	No change in ventilatory response to hypoxia or hypercapnea; decreased arousal as the result of hypercapnea
Carskadon et al., 1982	Elderly insomniacs (13)	Triazolam (0.25 mg); flurazepam (15 mg)	3	No change in respiratory variables in subjects (prescreened to rule out the sleep apnea syndrome)
Block, Dolly, and Slayton, 1984	COPD patients (20) without CO_2 retention, on theophylline	Flurazepam (30 mg)	1	Increase in frequency of DBEs and frequency, duration, and severity of episodes of desaturation
Guilleminault et al., 1984	Healthy elderly adults (10)	Flurazepam (30 mg)	1	Baseline apnea with an index of 5–7 had an increase in number and duration of apneas and decreased oxygen saturation

respiration during sleep. Dolly and Block (1982), in a study of 20 volunteers, found an increase in the number and duration of apneas and the degree of desaturation. Block, Dolly, and Slayton (1984) examined the effects of a single dose of 30 mg of flurazepam on 20 COPD patients without CO_2 retention, 18 of whom were also taking the respiratory stimulant theophylline. Flurazepam increased the frequency of sleep-related DBEs and the duration and severity of episodes of desaturation (defined as change in saturation greater than 4%). These changes were relatively small in magnitude, and major decreases in saturation were observed in only three subjects. These data should be considered very cautiously, however, insofar as the drug was given for only one night (major effects appeared only on the second night in the report by Mendelson et al., 1981a), and the patients were also receiving a respiratory stimulant. Hedemark and Kronenberg (1983), in a study of normal adults, reported no change in the ventilatory response to hypoxia or to hypercapnea, but found that the number of arousals to hypercapnea tended to decrease after 30 mg of flurazepam. Guilleminault et al. (1984) found that one night of 30 mg of flurazepam increased the mean number of apneas and decreased oxygen saturation in 10 elderly volunteers. On the other hand, studies of 15 mg flurazepam given to COPD patients (Cummisky et al., 1983) and elderly insomniacs prescreened to rule out apnea (Carskadon et al., 1982) did not find major respiratory effects. The possibility remains, then, that 30 mg flurazepam and, by implication, other long-acting benzodiazepine hypnotics, might further jeopardize the respiratory status of sleep apnea patients. Until guidelines are developed, it seems wise for sleep apnea patients to avoid their use.

Alcohol. There have been some differences in results on the effects of alcohol on sleep-related respiration in normal subjects. Taasan et al. (1981) reported that 2 ml/kg increased the number of apneic events and episodes of oxygen desaturation in asymptomatic subjects who were not prescreened by polysomnography. Scrima et al. (1982) studied six healthy snorkel divers who were, on average, 21 years younger than those in the Taasan et al. (1981) study and who were screened by polysomnography to rule out sleep disorders. They found little effect, after 0.8 g/kg. They did, however, report that 3 oz of 80-proof alcohol increased the incidence and severity of hypoxic events in obstructive sleep apnea patients (Fig. 6-9). Guilleminault et al. (1984) found that 0.6 g/kg of alcohol increased apneas in healthy elderly subjects who had baseline apnea indices of 5 to 7. Such data underscore the importance of cautioning these patients not to drink.

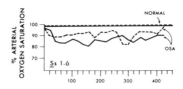

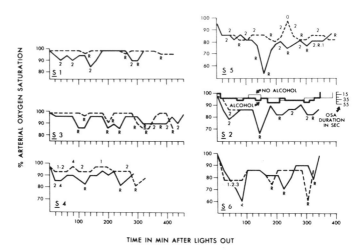

TIME IN MIN AFTER LIGHTS OUT

FIGURE 6-9. Percent lowest arterial oxygen saturation reached during 20-min intervals of sleep with (————) and without (– – –) alcohol. Left, mean arterial oxygen saturation values for obstructive apnea patients and healthy subjects. Note that the alcohol had no effect on the arterial oxygen saturation of healthy subjects. Below, means for each subject. For subject 2, the arterial oxygen saturation was recorded for only 60 min; therefore, apnea durations are also depicted for the no-alcohol (————) and alcohol (————) nights. Note the earlier occurrences of lower levels of arterial oxygen saturation on the alcohol night compared with the no-alcohol night in all subjects (paired t, $p < 0.01$). (From Scrima *et al.*, 1982. Reprinted by permission.)

Anesthesia

Since it appears likely that sleep apnea patients may be very sensitive to anesthesia, caution should be observed if surgery of any kind is required (Samuels and Rabinov, 1986). An additional complication is that these individuals often have short, thick necks, which may make intubation extremely difficult. Hill, Guilleminault, and Simmons (1978) mention that early in their studies the anesthesiologist involved in the tracheostomy surgery was unable to intubate two patients and emergency procedures had to be initiated.

Precautions Regarding Sleepiness

Obviously, those individuals who experience hypersomnolence should be cautioned with regard to driving. There are two related issues here. The first is that the degree of sleepiness varies greatly among these patients, from pathological hypersomnolence to virtually normal wakefulness. The second is that this author's impression is that these patients are very poor judges of their own degree of wakefulness. It is a common experience for a patient to believe that he is not impaired and then to find a sleep latency on the MSLT that indicates a major degree of sleepiness. One should determine the degree of impairment (and, hence, the appropriate precautions to be taken), based on objective measures of sleepiness from the MSLT.

QUESTIONS FOR THE FUTURE

It should be apparent that although we have some basic understanding of sleep apnea syndromes, many important questions remain unanswered. In terms of pathophysiology, one major issue will be the determination of the probably neural aspects of what we functionally describe as obstructive sleep apnea. It is clear that the respiratory cycle involves the coordination of a complex movement pattern of the diaphragm, chest wall, tongue, and pharyngeal musculature and that their relative activities vary with the state of consciousness. It is not hard to imagine how a deficit in organization of their behavior might lead to a functional obstruction. Insofar as many individuals with sleep apnea have apparent physical qualities that result in a smaller airway, sleep apnea then becomes a disorder resulting from the interaction of altered physiology with anatomical vulnerability. Other influences on respiration will also undoubtedly come to light. There is even evidence that the act of closing the eyes affects the respiratory rate.

Certainly, one intriguing aspect of sleep apnea is why it is often accompanied by personality changes and alterations in mood. Impotence is often a clinical complaint. As we have mentioned, there is growing evidence of an association between chronic pulmonary disease and sexual difficulty, but this does not appear to be the result of generally recognized endocrine causes, such as an androgen deficit. Whether impotence is somehow secondary to repeated hypoxic episodes remains to be determined. The genesis of sleepiness in sleep apnea and hypoventilation syndromes is also poorly understood. Many persons caring for these patients are struck with the degree of variation—some patients with relatively few DBEs may complain of sleepiness that seems disproportionate to the disorder, whereas other patients with a large number of DBEs seem relatively alert. Although there is some reported relationship to the degree of desaturation, this issue is poorly understood. Lugaresi et al. (1982) have reported elevated levels of homovanillic acid and 5-hydroxyindoleacetic acid in the cerebrospinal fluid, which declined after tracheostomy, in two apnea patients. In principle a central change in biogenic amine levels could produce sleepiness and alter respiration.

In terms of treatment, the mechanism of action of protriptyline remains uncertain. Originally, it was thought that this was largely secondary to REM sleep suppression, but further studies have indicated that its (limited) benefits occur when its effect on sleep stage is held constant. Hopefully, the future will see the development of new pharmacological treatments. Perhaps the study of receptors for benzodiazepines and other sedatives (see Chapter 4) may lead to the development of "inverse agonists" with both analeptic and respiratory stimulant qualities. Nonpharmacological therapies may also be developed. There is some evidence that respiration during sleep may be affected by conditioning techniques. In principle, respiration may be more easily altered than other motor behaviors in sleep because of the relative sparing of the diaphragm from the hypotonia of REM sleep (Badia et al., 1984). It seems likely that the next few years will see new and intriguing developments in some of these areas.

SUMMARY

During sleep there are a number of changes in respiration, including alterations in airway resistance, action of the diaphragm, intercostals, and pharyngeal musculature, and responsiveness to hypoxia and hypercapnea. Sleep apnea syndromes, relatively common disorders that are manifested as insomnia or excessive daytime sleepiness, are best understood in the context of these physiological changes. Complications include pulmonary and systematic hypertension, cor pulmonale, and impotence. Psychological manifestations may include difficulty concentrating, personality changes, and anxiety and depression. Cognitive deficits appear on neuropsychological testing. Sleep apnea occurs at all ages; the obstructive form is more common in males and during middle age, while the central form tends to occur in older persons. A growing body of evidence points to neurological aspects of the obstructive process, and it is possible that the apparently different forms have some common physiological origins. A range of treatment is available, including pharmacotherapy, low flow oxygen, CPAP, and surgical procedures. In addition, such adjunctive measures as weight loss and consideration of body position are important. Patients should be cautioned not to take alcohol or sedative–hypnotics, which greatly exacerbate respiratory difficulties.

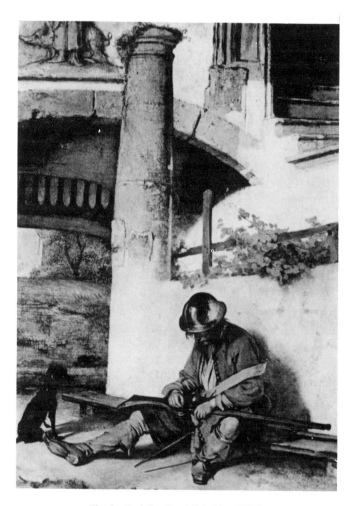

The Sentinel, by Carel Fabritius (1654).

CHAPTER 7

Narcolepsy and Disorders of Excessive Sleepiness

> Sleep may be produced by excessive direct or indirect debility; but such sleep is not salutary or refreshing, but what is termed morbid.
>
> —Thomas Ball, 1796

Narcolepsy is often considered to be an illness of excessive sleep; more precisely, it is a disorder manifested by brief, inappropriate episodes of sleep, in association with other "auxiliary" symptoms. Sleep attacks have been described by a number of nineteenth-century physicians, among whom the best known is Westphal (1877). Gelineau, in 1880, gave the name narcolepsy to a disturbance "characterized by an imperative need to sleep of sudden onset and short duration, recurring at more or less close intervals." As Zarcone (1973) points out, characters with symptoms suggestive of narcolepsy have appeared in many famous works of fiction, including Eliot's *Silas Marner*, Poe's "The Premature Burial," and Melville's *Moby Dick*.

DEFINITION

Yoss and Daly (1957, 1960a,b) considered narcolepsy to be comprised of a primary symptom—inappropriate attacks of sleep—to which may be added three auxiliary symptoms: cataplexy, hypnogogic hallucinations, and sleep paralysis. Other features, including disturbed nocturnal sleep and episodes of automatic behavior, have been emphasized by some authors. The clinical manifestations of each of these symptoms will be described in turn.

Excessive Daytime Sleepiness and Sleep Attacks

Patients with narcolepsy complain of chronic sleepiness, which is well documented in studies of daylong EEG and videotape recording (see, for example, Volk et al., 1984). They often describe irresistible "sleep attacks," brief episodes (often 15 min or less) of sleep that occur at any time of day. Some patients recognize that such an attack is imminent; others describe them as happening without warning. These episodes tend to occur during times of boredom or after meals, but they can also appear when least expected: during sexual intercourse, while engaged in a sports event, and so on. After these brief episodes of sleep, the patient may awaken completely refreshed. In many patients, there seems to be a refractory period of one to several hours before the next attack.

Cataplexy

This is a sudden loss of tone in the major striated muscles of the body, which may last from perhaps 30 sec to several minutes. Loss of muscle tone may be only partial, resulting in "buckling" of the knees or sagging of the head, or it may be more generalized, resulting in complete collapse. During these episodes, the patient remains conscious. Interestingly enough, the extraocular muscles are not affected; a patient experiencing a cataplectic attack can roll his eyes on command. When episodes last longer than 1 min, hallucinatory experiences may occur (Van den Hoed, Lucas, and Dement, 1979). Cataplexy (like sleep attacks) can result in injury to the patient. In contrast to sleep attacks, cataplectic episodes typically occur at moments of increased emotion. Thus, patients may report having a cataplectic attack in response to getting angry at a naughty child, hearing a funny joke, seeing a particularly exciting scene in a movie, and so on. It has been speculated that cataplectic episodes are triggered by changes in blood pressure or heart rate, which will be discussed in the section on propranolol. Cataplexy, incidentally, should be distinguished from catalepsy, the waxy rigidity of muscles as seen in catatonic schizophrenia.

Sleep Paralysis

These are episodes of paralysis of the striated musculature occurring in the transition period between wakefulness and sleep. The patient is fully conscious and may experience extreme anxiety or fear. Sleep paralysis at the onset of a nap was well described by a patient of Edward Binns, a physician writing in the 1850s, about what he termed "day-mares":

> During the intensely hot summer of 1825, I experienced an attack of this affection. Immediately after dining, I threw myself on my back upon a sofa, and, before I was aware, was seized with difficult respiration, extreme dread, and utter incapability of motion or speech. I could neither move nor cry, while the breath came from my chest in broken and suffocating paroxysms. During all this time I was perfectly awake; I saw the light glaring in at the windows in broad sultry streams; I felt the intense heat of the day pervading my frame; and heard distinctly the different noises in the street, and even the ticking of my own watch, which I had placed on the cushion beside me; I had, at the same time, the consciousness of flies buzzing around, and settling with annoying pertinacity on my face. During the whole fit, judgment was never for a moment suspended. I felt assured that I labored under incubus. I even endeavored to reason myself out of the feeling of dread which filled my mind, and longed, with insufferable ardour, for some one to open the door, and dissolve the spell which bound me in its fetters. The fit did not continue above five minutes: by degrees I recovered the use of sense and motion; and, as soon as they were so far restored as to enable me to call out and move my limbs, it wore insensibly away.

Episodes of sleep paralysis are often accompanied by hypnogogic hallucinations. A common experience is to perceive a frightening object or a person sitting on one's chest. Schenck (1969) has commented that this experience may be the basis of Henry Fuseli's famous painting, *The Nightmare*, in which such a situation takes place (Fig. 7-1). The woman pictured appears to be terrified by a demonic figure that is crouching on her chest, but she is unable to move.

Episodes of sleep paralysis usually last only a few seconds, but they can last up to 20 min. In contrast to cataplexy, the subject can be easily released from this state by calling his name or touching him. In addition to being part of the narcoleptic tetrad, sleep paralysis has been described as an isolated, benign experience occurring from time to time in nonnarcoleptics (Schenck, 1969; Penn, Kripke, and Scharff, 1981). Hufford (1982) found it in 23% of a college population in Newfoundland, where it is known as a visitation from the "Old Hag," the terror that comes in the night. Bell, Dixie-Bell, and Thompson (1986) found sleep paralysis to occur at least once a month in 27.3% of a black population in Chicago; about 15% of subjects with frequent episodes were noted to have panic disorder as well. These episodes were sometimes known as "the witch riding you."

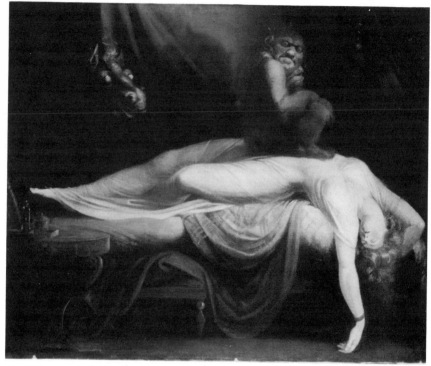

FIGURE 7-1. *The Nightmare*, Henri Fuseli (1741–1825). Courtesy of the Detroit Institute of Arts.

Hypnogogic and Hypnopompic Hallucinations

These episodes of auditory, visual, or tactile hallucinations occur during the transition between wakefulness and sleep. When these occur at sleep onset they are known as hypnogogic hallucinations; those that occur upon awakening in the morning are known as hypnopompic hallucinations. The general clinical impression is that hypnogogic and hypnopompic hallucinations carry more emotional impact and have more of a storylike quality than the relatively bland images that are often experienced by nonnarcoleptics. These hallucinations can be extremely frightening to the patient. In the unusual 5% of cases in which this is the dominant symptom, the patient may be mistakenly diagnosed as schizophrenic.

Disordered Nocturnal Sleep

Almost paradoxically, those patients who complain of excessive sleepiness during the day have very disturbed sleep at night (Rechtschaffen *et al.*, 1963). This is manifested polygraphically as an increase in the number of awakenings, wake time after sleep onset, and time in stage 1 sleep (Montplaisir and Godbout, 1986a). Narcoleptics may have more and longer awakenings than other patients with excessive sleepiness, but the distribution between REM and non-REM is similar (Zorick *et al.*, 1986). This has been taken to imply that narcolepsy involves a disorder of maintaining all the stages of sleep, as opposed to a selective disorder of REM sleep. Disturbed sleep has also been reported in animal models of narcolepsy (Kaitin, Kilduff, and Dement, 1986).

Automatic Behavior

Although not included in the original descriptions of narcolepsy, a number of patients exhibit episodes of automatic behavior—stereotyped repetitive actions that apparently occur without awareness. In a case cited by Zorick *et al.* (1979), the patient committed acts of shoplifting; although this is more dramatic than most, the common theme is behaviors in which poor judgment is shown. It is a good reminder that in cases of apparent automatic behavior the differential diagnosis should include narcolepsy.

Symptoms of narcolepsy may start at different times and occur in various combinations (Fig. 7-2). Perhaps the most typical pattern is the onset of sleep attacks, with other symptoms developing over the next few years. Although virtually 100% of narcoleptic patients have sleep attacks (by definition), only 10% have the complete tetrad. The most common auxiliary symptom is cataplexy, which occurs in combination with sleep attacks and other symptoms in perhaps 70% of patients. Hypnogogic hallucinations and sleep paralysis occur in combination with sleep attacks and other symptoms in 25% and 30% of patients, respectively (Sours, 1963; Yoss and Daly, 1957, 1960a; Bowling and Richards, 1961).

PSYCHOSOCIAL CONSEQUENCES

A number of studies have documented the profound effects of narcolepsy on a person's life. Broughton *et al.* (1981, 1983), comparing 60

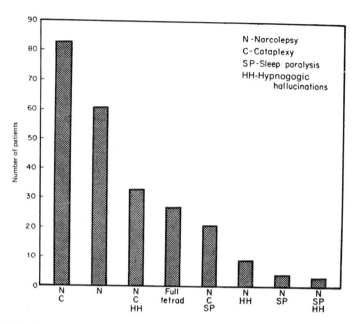

FIGURE 7-2. Frequency of various symptom combinations in the narcoleptic tetrad in 241 patients. (From Yoss and Daly, 1957. Reprinted by permission.)

patients each from North America, Asia, and Europe with matched controls, found that over 75% of patients had occupational problems because of the illness. They fell asleep at the wheel more often (66%) and had actual or near auto accidents more frequently (67%). Similarly, accidents in the home as the result of sleepiness (49%) or of sleepiness while smoking (49%) were more common. Interestingly, the differences in life effects in different cultures were relatively minor. Age, gender, or duration of illness had little effect on the prominence of life effects of narcolepsy. This may suggest that once the symptoms are established, there are major consequences in a person's life, which remain with little change. Patients with narcolepsy have also been compared to those with epilepsy without major organic pathology (Broughton, Guberman, and Roberts, 1984). Although both groups obviously had difficulties in many areas, the narcoleptics had higher frequencies of illness-related problems at work, poorer driving records, higher accident rates from smoking, and greater difficulty in planning recreation. The only areas in which epileptics had greater difficulties were in educational achievement and keeping a driver's license. Krishnan *et al.* (1984) found that about two-thirds of narcoleptic patients had psychiatric disorders meeting DSM-III criteria, including adjustment disorders, depression, alcohol dependence, and personality disorders but not psychotic disorders. Not surprisingly, psychopathology was more common in patients with both sleepiness and cataplexy than in those without cataplexy. Kales *et al.* (1982a) emphasized the difficulties such patients had in family life and interpersonal relations. They found that their patients were overly concerned with emotional control, which tended to lead to lack of expressiveness. This may be the basis for a report of difficulty achieving orgasm in narcoleptic women (Roy, 1977). From a behavioral point of view, it is understandable that the negative experience of a cataplectic episode after expressing emotion could lead to the avoidance of emotional situations. This implies that an important strategy in dealing with patients is to emphasize that feelings should be expressed before they reach intense levels.

PERFORMANCE DEFICITS

A number of studies have assessed the effects of narcolepsy on various measures of daytime performance. Narcoleptics have been found to do poorly on the Wilkinson auditory vigilance task and the four-choice serial reaction time (Valley and Broughton, 1981). Subjective measures of sleepiness were greater in narcoleptics, but there was no good correlation between perceived sleepiness and performance. During the auditory vigilance task, EEGs indicated that narcoleptics were more likely to show theta activity or actually enter stage 2 sleep (Valley and Broughton, 1983). Although performance deteriorated during those times, they also had poorer scores during wakefulness. This calls into question the common notion that their difficulties are the result of brief periods of microsleep. Auditory evoked-potential studies during the vigilance task also showed changes similar to those seen in drowsiness in normal subjects, even when performance was normal and visual evaluation of the EEG showed wakefulness (Broughton *et al.*, 1982). Narcoleptics have been found to have lower values on the critical flicker fusion test but not on the continuous vernier visual acuity test (Levander and Sachs, 1985). Their skin conductance was lower, although there were no differences in spontaneous fluctuations or in heart rate. Stimulants improved the critical flicker fusion results; they did not alter the basal skin conductance but did decrease the spontaneous fluctuations seen during monotonous tasks. The authors speculated that narcoleptics have a deficit in time resolution of stimulus input which is not related to lower arousal, but which is correctable by

stimulants. In studies of the choice reaction time task, there was either
no change in (Levander and Sachs, 1985) or decreased performance
(Godbout and Montplaisir, 1986). Narcoleptics also often complain of
memory impairment. A study of formal memory tests found no difference from normal subjects, during short testing sessions (Aguirre,
Broughton, and Stuss, 1985). This suggests that they do not have an
actual organic memory deficit, although they are distressed by subjective sleepiness during testing sessions. In summary, the performance
of narcoleptics on certain types of tests is decreased, and there is EEG
evidence of brief periods of light sleep during which performance de-
teriorates. However, the performance of narcoleptics may be impaired
even during EEG-define wakefulness, and not all their difficulties can
be attributed to lower arousal.

DISORDERED PHYSIOLOGY

Narcolepsy appears to be associated with a variety of alterations in
physiology, although which are consequences and which are
predisposing factors is not clear. As we will see later, REM sleep appears inappropriately early in sleep in these patients, and many
aspects of narcolepsy may be viewed as a dysregulation of REM sleep.
Among other processes which are altered is the sleep-related secretion
of growth hormone (GH) (see Chapter 5). In narcoleptics the peak that
usually appears early in sleep, during slow-wave sleep, is absent
(Higuchi et al., 1979). In the daytime, the GH response to an amphetamine challenge may also be decreased (Parkes et al., 1977). In contrast
to normal volunteers, narcoleptics may also have increased cerebral
blood flow at sleep onset (Sakai et al., 1979; Meyer et al., 1980). Alterations in carotid sinus response to variations in blood pressure have also
been postulated (Scrima, 1981). Studies of 24-hr rectal temperature indicate that narcoleptics may have a higher mean and earlier occurrence
of the circadian minimum value compared to controls (Mosko,
Holowach, and Sassin, 1983). They may also have a higher incidence of
abnormal glucose tolerance tests than the general population (Honda et
al., 1986b). Whether any of these findings are critical to the nature of
the disorder is not clear. One observation of particular interest is that
in human cerebrospinal fluid there may be alterations in dopamine
metabolites (Montplaisir et al., 1982; Faull et al., 1986b). This finding is
consistent with neurochemical studies in narcoleptic dogs, in which
decreased utilization, or turnover, of dopamine has been reported
(Mefford et al., 1983). Because of the possible role of dopamine in
sleep–waking regulation, this seems an important area to pursue.

NATURAL HISTORY

Symptoms of narcolepsy usually begin when patients are between 10 and 20 yr old—5% of the cases may appear before age 10 and 25% after age 20 (Zarcone, 1973). Kessler, Guilleminault, and Dement (1974) found a mean age of onset of 19.4 yr. Both sexes are affected approximately equally (Yoss and Daly, 1960a,b). A classical history would be a teenager who complains of the gradual onset of sleepiness, for which no obvious cause is found. Within a few years, cataplexy or other secondary symptoms appear, at which time the diagnosis becomes clearer. Carskadon, Harvey, and Dement (1981) described this progression in a pubertal girl with a narcoleptic parent. At age 12, when she had no sleep complaints, the multiple sleep latency test (MSLT) (a measure of daytime sleepiness to be discussed later) showed a normal mean sleep latency of 14.1 min; within 3 yr, some symptoms had appeared, and the mean sleep latency dropped to 3.8 min, which is considered to indicate pathological sleepiness. At the same time, episodes of REM-onset sleep, the hallmark of narcolepsy, appeared on her EEG. Once the illness develops, it usually lasts for most of one's life, although the clinical impression is that symptoms may decrease in old age.

EPIDEMIOLOGY AND GENETICS

The prevalence of persons with episodes of excessive sleepiness was reported to be about 0.02–0.03% in a Yugoslavian study (Bruhova and Roth, 1972). In the San Francisco Bay Area, the prevalence of sleep attacks and cataplexy was found to be 0.097% (Dement, Carskadon, and Ley, 1973a). The latter figure indicates that as many as 100,000 persons in the United States may have these symptoms (Guilleminault, Carskadon, and Dement, 1974).

Nevsimalova-Bruhova (1973), examining the first- and second-degree relatives of 64 probands with sleep attacks plus an auxiliary symptom, found various types of sleep disorders in 34.4%. Kessler *et al.* (1974) reported that 52% of first- or second-degree relatives of REM narcoleptics had either narcolepsy or a disorder of excessive sleep and that 9.2% of parents, siblings, or children of probands were affected. Symptoms of narcolepsy itself were found in 2.5%; this familial prevalence would be about 60 times the rate expected in the general population. In a British study of 50 narcoleptic patients 52% had a first-degree relative with some form of sleep-related disorder, whereas 16% had both sleep attacks and cataplexy (Baraitser and Parkes, 1978). In a large multicenter study, narcolepsy was the second most common diagnosis (after sleep apnea) among patients complaining of excessive sleepiness (Coleman et al., 1982; Fig. 6-1).

The mode of inheritance of narcolepsy is unclear from clinical studies. Baraitser and Parkes (1978) felt that their data were most consistent with a single dominant gene. As we will see later, studies of Labrador retrievers and Doberman pinschers with narcolepsy indicate a single-gene recessive mechanism (Baker et al., 1982). Nevsimalova-Bruhova (1973) and Kessler et al. (1974) saw no simple Mendelian mechanism; the latter authors suggested that the high frequency of other disorders of excessive sleepiness in relatives of narcoleptics implies a single continuous distribution of liability to these disorders with one or more thresholds. Leckman and Gershon (1975) determined that the data from the Kessler et al. (1974) study are compatible with a two-threshold multifactorial model. The principal implication is that disorders of excessive sleepiness and narcolepsy may have a common genetic origin and that narcolepsy is the more severe, less frequent manifestation.

The discovery that certain leukocyte histocompatibility antigens (HLA) may be associated with narcolepsy afforded a valuable new approach. Laboratories in Japan (Juji et al., 1984), France (Billiard and Seignalet, 1985), and Britain (Langdon et al., 1986a) found the HLA DR2 complex in virtually 100% of narcoleptics, whereas it appears in 21 to 49% of controls. The DQ1 antigen also is present in most patients (Billiard and Seignalet, 1985; Honda et al., 1986a; Langdon et al., 1986a). Data about other antigen complexes, including B7, are conflicting. The issue is growing more complex, insofar as case reports of patients with narcolepsy who are DR2 negative have appeared (Guilleminault, 1986; Othman, Rundell, and Orr, 1987).

Certainly, one use of these observations concerning HLA antigens is the facilitation of studies of the mechanism of transmission. Thomson (1985) found that the Japanese and British studies were most consistent with an additive or dominant model, with possible incomplete penetrance. Billiard et al. (1986a), analyzing the French patients, also believed this to be likely. The HLA findings provide new ways of looking at narcolepsy. At least two other illnesses—Goodpasture's syndrome (Rees et al., 1978) and multiple sclerosis (Cohen et al., 1984)—have been associated with HLA DR2, and both are associated with alterations in immunological systems. This implies that such changes should be explored in narcolepsy. Although earlier work was not promising (see, for example, Honda et al., 1986a), Langdon et al. (1986a) have noted increased immunoglobulin concentrations in the cerebrospinal fluid of some patients. At the least, the HLA findings indicate that the DR2 complex, or one which is associated with it, may produce some abnormality of enzyme or receptor function that is involved in narcolepsy.

ETIOLOGY

The precise etiology of narcolepsy is unknown, although a number of possible causes have been proposed. It has been considered to be an epileptic equivalent (Roth, 1946) or a manifestation of psychodynamic conflicts (Levin, 1959). In 1963, Rechtschaffen et al. suggested that the syndrome of sleep attacks plus auxiliary symptoms may represent a defect in the control of REM sleep. They obtained 18 recordings of nocturnal sleep on nine patients with sleep attacks, eight of whom had at least one other symptom. In 11 recordings (in seven of nine patients) it was found that episodes of REM sleep occurred either at or within 11 min of sleep onset. In contrast, there were approximately 90 min of non-REM sleep before the first REM period in normal subjects. Narcoleptic patients did not differ from controls in the total percentage of REM sleep during the night. Their sleep was disturbed, however, as manifested by an increased number of body movements and decreased amounts of large slow-wave activity.

Dement, Rechtschaffen, and Gulevich (1966b) demonstrated that in patients with cataplexy, sleep attacks were also characterized by REM at sleep onset. Subsequent studies showed that daytime naps of similar patients contained at least some episodes of REM-onset sleep (Fig. 7-3). Roth, Bruhova, and Lehovsky (1969), for example, found REM-onset sleep during afternoon naps in 47% of 70 recordings obtained from 50 patients with sleep attacks plus cataplexy or sleep paralysis. Similarly, Wilson et al. (1973) recorded daytime naps from 49 patients with sleep attack plus one or more auxiliary symptoms; 90% of the patients had at least one episode of REM-onset sleep. Of the 24- or 36-hr recordings from six patients studied by Guilleminault et al. (1973c), there were 55 episodes of sleep, of which 48 were of the REM-onset type. Billiard et al. (1986b) found 94 REM-onset sleep episodes and 60 non-REM-onset sleep episodes in 36 narcoleptic patients studied over 34 hr. REM-onset sleep episodes were most frequent between 12:00 PM and 2:00 PM. There is also some tentative data indicating that nighttime REM periods in narcoleptics occur with the same periodicity as the preceding daytime episodes, which suggests that they are responsive to an underlying ultradian rhythmicity (De Koninck et al., 1986).

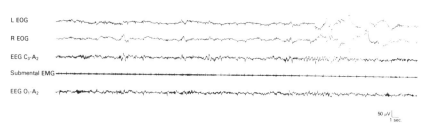

FIGURE 7-3. REM-onset sleep in a 28-year-old male with excessive daytime sleepiness and cataplexy.

It seems likely, then, that patients with sleep attacks plus one or more auxiliary symptoms suffer from a disorder of REM sleep regulation. Viewed in this way, it could be argued that the auxiliary symptoms of narcolepsy represent the intrusion into wakefulness of the tonic inhibition of muscle tone ordinarily observed in REM sleep (Guilleminault, Smythe, and Dement, 1973e; Dement, Guilleminault, and Mitler, 1973b). Further support for this view comes from studies of the H-reflex, which is determined by stimulating an afferent nerve and measuring the resulting muscle contraction. A decreased H-reflex is thought to represent increased descending inhibition of this system. It is greatly decreased or absent in normal subjects during REM sleep (Hishakawa and Kaneko, 1965) and in patients during cataplectic attacks (Guilleminault *et al.*, 1973e). Guilleminault *et al.* (1974) have pointed out that during cataplectic attacks patients can voluntarily move their extraocular muscles; this, too, is similar to what happens during REM sleep, when the tone of major striated muscle groups is decreased, but rapid eye movements occur. Sleep paralysis and hypnogogic hallucinations can also be viewed as episodes of REM-associated events (decreased muscle tone and dreaming) occurring in other states of arousal.

There has also been interest in the possible role of blood pressure dysregulation in narcolepsy. In 1954, Bonvallet, Dell, and Hiebel reported that carotid sinus distention induced slow-wave sleep, which led Kleitman (1963) to suggest that abnormalities of blood pressure regulation might be critical in narcolepsy. Scrima (1981) suggested that cataplexy, at least in part, is a response of hypersensitive baroreceptors to momentarily increased blood pressure during the expression of emotion. The atonia could possibly result from this response and from the loss of muscle tone usually seen in REM sleep. This is the rationale for efforts to treat narcolepsy with such agents as propranolol, to be mentioned later. Scrima, too, emphasized that narcolepsy may depend on several factors working together, including a genetic predisposition and environmental stress.

In summary, a great deal of data suggests that sleep attacks and auxiliary symptoms of narcolepsy represent the intrusion into wakefulness of various physiological components of REM sleep. There is no clear understanding of the control system that might be disturbed to produce these symptoms. Some new insights, however, are coming from studies of animals with narcolepsy.

ANIMAL MODELS OF NARCOLEPSY

Narcolepsy has been found in dogs (Mitler and Dement, 1977), horses (Sweeney et al., 1983; Dreifuss and Flynn, 1984), and Brahman bulls (Strain et al., 1984). The 24-hr totals of wakefulness, light sleep, and slow-wave sleep in narcoleptic dogs were similar to controls, although REM sleep was decreased. Cataplectic attacks were indistinguishable from REM sleep (Mitler and Dement, 1977). Later EEG studies also described an early period resembling wakefulness with loss of muscle tone, a REM-like state, and then a transition into waking or non-REM sleep (Kushida, Baker, and Dement, 1985). These animal studies suggested both genetic and neurological mechanisms that might lead to narcolepsy. In Doberman pinschers and Labrador retrievers there may be a single autosomal recessive gene, as well as nongenetic mechanisms, possibly developmental or traumatic (Baker et al., 1982). The mode of transmission in smaller dogs such as poodles is more complex and less clear.

Narcoleptic dogs have been used in biochemical as well as genetic studies. Faull et al. (1982) reported decreased dopamine and serotonin metabolite levels in the cerebrospinal fluid. After probenecid administration, all the metabolites increased, but 5-hydroxyindoleacetic acid (5-HIAA) and 3-methoxy-4-hydroxyphenylglycol (MHPG) (see Chapter 2) were still lower than in controls. Mefford et al. (1983) have found evidence of a defect in utilization or turnover of CNS dopamine in such animals. A later study reported elevations of dopamine, norepinephrine, and epinephrine in many brain areas, which suggests that the release of all three catecholamines might be defective (Faull et al., 1986a). Interestingly, serotonin and 5-HIAA concentrations did not differ from controls. Muscarinic cholinergic receptors may be increased in the brain stem (Boehme et al., 1984; Kilduff et al., 1986). This could mean that cholinergic system hypersensitivity might be involved in some manifestations of narcolepsy. Because of the possible role of benzodiazepine receptors (Chaper 4) in the action of sedative agents, it seemed appropriate to determine if these receptors are changed in narcolepsy; a study by Bowersox et al. (1986) found no significant difference in number or affinity of benzodiazepine receptors in narcoleptic and control dogs.

DIAGNOSIS

Sleep Laboratory Findings

Nocturnal recordings confirm patients' complaints of both excessive sleepiness and disturbed nighttime sleep. In narcoleptics, sleep latencies tend to be shorter and there is often less total sleep and increased wake time after sleep onset (Richardson et al., 1978). Episodes of REM-onset sleep sometimes appear, although in about one of five patients the REM latency may actually be prolonged (Mosko, Shampain, and Sassin, 1984). For this reason, it is best to perform the MSLT, in which the patient lies quietly in a dark room for four or five 20-min periods at 2-hr intervals across the day. Two types of information are obtained: an objective measure of sleepiness as reflected in the sleep latency (Fig. 7-4) and the presence of REM-onset sleep. When naps are looked at individually, there is often a tendency for narcoleptics and sleep apnea patients to have latencies that are slightly longer in the last nap (Walsh et al., 1982), possibly due to circadian reasons or because of improved wakefulness as a result of the small amount of accumulated sleep during the study. A mean sleep latency of 5 min is often considered the criterion for pathological sleepiness. In a study of 144 patients with excessive daytime sleepiness, 61 appeared to have narcolepsy by clinical criteria; this standard had a sensitivity of 57% and a specificity of 94% (Amira, Johnson, and Logowitz, 1985). The relationship of MSLT measures of sleepiness to nocturnal sleep has also been examined, and there is some indication that the nocturnal REM latency is positively correlated with the mean sleep latency on the MSLT (Browman et al., 1986).

The incidence of REM-onset sleep episodes during the MSLT has been examined in several studies (Richardson et al., 1978; Mitler et al., 1979a; Walsh et al., 1982; Amira et al., 1985). In the latter study, the finding of two or more REM-onset sleep episodes was found to have a sensitivity of 84% and a specificity of 99%. It is probably important to look for at least two episodes, since a single REM-onset sleep can appear fairly frequently. Such occurrences may be associated with alcohol or drug withdrawal, circadian sleep disturbances, and sleep apnea syn-

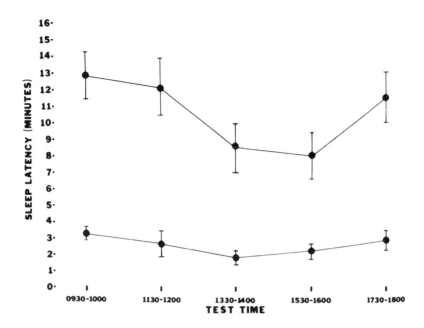

FIGURE 7-4. Mean ($\pm$ SEM) sleep latencies for control (upper curve) and narcoleptic (lower curve) subjects. For each opportunity to sleep, narcoleptics fell asleep significantly more quickly than did control subjects. (From Richardson *et al.*, 1978. Reprinted by permission.)

dromes. Walsh *et al.* (1982) found that all 13 narcoleptic patients in their series had at least two REM-onset sleep periods and that of their obstructive sleep apnea patients, 57% had at least one episode and 28% had two or more (Table 7-1). The presumption has been that this is a consequence of partial REM sleep deprivation as the result of the apneic episodes.

Other objective measures of daytime sleepiness are also available. The maintenance of wakefulness test (MWT) or repeated test of sustained wakefulness (RTSW) are conducted similarly to the MSLT except that the patient is instructed to try to remain awake (Hartse, Roth, and Zorick, 1982) and may be in a sitting position (Mitler, Gujavarty, and Browman, 1982). Sleep latencies for narcoleptics generally increase, compared to the MSLT, but remain shorter than for normal subjects.

Pupillometry has also been used as an objective measure of sleepiness, and it has been suggested that this approach may even distinguish between narcolepsy and CNS hypersomnolence (Schmidt, 1982). Pupil diameter may change rhythmically in the dark in narcoleptics, so

TABLE 7-1. Number (and Percent) of REM-Onset Sleep Episodes for
Narcoleptic and Obstructive Sleep Apnea Patients

	Time of nap				
	10.00	12.00	14.00	16.00	18.00
Narcoleptic	11/13 (85%)	9/13 (69%)	10/13 (77%)	10/13 (77%)	7/13 (54%)
Obstructive sleep apnea patients	1/14 (7%)	6/14 (43%)	0/14 (00%)	3/14 (21%)	3/14 (21%)
X	14.34	1.95	17.10	8.13	3.04
$p<$	0.01	(NS)	0.01	0.01	(NS)

(From Walsh, Smitson, and Kramer, 1982. Reprinted by permission.)

that serial measures are necessary in such studies (Pressman *et al.*, 1984). Broughton *et al.* (1986) have also suggested that complex cerebral evoked potentials may provide objective measures of sleepiness in narcoleptics.

In summary, sleepiness may be measured by several objective techniques, of which the most widely used are sleep latencies on the MSLT and MWT. Sometimes these objective measures differ from narcoleptic patients' reports of ability to stay awake after treatment, suggesting that symptom control does not always correlate with ability to maintain wakefulness (Mitler *et al.*, 1982).

Narcolepsy with Other Sleep Disorders

Nocturnal sleep studies of narcoleptics often find other concurrent disorders as well. Mosko *et al.* (1984) found significant myoclonic activity, defined as episodes lasting 45 min or 15% of total sleep, in 48.9%, and sleep apnea (more than five disordered breathing events per hour) in 9.8% of their subjects. Baker *et al.* (1986) found that 46% of narcoleptics had more than 40 periodic leg movements, and 13% had more than five disordered breathing events per hour. One study found some apneas in 69% of 16 patients (Chokroverty, 1986). The occasional long REM latency sometimes seen in narcoleptic patients could conceivably be the result of disturbances of the preceding non-REM sleep by these other disorders. It may be hypothesized that either narcolepsy or sleep apnea syndrome is involved in the etiology of the other, but it seems more likely that both are due to a central defect in the regulation of both sleep and respiration (Guilleminault *et al.*, 1972a).

Clinical Evaluation

When a patient presents with a complaint of excessive daytime sleepiness, a carefully detailed history is mandatory. A history of excessive sleepiness going back to teenage or young adult years, brief periods of sleep that leave the patient temporarily refreshed, the occurrence of auxiliary symptoms, disturbed nocturnal sleep, and automatic behavior strongly suggest narcolepsy.

One should also look for symptoms that suggest other disorders of excessive sleepiness. The patient should be questioned thoroughly about a history of loud snoring, hypertension, and other symptoms suggestive of obstructive sleep apnea. Although obstructive sleep apnea may occur at any age, and in either sex, the most typical history would be symptoms of a few years duration in a middle-aged, possibly overweight male. In sleep apnea, "sleep attacks," although a serious problem, often do not have the irresistible quality of those in narcolepsy. Hypnogogic hallucinations and automatic behavior, which are usually associated with narcolepsy, may sometimes appear in sleep apnea (Guilleminault *et al.*, 1978). A complete diagnosis requires an all-night polysomnogram, which includes determinations of nasal and oral air flow, chest and abdominal expansion, arterial oxygen saturation, and other measures (Chapter 6).

Patients should be questioned regarding a history of depression, abuse of stimulants or other drugs, seizure disorder, and kicking movements during sleep suggestive of nocturnal myoclonus. It is important to distinguish between sleep attacks and episodes of syncope that result from cardiac disorders, orthostatic hypotension, or carotid sinus dysfunction. A physical examination should be performed, and any suggestions of neurological, metabolic, or endocrine disease should be followed up with appropriate testing. Hypothyroidism, in particular, should be considered, with T_3 and T_4 determinations, if indicated. Hypoglycemia as the result of tumors of the pancreas may produce episodes of sweating, palpitations, and decreased level of consciousness. If hypoglycemia is suspected, blood sugar determinations should be performed during prolonged fasting.

OTHER DISORDERS OF EXCESSIVE DAYTIME SLEEPINESS

A whole range of other disorders produce excessive sleepiness, and a well-formulated list is found in the ASDC nosology (1979). Prominent among these are sleepiness related to nocturnal myoclonus

(Chapter 11), sleep apnea syndrome (Chapter 6), depression (Chapter 9), and drug or alcohol dependence (Chapter 8). Several other disorders will be briefly summarized here.

Idiopathic Central Nervous System Hypersomnolence

Some patients may have severe daytime sleepiness, with no auxiliary symptoms. The MSLT usually will confirm the hypersomnolence but does not show REM-onset sleep episodes (Hishikawa and Kaneko, 1965; Roth et al., 1969). Such patients have been characterized as having independent narcolepsy, non-REM narcolepsy, or idiopathic CNS hypersomnolence. The general clinical impression is that the sleep attacks are less discrete than in narcolepsy and the need to sleep can be resisted somewhat. When inappropriate episodes of sleep do occur, they are often of longer duration (Guilleminault et al., 1974). Upon

TABLE 7-2. Periodic Leg Movements and Sleep Apneas in
Narcolepsy and Idiopathic CNS Hypersomnolence

Variable	Narcolepsy		Idiopathic CNS hypersomnia		$(p < 0.05)^a$
Periodic leg movements Total/night (non-REM)	58.3	8.1	19.6	7.3	0.001(t)
Number/night with no arousal (non-REM)	36.5	5.7	14.0	5.5	0.005(t)
Number/night with arousal but no waking (non-REM)	18.8	3.5	4.8	1.8	0.000(t)
Number/night with arousal and waking (non-REM)	2.6	0.5	0.5	0.2	0.000(t)
Sleep apnea index (overall)	2.7	0.6	1.1	0.2	0.008(t)
Obstructive sleep apnea Number/night	10.4	2.8	1.9	0.8	0.004(t)
Obstructive sleep apnea index Non-REM	1.6	0.50	0.3	0.11	0.009(t)
REM	2.2	0.56	0.7	0.43	0.031(t)
Transitional	1.7	0.51	0.3	0.14	0.008(t)
Central sleep apnea index (REM)	6.1	2.9	3.4	1.2	0.007(W)
Hypopnea Hypopnea index (REM)	4.2	1.0	2.3	0.9	0.007(W)

(From Baker et al., 1986. Reprinted by permission.)
^{a}All values given are means ± SE. Statistical tests: (t) Student's t test; (W) Wilcoxon rank sum test.

awakening, the patient with CNS hypersomnolence may still feel lethargic, in contrast to the brief, refreshed state that often (but not always) follows an attack in narcolepsy. The nocturnal sleep in idiopathic CNS hypersomnolence seems to be relatively normal (Passouant *et al.*, 1968), with longer total sleep and less awakenings and wake time after sleep onset than is seen in narcoleptics (Montplaisir and Godbout, 1986). Although apneas and myoclonus have been observed in these patients (Table 7-2), it is not clear that their incidence is higher than in the general population (Baker *et al.*, 1986). There may be a familial form of this disorder, which is often associated with such other symptoms as headaches and fainting spells, or the disorder may occur in isolation. In both idiopathic hypersomnolence and narcolepsy there may be decreased concentrations of CSF dopamine and indoleacetic acid, a metabolite of tryptamine (Montplaisir *et al.*, 1982). Faull *et al.* (1986b) found that MHPG in the cerebrospinal fluid of these patients did not correlate with other biogenic amine metabolites, which raised the possibility of noradrenergic dysfunction.

Studies of HLA antigens in idiopathic CNS hypersomnolence are contradictory. Honda *et al.* (1986a) found an increased incidence of HLA DR2-positive reports in patients with excessive sleepiness and secondary symptoms but not cataplexy. Poirier *et al.* (1986) found increased HLA Cw2, DR5, and B27 in hypersomnolence patients; these antigens are in linkage dysequilibrium with DR2, which might suggest that narcolepsy and CNS hypersomnolence are different disorders.

Sleep Drunkenness

Some patients with a history of hypersomnia complain that upon awakening in the morning they are disoriented and confused for some time (Roth, Nevsimalova, and Rechtschaffen, 1972). Nocturnal sleep is not disturbed but is described as excessively "deep." Further descriptions and EEG data will determine whether this unusual condition should be classified as a discrete symptom complex; it seems more likely, however, that sleep drunkenness is only one manifestation of idiopathic CNS hypersomnolence.

Insufficient Sleep Syndrome

Patients with a life-style that leads to an insufficient number of hours in bed will often complain of sleepiness. Typically they do not understand that their habits contribute to their difficulties. It is very useful to have these patients keep a careful sleep diary. A polygraphic study usually reveals relatively efficient sleep and a prolonged sleep time, in contrast to the disturbed sleep of narcolepsy. These patients generally have more slow-wave and REM sleep than narcoleptics, although not necessarily more than normal subjects (Zorick *et al.*, 1982).

Hypersomnolence Associated with Medical or Toxic Conditions

Excessive sleepiness is found in a variety of organic conditions, including brain tumors, encephalitis, hypoglycemia, severe anemia, left-ventricular cardiac insufficiency, hypothyroidism, and early stages of narcotic withdrawal. Hypersomnolence may also develop months after head trauma (Zarcone, 1973). Studies of patients with definable organic states leading to hypersomnia generally find that daytime sleep episodes begin with non-REM sleep. Clinically, daytime sleep in these patients lasts longer than the sleep attacks of narcolepsy.

"Secondary Narcolepsy"

There have been some reports of organic lesions resulting in both sleep attacks and auxiliary symptoms (Nevsimalova-Bruhova, 1973; Roth and Nevsimalova, 1975), but these authors did not provide detailed analysis of EEG data. Such cases have been described with midbrain tumors (Stahl *et al.*, 1980), pontine gliomas (Schoenhuber, Angiari, and Peserico, 1981), and pontine and hypothalamic gliosis (Erlich and Itabashi, 1986). The possibility of such neuropathology should be kept in mind, although such clearly defined lesions in patients with narcolepsy are very unusual.

Excessive Sleepiness in Depression

Excessive sleepiness is often seen in patients suffering from an affective disorder, particularly bipolar depression (Chapter 9). Parenthetically, many physicians have the impression that there is a higher incidence of depression among narcoleptics than might be expected by chance. The relationship (if any) between the two disorders is not well understood, but a number of intriguing similarities are seen. These include some reports of decreased REM latency in depressed patients, the use of REM deprivation as a treatment for depression, and the use of tricyclic antidepressants to treat both narcolepsy and depression.

PHARMACOTHERAPY OF NARCOLEPSY

Stimulants

Since the first reports of therapy with amphetamine sulfate (Prinzmetal and Bloomberg, 1935) and methylphenidate (Daly and Yoss, 1956), stimulants have been widely used in the treatment of narcolepsy. Dextroamphetamine has been found to be more potent than L-amphetamine (Parkes and Fenton, 1973), although in equipotent doses, both decrease daytime sleepiness. Pemoline, which has a somewhat longer half-life, is often used. There is some preliminary evidence of benefits from the stimulants mazindol and fencamfamin (Shindler et al., 1985; Vespignani et al., 1984). In general, stimulants are relatively ineffective in the treatment of auxiliary symptoms (Parkes and Fenton, 1973; Guilleminault et al., 1974), although one study suggests that mazindol may also ameliorate cataplexy (Iijima et al., 1986). Methylphenidate may be relatively more effective in improving wakefulness than daytime performance, whereas pemoline may be more effective in improving performance (Mitler et al., 1986a).

Complications from taking stimulants include abuse, insomnia, and "paradoxical" increased sleepiness (Guilleminault et al., 1974). It should be borne in mind that amphetamines are secreted in human milk in concentrations three to seven times those found in blood (Steiner et al., 1984). Questions have been raised as to whether it is wise to withdraw amphetamines in patients experiencing myocardial infarction; in one case report, this was done with no difficulties except increased sleepiness (Orzel, 1982).

Symptoms of depression may occur when dextroamphetamine is discontinued in narcoleptic patients. Guilleminault et al. (1974) found that this can be alleviated by changing the patient to a tricyclic antidepressant plus methylphenidate, and withdrawing slowly. In this latter procedure, a wait of at least 24 hr between the last dose of amphetamine and the first dose of antidepressant is recommended, in order to avoid a possible toxic interaction.

Antidepressants

Tricyclic antidepressants are the most commonly used treatment for auxiliary symptoms; they are relatively ineffective for sleep attacks. Imipramine is probably the most widely used agent (Akimoto, Honda, and Takahashi, 1960; Guilleminault et al., 1974). Chlorimipramine, which is available only for research in the United States, may be more effective than imipramine, however (Guilleminault *et al.*, 1974; Chen, 1980). Shapiro (1975) found that the auxiliary symptoms of patients treated with chlorimipramine improved within 48 hr and that most patients continued to do well up to 21 months of follow-up.

Difficulties with the use of tricyclics include such anticholinergic effects as dry mouth and blurred vision. Impotence develops in many male patients (Karacan, 1986). The REM-suppressing effects of this group of drugs have been cited as evidence that these symptoms are "attacks" of some components of REM sleep.

Newer antidepressants have also been employed in narcolepsy. Trazodone was found to help one patient's sleep attacks and cataplexy (Sandyk, 1985). Nomifensine was reported to worsen symptoms in another case report (Sandyk and Gillman, 1985b).

Monoamine Oxidase Inhibitors

Wyatt *et al.* (1971b) administered phenelzine (60–90 mg/24 hr) for 1 yr to seven narcoleptic patients who had previously had unsatisfactory responses to more conventional therapies. All noted improvement in cataplectic and sleep attacks, although three continued to experience drowsiness. The patients' vocational and personal life seemed better. Side effects included hypotension, edema, and impaired sexual function. If medication was abruptly discontinued, depression, anxiety, and sometimes hallucinations occurred. When phenelzine was slowly withdrawn over one to three weeks, narcoleptic symptoms reappeared, but there were no severe psychological disturbances. Polygraphic recordings during treatment showed a decrease in daytime sleep. REM sleep was greatly decreased for periods of over a year in some cases.

Serotonin Antagonists and Agonists

Wyler, Wilkus, and Troupin (1975) gave the serotonin receptor blocker methysergide (2–4 mg/24 hr) to four patients with narcolepsy and one patient with sleep attacks. All five patients had a reduction in sleep attacks comparable to that seen in previous treatment with dextroamphetamine. Cataplexy, however, was less well controlled. Calf muscle claudication was a problem in two patients. The use of methysergide in narcolepsy should await further studies with appropriate controls. Reports of retroperitoneal fibrosis in a small percentage of patients who take methysergide for periods of a year or longer argue against its long-term use.

Ergotamine, which has serotonin blocking properties, has also been reported to benefit a narcoleptic in a single case report (Kaneko *et al.*, 1978). On the other hand, fluvoxamine and clomipramine (Schachter and Parkes, 1980), zimelidine (Montplaisir and Godbout, 1986b), and fluoxetine (Langdon *et al.*, 1986b), which might be expected to enhance serotonergic activity, may improve cataplexy, but not sleepiness. Similarly, L-tryptophan was thought to benefit three patients with isolated sleep paralysis (Snyder and Hams, 1982). A study of 5-HTP described little or no improvement (Autret *et al.*, 1977).

Gamma-Hydroxybutyrate

Several studies have indicated the usefulness of gamma-hydroxybutyrate (GHB) for both excessive sleepiness and cataplexy (Broughton and Mamelak, 1975, 1980; Mamelak and Webster, 1981; Scharf *et al.*, 1985; Mamelak, Scharf, and Woods, 1986). The mechanism of action of GHB, which has also been proposed for use as a hypnotic (Mamelak, Escriu, and Stokan, 1977), is not clear. It was originally thought to be converted to GABA, although some evidence suggests that its contribution may be negligible (Mohler, Patel, and Balazs, 1976). Daytime sleepiness in narcolepsy may still be evident, but lower doses of stimulants have been found to be adequate (Scharf *et al.*, 1985). In a case report of a patient with both narcolepsy and central sleep apnea, the narcolepsy improved, with no evidence of any worsening of ṭpneic episodes (Mamelak and Webster, 1981). One difficulty with oral GHB is that its short half-life necessitates its administration two or three times during the night. When it is administered intravenously, a number of side effects, which include drowsiness, slurred speech, ataxia, and nystagmus (Price *et al.*, 1981) occur, so it seems clear that the oral route is preferred.

Propranolol

Kales *et al.* (1979) found that propranolol given for 12 days improved daytime wakefulness, although its effects on cataplexy were mixed. A larger study by Meier-Ewart, Matsubayashi, and Benter (1985), in which half the patients were also receiving tricyclics, reported an initial improvement in both sleepiness and cataplexy, although its effectiveness decreased after six months; after 26 months, very few patients receiving propranolol alone were helped. The authors pointed out that improvement in cataplexy as the result of propranolol administration would be consistent with Scrima's (1981) hypothesis that carotid sinus baroreceptor hypersensitivity is involved in the genesis of cataplexy. This topic should be explored further. On the other hand, patient studies have found no clear change in heart rate in the triggering of cataplexy (Guilleminault et al., 1986a); animal model studies have found no clear blood pressure change, although heart rate has been reported to increase just before cataplectic episodes (Siegel et al., 1986).

Viloxazine, a derivative of propranolol, has also been used to treat narcolepsy (Guilleminault et al., 1986b). The patients reported fewer sleep attacks, although objective measures of wakefulness did not improve.

Opiates

The opiates codeine, pentazocine, and naloxone have been reported to help individual patients (Harper, 1981; Sandyk and Gillman, 1985a). Salin-Pascual, de la Fuente, and Fernandez-Guardiola (1985) found an improvement in two patients. Interestingly, tolerance to the REM-suppressing effects of opiates developed, although the beneficial effects continued; this raises the possibility that the therapeutic mechanism may not necessarily involve REM suppression. Fry et al. (1986) reported that codeine induced subjective improvement, but without objective evidence of improved wakefulness.

Other Treatments

A case report of delta sleep-inducing peptide (DSIP) administration described decreased sleep attacks and enhanced daytime alertness (Schneider-Helmert, 1984, 1985). Trials with amantadine (Ersmark and Lidvall, 1973) and L-DOPA (Gunne, Lidvall, and Widen, 1971) have shown no improvement. Although thyroid extract is frequently given, it is probably of no benefit (Yoss and Daly, 1960a,b). Similarly, L-histidine does not appear to be useful in the treatment of narcolepsy (Gillin et al., 1975a).

Several nonpharmacological steps are also important in the management of the narcoleptic patient. Clinical lore suggests that brief naps during the day improve wakefulness. A study of the effect of naps on the MSLT found that a 15-min nap in the late afternoon improves wakefulness as measured 15 but not 30 min later (Roehrs et al., 1986a). Increasing the nap length was not of further benefit. Napping has also been reported to improve performance on most aspects of the choice reaction time task (Godbout and Montplaisir, 1986).

It seems clear from the many psychosocial consequences of narcolepsy that counseling is very important. Many patients have achieved much less in their lives than their true capabilities would have allowed. The clinical impression that is often given is of chronic, low-grade dysphoria. Educating patients about their disorder and encouraging them are an important part of the treatment. Behavioral approaches are also being developed (Kolko, 1984).

SUMMARY

Narcolepsy is characterized by sleep attacks plus one or more auxiliary symptoms including cataplexy, hypnogogic hallucinations, and sleep paralysis. These symptoms may represent intrusions of some components of REM sleep into wakefulness. There is some preliminary evidence that abnormal blood pressure regulation may be involved in the genesis of cataplexy. The finding of certain HLA antigens in most narcoleptics has opened up new ways of studying its etiology. A number of intriguing questions remain, including suggestions that there may be performance deficits unrelated to sleepiness and that perceived benefits of medication may not always correlate with objectively measured improvement in wakefulness.

The differential diagnosis of narcolepsy includes other disorders of excessive sleepiness, such as sleep apnea syndrome, nocturnal myoclonus, depression, drug and alcohol abuse, and idiopathic CNS hypersomnolence. When a diagnosis is made, tricyclic antidepressants are effective for the auxiliary symptoms of narcolepsy; the stimulants dextroamphetamine, methylphenidate, and pemoline are of benefit in the treatment of sleep attacks. Monoamine oxidase inhibitors may be of use in patients resistant to other forms of therapy. Serotonin antagonists, propranolol, GHB, opiates, and other agents have been shown to benefit some patients, but they require further evaluation.

CHAPTER 8

Alcohol, Alcoholism, and the Problem of Dependence

Investigators of sleep physiology and of alcoholism have several common interests. Ethanol ingestion affects EEG sleep stages. It may also modify the metabolism of the biogenic amines, which are thought to play an important role in the regulation of sleep (see Chapters 1 and 2). Finally, there is some evidence that a disorder of sleep stage regulation may be involved in ethanol withdrawal syndromes. Each of these areas will be discussed here, in terms of knowledge gained from animal studies and effects of ethanol on sleep in normal volunteers and alcoholics.

ANIMAL STUDIES

Ethanol and the Sleep EEG

One of the earliest animal studies on the effects of ethanol on sleep was performed by Yules et al. (1966). They found that oral administration of 1.0 g/kg produced a small but significant (8–14%) decrease in REM sleep time during 7-hr recordings of cats. This effect, which was most pronounced during the first half of the night, was the result of decreases in the mean duration of REM sleep episodes, with no systematic changes in the number of episodes or REM latency. During successive nights of ethanol administration, the percentage REM time rose until it returned to normal on the fourth night. As will be seen later, the decrease in percentage REM sleep resulting from the shortening of mean duration of episodes, with a return to baseline values on subsequent nights, is consistent with data obtained from normal human subjects.

Two studies have examined the problem of whether the sleep EEG effects of ethanol are dose related. Branchey, Begleiter, and Kissin (1970) gave acute intraperitoneal injections of 0.5 or 1.5 g/kg of ethanol to 12 chronically implanted rats, and the EEG was recorded for 24 hr. Non-REM sleep increased at both doses, particularly in the first few hours after injection. At the lower dose, the percentage of REM sleep was unchanged, but after 1.5 g/kg of ethanol, it decreased during the first 6 hr. Mendelson and Hill (1976) injected ethanol in doses of 1.1–2.5 g/kg intraperitoneally to groups of six rats each, and obtained 7-hr EEG recordings. Sleep latency was decreased. As the dose of ethanol was increased, the percentage of non-REM sleep rose, and the percentage of REM sleep decreased (Figs. 8-1 and 8-2). These effects were seen most strongly in the first 3.5 hr of recording. The number of awakenings did not change in a systematic manner in the recordings as a whole. They did, however, increase with higher doses of ethanol during the second 3.5-hr period. Interestingly, the percentage of sleep in the total recording was unchanged. As will be seen later, a shortened

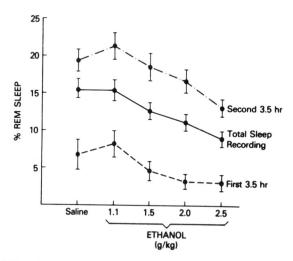

FIGURE 8-1. Effect of four doses of ethanol on percentage of REM sleep in the rat. (From Mendelson and Hill, 1978. Reprinted by permission.)

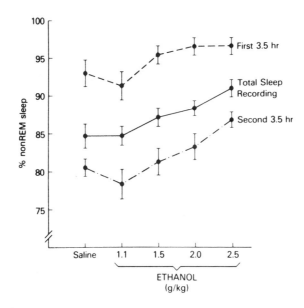

FIGURE 8-2. Percentage non-REM sleep in the same study as Figure 8-1.

sleep latency with enhanced awakenings and little change in total sleep is a common observation in studies of ethanol administration in normal human subjects.

Sleep in rats has also been used as a model of ethanol withdrawal. Mendelson *et al.* (1978) gave oral ethanol for four days at a rate determined by degree of behavioral impairment. On days one and three of administration, sleep latency declined and total sleep increased. On the first day of withdrawal, sleep latency and intermittent waking time increased, while total sleep decreased to less than half of baseline (Fig. 8-3). By the fourth day total sleep time had returned to normal values, and REM sleep had increased substantially above baseline (Fig. 8-4). These findings of initial sleep loss and a REM sleep rebound during withdrawal are similar to those seen in clinical alcohol withdrawal syndromes, as we will see later.

Effects of Prior Exposure to Ethanol

Gitlow *et al.* (1973) stressed the possibility that ethanol may alter the sleep EEG long after administration has been discontinued. They gave a total dose of 4–9 g/kg of ethanol orally to rats daily for four to six weeks. The animals were then housed and fed normally for six to

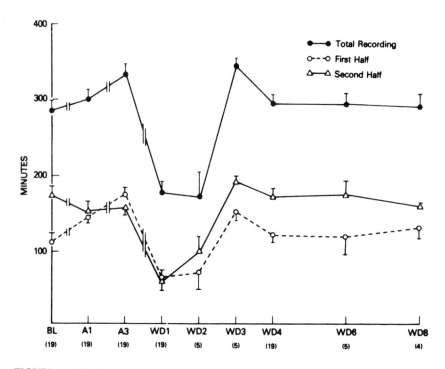

FIGURE 8-3. Total sleep time of rats given ethanol for four days. BL, baseline; Al and A3, first and third days of ethanol; WD, withdrawal. (From Mendelson *et al.*, 1978. Reprinted by permission.)

eight months. New recordings showed no change in total minutes of REM sleep or in number of REM sleep episodes, compared to saline-fed controls. The postethanol rats, however, respoŋded quite differently than controls to 4 g/kg of ethanol. After ethanol, total minutes of REM sleep and the number of REM sleep episodes were reduced in both groups. In the group that had received ethanol several months earlier, however, this effect was much more pronounced. Thus, there was a persistent abnormal REM sleep response to ethanol months after chronic administration had been discontinued. Gitlow, Dziedzic, and Dziedzic (1977) found that six months after a six-week course of ethanol administration rats had less motor sedation after an acute ethanol challenge. It has also been reported, incidently, that prior thiamine deficiency without ethanol exposure may decrease behavioral impairment resulting from ethanol administration seven months later (Martin *et al.*, 1985). It is not clear whether prenatal exposure in-

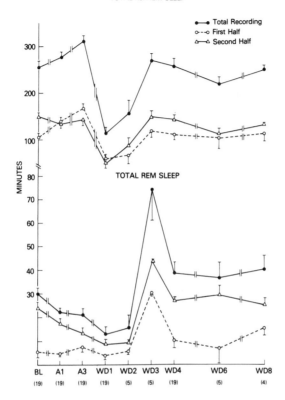

FIGURE 8-4. Non-REM and REM time in the same study as Figure 8-3.

fluences response to ethanol later, although a study of loss of the righting reflex in mice showed little effect (Randall *et al.*, 1983).

Behavioral Measures of Sleep in Long- and Short-Sleeping Mice

In addition to EEG studies, behavioral observations of ethanol-induced sleep have provided interesting insights. Mice can be selectively bred to develop strains that differ in length of behaviorally defined sleep in response to acute injections of ethanol (Heston *et al.*, 1974; Randall and Lester, 1974; Camjanovich and MacInnes, 1973). Camjanovich and MacInnes (1973) concluded that differences in blood ethanol clearance accounted for differences in sleep time; but Heston *et al.* (1974) found similar clearance rates in long-sleeping and short-sleeping strains and concluded that the disparity in sleep time was related to a different CNS sensitivity to ethanol. A study of long- and short-sleeping strains found similar degrees of binding of norepinephrine and GABA in the cortex and cerebellum and of choline in striatum and cortex (Howerton, Marks, and Collings, 1982). Ethanol inhibited neurotransmitter uptake to a similar degree in both strains. It is, then, less likely that this is the mechanism of behavioral sedation by ethanol. Randall and Lester (1974) found that strains that differ in sleep time after ethanol had similar sleep times in response to phenobarbital. Thus, the hypnotic effect of ethanol in a strain was specific to that agent and could not be generalized to other sedatives.

ETHANOL AND NEUROTRANSMITTERS

Ethanol-induced sleep time may be influenced by pharmacological manipulation of various transmitters. Pretreatment with the catecholamine synthesis inhibitor alpha-methyl-paratyrosine (Fig. 2-10) enhances the ethanol sleep time response (Erikson and Matchett, 1974), and this effect is decreased by L-DOPA administration (Blum et al., 1972). Parachlorophenylalanine, which decreases serotonin synthesis (Fig. 2-1), has been reported to increase ethanol-induced sedation (Erickson and Matchett, 1974), although other studies have not confirmed this finding (Blum et al., 1972; Sutoo and Sano, 1984). Although the serotonin precursors tryptophan and 5-hydroxytryptophan (5-HTP) (Fig. 2-1) have been reported to have no effect on ethanol sleep time (Blum et al., 1972), serotonin itself has been reported to increase it (Merritt and Geller, 1973). The GABA agonist muscimol may potentiate, and picrotoxin may block, ethanol-induced reduction in motor activity (Liljequist and Engel, 1982). Similarly the anticonflict actions of ethanol, a model for antianxiety effects (Chapter 4), may be blocked by picrotoxin but not by bicuculline (Liljequist and Engel, 1984). Ethanol-induced sleep time may be shortened by physostigmine, which enhances cholinergic activity (Erickson and Burnam, 1971). Studies of rat hippocampal pyramidal cells in situ, however, indicate that systemic ethanol may increase excitatory responses to iontophoresis of acetylcholine (Mancillas, Siggins, and Bloom, 1986). In the same study, ethanol also enhanced inhibitory responses to somatostatin-14 (see Chapter 5) and had no significant interaction with GABA, norepinephrine, or serotonin.

Ethanol alters the metabolism of a variety of neurotransmitters; indeed, its effects are so widespread that the difficulty is in determining which effect mediates its pharmacological properties. Studies of effects of ethanol on neurotransmitters have been reviewed by Hoffman and Tabakoff (1985). In general, many of these actions are biphasic, depending on the dose of ethanol employed; they differ in various brain regions and depend on the strain or species studied. Often these effects diminished over the course of chronic administration, showing a biochemical tolerance not unlike the well-described behavioral tolerance. At low doses, ethanol may increase norepinephrine turnover in the rat, whereas high doses may decrease it (Hunt and Majchrowicz, 1974). Turnover may remain high after chronic treatment and in withdrawal (Pohorecky, 1974). Serotonin concentrations after acute administration have been reported to be decreased (Gursey and Olson, 1961) or unchanged (Pscheidt, Issekuty, and Himwich, 1961) in rabbits, and increased in mice (Erickson and Matchett, 1974) and rats (Palaic *et al.*, 1971). Ethanol may not affect tryptophan or serotonin metabolism in the brain, although it may inhibit 5-hydroxyindoleacetic acid (5-HIAA) transport (Tabakoff and Hoffman, 1983; Tabakoff, Ritzmann, and Boggan, 1975). In a study using *in vivo* dialysis cannulae in the corpus striatum, ethanol induced serotonin release as reflected in increased 5-HIAA in the perfusion samples (Holman and Snape, 1985). After pretreatment with a DOPA decarboxylase inhibitor, acute low (<2 g/kg) doses of ethanol may decrease striatal dopamine release, whereas high doses may enhance synthesis and release (Kiianmaa and Tabakoff, 1983). In the rat, ethanol also acutely inhibits spontaneous acetylcholine release from brain slices and *in vivo* (Hunt and Dalton, 1976). Low acute doses of ethanol may reduce aminooxyacetic acid-induced GABA accumulation (an indirect measure of GABA turnover; see Chapter 2) with consequent increases in GABA concentrations (Wixon and Hunt, 1980). It was suggested that the resulting decrease in GABAergic acitivity might be associated with the excitatory behavioral effects seen at low doses. There was little effect at higher doses of ethanol, which made it appear somewhat less likely that changes in GABA function are responsible for the sedative effects of ethanol.

There has also been interest in the possibility that some of the pharmacological properties of ethanol may be mediated by prostaglandins. Linnoila *et al.* (1974) demonstrated that indomethacin may cause deficits in coordination and attention and that these effects are partially blocked by ethanol. George, Elmer, and Collins (1982) suggested that some of the pharmacological actions of ethanol may be mediated by changes in the membrane-bound arachidonic acid cascade. Although the actions of prostaglandins in the central nervous system are less clear, prostaglandins are involved in neurotransmitter regulation in the peripheral nervous system. Hence, changes in prostaglandins could conceivably be a mechanism by which ethanol inhibits transmitter release.

Davis and Walsh (1970) and Davis (1973) have suggested that one effect of ethanol on biogenic amine metabolism may help explain the development of dependence and cross-dependence with other drugs. Davis noted that ethanol (via its metabolite acetaldehyde), chloral hydrate, and barbiturates may modify catecholamine metabolism to produce tetrahydroisoquinoline alkaloids. These compounds, which are intermediates in the biosynthesis of morphinelike substances, might play a role in the pharmacological effects shared by these drugs. This hypothesis has been challenged on a number of grounds, however (see, for example, Halushka and Hoffman, 1970), and is best considered as speculative. Tetrahydroisoquinolines have also been reported to block the development of environment-dependent tolerance to ethanol (Melchior, 1982).

Ethanol also interacts with drug receptors. In a mouse neuroblastoma–rat glioma hybrid cell line, ethanol acutely inhibited opiate binding; after long-term exposure, the tissue showed evidence of an adaptive increase in the number of sites (Charness, Gordon, and Diamond, 1984). As discussed in Chapter 4, ethanol is thought to interact with the benzodiazepine receptor complex. It enhances binding of diazepam to the benzodiazepine recognition site, probably indirectly by way of a site near the chloride channel (Davis and Ticku, 1981). Behavioral effects of ethanol such as the loss of the righting reflex, may be partially blocked by agents acting at or near the chloride channel (Mendelson et al., 1985). Ethanol may stimulate GABA receptor-mediated chloride transport in synaptosomes (Suzdak et al., 1986), which could conceivably be involved in its sedative properties.

Ethanol may also alter calcium flux across membranes. Intraventricular administration of calcium potentiates, and calcium chelating agents inhibit, the ethanol-induced loss of the righting reflex (Erickson et al., 1980). This effect of calcium may be blocked by parachlorophenylalanine (PCPA), alpha-methyl-paratyrosine (AMPT), and diethyldithiocarbamate, which reduce serotonin, norepinephrine, and dopamine synthesis, respectively (Sutoo and Sano, 1984). Calcium binding to synaptic membranes has been reported to be decreased (Ross, Kibler, and Cardenas, 1977) or increased (Michaelis and Myers, 1979) by ethanol. Ethanol at 80 mM may acutely enhance calcium uptake into synaptosomes, with some tolerance occurring after chronic exposure (Friedman, Erickson, and Leslie, 1980). Other studies have described decreased uptake at ethanol concentrations as low as 45 mM

(Harris and Hood, 1980; Stokes and Harris, 1982). Ethanol may also interfere with the maintenance of other ionic gradients across membranes. In rat brain preparations, ethanol has been reported to inhibit Na^+-K^+-dependent ATPase in the presence of norepinephrine (Rangaraj and Kalant, 1979).

In summary, ethanol has a variety of biochemical and neurophysiological effects, including alterations of biogenic amine uptake and metabolism, and interactions with drug receptors and ion flux. Many seemingly opposite effects have been reported in the literature; these may be explained, in part, by the wide range of doses employed. It is also not clear which of these many effects may relate to specific pharmacological properties of ethanol. Ethanol has long been known to increase membrane fluidity (e.g., Chin and Goldstein, 1977), which might be expected to have wide-ranging effects on cellular function (Hunt, 1985). These might include some of the alterations in neurotransmitter action which we have described. Before this is accepted as the fundamental mechanism, several problems need to be solved. As Hunt (1985) points out, older animals are more susceptible to sedation from ethanol, yet they tend to have less disordered membranes. Hyperthermia tends to disorder membranes, yet does not in itself have intoxicating effects. It is always possible, of course, that changes in temperature do not affect membranes in the same way as ethanol does. Whether this, or some other effect, is the primary mechanism by which ethanol induces sedation is not clear.

ETHANOL IN NORMAL HUMAN SUBJECTS

Studies of acute ethanol administration in normal volunteers are outlined in Table 8-1. There is generally a sedative effect, which is demonstrated more consistently by a shorter sleep latency than by changes in total sleep time. REM sleep is decreased in the first half of the night. This may occur even when ethanol has been consumed some hours before sleep, so that blood ethanol concentrations at sleep onset are only 5 mg% (Yules, Lippmann, and Freedman, 1967), which is below the level at which inebriation is evident (Mirsky et al., 1941). Sometimes the evidence of the initial REM sleep suppression is "washed out" by increased amounts of REM sleep in the second half of the night. Thus, in some studies (Gresham, Webb, and Williams, 1963; Yules, Freedman, and Chandler, 1966; Williams, MacLean, and Cairns, 1983) REM sleep decreases for the whole night, whereas in other studies (Williams and Salamy, 1972; MacLain and Cairn, 1982) to-

TABLE 8-1. Effects of Ethanol on Sleep of Normal Subjects

References	Subjects	Dose	Days of administration	Sleep stages, first night of administration			Sleep stages, subsequent nights of administration			Sleep stages during withdrawal			Comment
				%REM	%SWS	%Waking	%REM	%SWS	%Waking	%REM	%SWS	%Waking	
Gresham et al., 1963	7	1 g/kg	5	↓	—	—	—	—	—	—	—	—	
Yules et al., 1966	3	1 g/kg	5	↓	↑	↑	↑	↑	—	↑	↑	↑	
Yules et al., 1967	4	1 g/kg	3	↓	↑ (stage 4)		↑			↑	↓ (stage 4)	↑	Administered 4 hr before sleep
Knowles et al., 1968	1	3.5, 6.0 oz	27	↓	—	↑	↑	—	↑	↑	—	↑	
Williams and Salamy, 1972	6	0.87 g/kg	3	↓	↑		↓	↑	↑	↑	↑	↑	
Rundell et al., 1972	7	0.9 g/kg	3	↓	↑	↑	↑	↑	↑	↑	↑	↑	
Williams and Salamy, 1972	10	0.87 g/kg	1	0	0ᵃ	→				↑	↑	↑	
Rundell et al., 1972	10	0.9 g/kg	1	→	↑	↑				↑	↑	↑	
MacLean and Cairns, 1982	10	0–1 g/kg	1	0	0ᵃ	0							
Williams et al., 1983	11	0–.75 g/kg	1	→	0ᵃ	↑							

ᵃIncrease during first half of night.

tal REM sleep is unchanged. The biphasic effect of REM sleep has been thought of as a "partial drug withdrawal" phenomenon. As evidence to support this view, it has been pointed out that ethanol is initially cleared from the blood in a linear manner, at about 10-20 mg%/hr in both waking and sleeping subjects (Knowles, Laverty, and Kuechler, 1968; Williams and Salamy, 1972). [After a few hours its metabolism follows first-order kinetics, again with no difference between waking and sleep (Madsen and Rossi, 1980).] Thus, the blood level of 80 mg% seen in many of these studies would have decreased to 40 mg% after the first 4 hr of an 8-hr sleep study. It follows then that with a higher initial dose, REM sleep may be suppressed for a longer period of time. Knowles *et al.* (1968), in one of the rare multiple dose studies, demonstrated such a dose-related phenomenon. After the administration of 3.5 oz of ethanol to a subject, the familiar pattern of initial decreases in REM sleep followed by later increases occurred; at a high dose (6 oz), REM sleep was clearly suppressed for the whole night. The biphasic effect on REM sleep is not at all unique to ethanol, it has also been reported with short-acting hypnotics (Kales *et al.*, 1969b).

Decreased percentages of REM sleep following ethanol administration in normal subjects seem to be largely the result of a decreased mean duration of REM sleep episodes rather than changes in periodicity (Yules *et al.*, 1966; Williams and Salamy, 1972; Rundell *et al.*, 1972); a single study (Rundell *et al.*, 1972) also reported a small but significant decrease in REM-to-REM periodicity during repeated administration. Data on "compensatory increases" in other stages during the period of decreased REM sleep have varied. Yules *et al.* (1967) found that stage 2 sleep increased in subjects who had received ethanol immediately before sleep, and stage 2 and stage 4 sleep increased in subjects who drank 4 hr before sleep. Williams and Salamy (1972) noted a tendency for slow-wave sleep to increase during the decrease in REM sleep, but this did not reach statistical significance.

When ethanol is given chronically to normal subjects, REM sleep gradually returns to normal (Yules *et al.*, 1967) or to slightly above normal (Yules *et al.*, 1966; Williams and Salamy,1972). Upon withdrawal, there may be an initial "rebound" increase in REM sleep above baseline levels (Yules *et al.*, 1966, 1967; Knowles *et al.*, 1968) that lasts a few days. This finding has not been constant, and was not observed during withdrawal in normal subjects in at least two studies (Williams and Salamy, 1972; Rundell *et al.*, 1972). The rebound phenomenon, in which total REM sleep time during withdrawal may be greater than the amount "lost" during ethanol administration (Yules *et al.*, 1966), has been the basis of two concepts seen throughout the literature on ethanol and sleep. The first is that ethanol may produce a "self-sustaining disregulation" of control of sleep stages, which may persist long after the drug is no longer present (Yules *et al.*, 1966, 1967). The second is that the rebound phenomenon may be characteristic of addictive drugs (Oswald, 1969a; Kales *et al.*, 1969a). (This latter concept has been developed from studies of a variety of agents, including morphine, barbiturates, and amphetamines.)

In analyzing data from ethanol studies in normal subjects, several methodological points should be considered. The first is that although changes in sleep as the result of ethanol administration may be dose related, there has been very little EEG work that carefully evaluates the dose–response relationship. It should also be noted that interpretation of sleep studies has been greatly complicated by the rapid clearance of ethanol from the blood. One approach that might be of help would be to follow the sleep EEG in subjects with relatively constant ethanol blood levels maintained by continuous infusion. A final difficulty is that studies on normal subjects usually involve the administration of a single dose of ethanol each day. In contrast, studies of chronic alcoholics usually have been designed so that the patient receives a cumulative dose of ethanol over many hours. The rationale for the latter design is that it more closely simulates the normal drinking pattern of the patient. The result of these different methods of administration is that comparisons of studies on normal subjects with those on alcoholics must be made with great caution.

EFFECTS OF ETHANOL IN CHRONIC ALCOHOLICS

Sleep in "Dry" Alcoholics

After the acute withdrawal symptoms have passed, alcoholics often complain of anxiety, sleeping problems, and autonomic disturbances for four to eight weeks or longer, often followed by mood disturbances during the next months (Mossberg, Liljeberg, and Borg, 1985). Relapses often occur during these periods of mood changes, which can include depressive symptoms. Studies of sleep in dry alcoholics are summarized in Table 8-2. Lester *et al.* (1973) performed one of the few studies in which alcoholics were directly compared with age-matched controls. It was found that alcoholics who had been abstinent for at least three weeks had more stage 1 and REM sleep, and less stage 3 sleep, than controls. Younger alcoholic subjects (24–39 years old) had less stage 4 sleep; this difference was not observed among older alcoholics, presumably because the older control subjects displayed the decreased stage 4 sleep that is observed in normal aging (Feinberg and Carlson, 1968). The increased REM sleep in alcoholics was related to a greater number of REM cycles, rather than longer REM episodes. The sleep of alcoholics appeared to be disturbed, as shown by an increased number of arousals and more changes in sleep stages.

The decreased slow-wave sleep and increased number of stage changes in alcoholics have been seen up to one or two years of abstinence (Adamson and Burdick, 1973). Wagman and Allen (1974) found that 200 weeks of abstinence were required for complete recovery of slow-wave sleep (defined as 18% of total sleep). Significant variables in slow-wave sleep recovery included age and the logarithm of duration of abstinence. Gross et al. (1973) observed decreased slow-wave sleep during acute withdrawal and suggested that the return of slow-wave sleep may be used as an indication of physiological recovery.

Smith, Johnson, and Burdick (1971) suggested that the disturbed sleep pattern with decreased slow-wave sleep seen in alcoholics is similar to that seen in the elderly. They also provided psychological testing results in which alcoholics obtained scores that might be expected of senile patients or patients with diffuse cortical damage. There are, of course, specific syndromes involving memory disorders among alcoholics, such as Wernicke's encephalopathy. Studies of dry alcoholics who do not have one of these specific disorders, however, indicate that few deficits are observed, that they are subtle, and that they may be reversible (Goodwin and Hill, 1975). Tarter and Edwards (1985), for instance, argued that impairments are not very striking on standard clinical tests of learning and memory and that in laboratory-based tests they are obvious only when the task is demanding.

Lester et al. (1973) observed that the increased REM sleep periodicity, disruption of REM sleep episodes, and decreased slow-wave sleep seen in alcoholics are similar to the effects seen with reserpine (Coulter et al., 1971). This is particularly interesting in the light of a long-standing impression that ethanol may have biochemical effects similar to those of reserpine (Williams and Salamy, 1972).

Gillin et al. (1986) examined abstinent primary alcoholics in the first and fourth week of treatment and at a three-month follow-up. REM latencies were relatively short at all three times, with values of 55.0 ± 29.0, 68.0 ± 35.0, and 46.0 ± 30.0 min, respectively. Half of the patients had values of less than 45 min. The consistency of short REM latencies across all three time points implies that this is not the result of withdrawal and that primary alcoholics may be added to the list of groups who may be prone to short REM latencies (see Chapter 9).

TABLE 8-2. Effects of Ethanol on Sleep of Chronic Alcoholics

References	Subjects	Dose[a]	Days of administration	Sleep stages when drinking compared to abstinence			Sleep stages during withdrawal compared to abstinence			Comment
				%REM	%SWS	%Awake	%REM	%SWS	%Awake	
Studies with data on abstinence and drinking										
Greenberg and Perlman, 1967	3	0.4–2.1 oz of 4 hr	4–10	↓	—	—	↑	—	—	
Mello and Mendelson, 1970	12	4.4 oz	14–32	—	—	↑	—	—	↑	Behavioral data only
Gross et al., 1973	4	3.1 mg/kg	15	↓	↑	↑	↑	↓	↑	Changes, first half of night
Lester et al., 1973	17	150 mg%[c] at bedtime	2	↓	↑	↓	↑	↑ (Stage 3)	↑	
Wolin and Mello, 1973	14	50–300 mg%[c]	12	↓ (decrease in 36%)	—	—	↑ (increase in 29%)	—	—	Data estimated from individual patient graphs
Zarcone et al., 1977	9	39 g/kg	1	↓	↑	—				
Studies comparing sleep during drinking with withdrawal										
Johnson et al., 1970	14	150 mg%[c]	2				↑	↑	↑	Decreased intermittent waking
Allen et al., 1971b	6	8 oz	3–7				↑	↑	↑	

Sleep stages compared to normal values %REM %SWS %Awake

Studies of abstinent alcoholics

		Days of abstinence				
Adamson and Burdick, 1973	10	1–2 yr	↑	→	↑	Uncontrolled
Lester et al., 1973	17	3 weeks minimum	←	→	↑	
Snyder et al., 1984	126	24 days	↑	↑	↑	
Touchon et al., 1981	20	—	—	→	—	
Gillin et al., 1986	11	8 days–4 months	—[b]	→	←	

Studies comparing sleep during acute withdrawal to normal values

		Days since drinking				
Gross et al., 1966	4	0–4	←	→	←	Uncontrolled
Greenberg and Perlman, 1967	14	0	←	—	←	Uncontrolled

[a]Method of presentation of dosage varies in different studies. When sufficient information was provided, this was converted to g/kg; otherwise, it is listed as presented in the papers.
[b]Half of patients had REM latency <45 min.
[c]Blood alcohol concentrations.

Response to Ethanol

Although the sleep of abstinent alcoholics differs greatly from that of normal subjects, both groups have some similarities in their response to ethanol. Sleep latency and percentage REM sleep decrease, whereas slow-wave sleep may increase (see, for example, Zarcone *et al.*, 1977). Lester *et al.* (1973) noted that ethanol administration in alcoholics decreased the inter-REM interval. This was reported in one study of normal subjects (Rundell *et al.*, 1972), but most evidence has been that normal subjects respond to ethanol with decreases in mean REM period duration. Mello and Mendelson (1970) observed that the distribution of behaviorally defined sleep over the 24-hr day changes when alcoholics spontaneously consume ethanol. They found that ethanol consumption resulted in a tendency to sleep in a series of relatively brief episodes, although total sleep time over 24 hr might be increased.

Many alcoholics are given disulfiram to help keep them from drinking. In a study of disulfiram in alcoholics, there were no effects on sleep latency or total sleep, but a reduction in REM sleep time was noted (Snyder, Karacan, and Salis, 1981).

Sleep during Acute Withdrawal

During withdrawal, REM sleep may increase. Johnson, Burdick, and Smith (1970) found that this was the result of an increased number of REM periods and shorter inter-REM intervals, with no change in mean duration of REM episodes compared to measurements during drinking. Allen *et al.* (1971b) reported that there is first an initial decrease in REM, followed by an increase. This implies that there is an oscillating system rather than a simple rebound in response to the previously decreased REM. As mentioned earlier, a decrease in the percentage of slow-wave sleep occurs in alcoholics during acute withdrawal (Gross *et al.*, 1973), as well as during chronic abstinence.

Psychotic episodes during ethanol withdrawal are associated with an increased number of REM sleep episodes and percentage REM sleep. In some cases REM sleep may make up over 90% of the sleep time (Greenberg and Perlman, 1967). Waking hallucinations may occur during this time, with a predominant alpha rhythm and active rapid eye movements (Gross *et al.*, 1966). Greenberg and Perlman (1967) found that this elevation and fragmentation was similar in kind, but quantitatively greater in alcoholics who developed delirium tremens

than in those who developed nonpsychotic abstinence syndrome.*
Wolin and Mello (1973) reported that although the relationship of REM
rebound to hallucinations during withdrawal was not inevitable in all
subjects, there was at least some positive relation. In a group of five
subjects who developed hallucinations, three had rebounds; of six subjects who had vivid dreams only, one had rebound; of three subjects
who had no change in dreaming, there were no rebounds.

REM Sleep Rebound

It has been speculated that increased REM sleep during ethanol
withdrawal syndromes leads to hallucinations and that this increase may
represent a basic mechanism of drug dependence. These hypotheses
will be discussed.

The REM intrusion hypothesis, which has been reviewed by Vogel
(1968), suggests that hallucinations reflect intrusions of REM sleep into
the waking state. This concept was anticipated by Lasegue, who in
1881 wrote a paper entitled "Alcoholic Delirium is not a Delirium, but
is a Dream." A similar concept has been invoked in studies of
schizophrenia (see Gillin and Wyatt, 1975). Several possibilities exist: It
may be that hallucinations during alcohol withdrawal do in fact represent the intrusion of REM sleep into waking, there may be no relationship between the two, or finally both may reflect some more basic
phenomenon. An effective hypothesis would have to be consistent
with observations of hallucinations in alcoholics when REM sleep is
normal (Wolin and Mello, 1973) and of REM rebound in both alcoholics
(Wolin and Mello, 1973) and normal subjects (Yules et al., 1966) with no
evidence of psychosis. As mentioned earlier, it may be that there is a
quantitative difference in REM sleep between alcoholics who develop
hallucinations and those who do not. An alternative is that an additional, as yet unknown, change in CNS function must also be present
if hallucinations are to occur. Feinberg (1969) speculated that impairment of the mechanisms that govern stage 4 sleep may be the second
factor. Clearly, the relation of increased REM sleep to the occurrence of
hallucinations is not a simple one.

---

*It is not clear in this article whether the amount of REM sleep is higher in those patients
with hallucinations only, or in those with the complete syndrome of delirium tremens.
The latter state is usually thought to include not only hallucinations but also disorientation and autonomic changes.

A second unanswered question that differs somewhat from the problem of whether the REM rebound causes hallucinations during withdrawal is whether the effects of ethanol on REM sleep are related to the development of dependence. Oswald (1969a) and Kales *et al.* (1969a) pointed out that this pattern—initial REM suppression during administration, later return to normal, and a large increase upon withdrawal—is seen not only with ethanol but also with a variety of drugs generally considered to be addicting, such as the amphetamines, morphine, and the barbiturates. It has been suggested that psychoactive drugs not generally considered to be addictive, such as lithium and chlorpromazine, acutely suppress REM sleep but have little or no rebound effect upon withdrawal.

As with hallucinations, the relation between changes in REM sleep and the addictive process could be formulated several ways. REM suppression and withdrawal rebound could be involved in the etiology of dependence. Alternatively, these changes may reflect a more basic mechanism, an example of tolerance and dependence in a particular physiological system. Finally, of course, the two processes may be unrelated. In evaluating these alternatives, several points should be mentioned. First, since the time this relationship was first formulated, a number of contradictory observations have been reported. An increase in REM sleep does not always occur during withdrawal from dependence-inducing substances. There have been reports of no REM rebound, for instance, after 200 mg phenobarbital for five nights, 200 mg of secobarbital for eight nights (Feinberg *et al.*, 1974a), 100 mg of secobarbital for two weeks (Kales *et al.*, 1976a), 1 mg of flunitrazepam or 10 mg of nitrazepam for one week, or 0.5 mg of triazolam for two weeks (Kales *et al.*, 1978). During withdrawal from these agents, however, sleep was disturbed, with increased sleep latency and intermittent waking time in the absence of REM rebound. Moreover, the REM rebound in ethanol withdrawal is inconsistent; Wolin and Mello (1973) described patients with signs of clinical withdrawal whose REM sleep was not increased. It should also be mentioned that REM sleep enhancement during drug withdrawal need not be associated with prior suppression during drug administration. This has been seen in several subjects receiving amphetamines (Feinberg *et al.*, 1974b) and in a subject taking the antihistamine chlorpheniramine maleate (Kales *et al.*, 1969b).

A second difficulty with relating the REM sleep rebound to withdrawal symptomatology is the timing of the processes. Several studies (e.g., Yules *et al.*, 1966) have described tolerance to the REM-suppressing effects of ethanol, and withdrawal rebound, after only a few days of administration of moderate amounts to normal volunteers.

This is a very different time course from the time-course required for the development of clinical tolerance and dependence. Finally, by selectively awakening subjects, one can produce REM suppression and later rebound. Although this was initially thought to produce psychotic changes, it appears that it probably has little harmful effect on humans and certainly does not produce changes similar to drug withdrawal syndromes (Vogel, 1968; see Chapter 1). Indeed, in some situations, notably depression, REM sleep deprivation has actually been found to have beneficial effects (see Chapter 9). During studies of normal subjects who have been REM sleep deprived, the recovery nights during which REM sleep is increased are often described as restful. In summary, although disturbed sleep is very much a part of the withdrawal process from ethanol and other drugs of dependence, the role of the REM sleep rebound itself is very uncertain.

EXPERIMENTAL APPROACHES TO ETHANOL TOXICITY AND WITHDRAWAL

The traditional therapy for ethanol withdrawal includes the use of minor tranquilizers, supplemental nutrition, and hydration if indicated (Rothman, 1984). Drugs such as chlordiazepoxide that have cross-tolerance to ethanol can help prevent delirium tremens (Kaim, Klett, and Rothfeld, 1969). Studies with mice support this practice, insofar as ethanol and chlordiazepoxide combined do not alter tolerance, but may decrease the effects of withdrawal syndromes, compared to ethanol alone (Chan et al., 1982). The ameliorative effect of diazepam on the ethanol withdrawal syndrome in rats is reduced by RO 15-1788, a benzodiazepine receptor blocker, suggesting that this is the site of action of its effect (Adinoff et al., 1986). The blocker by itself had no effect on the withdrawal syndrome, which argues against the possibility that the syndrome is the result of an endogenous ligand acting at the benzodiazepine recognition site.

In the treatment of delirium tremens, there may be little difference in outcome between patients treated with drugs that have a cross-tolerance and drugs, such as the phenothiazines, that do not (Kaim, 1974). Interestingly enough, none of these compounds seems to decrease the duration of delirium tremens to less than the three days described in untreated patients of the last century (Ware, 1841).

Results from such biochemical and sleep studies as those outlined in this chapter have led to various experimental approaches. Those mentioned here are of interest in that they were derived from observations on the metabolism of alcohol and its effects on sleep.

Bates (1972), noting reports of decreased total sleep time in alcoholics and studies showing psychotic states resulting from sleep deprivation (see Chapter 1), used "sleep therapy" for alcohol withdrawal. In a manner reminiscent of sleep therapies for depression (Klasi, 1922), thirty-two subjects who experienced hallucinations during withdrawal were given continuous infusions of pentobarbital, which produced sleep for 12–24 hr. This may have reduced the duration of psychotic withdrawal phenomena to about 30 hr, which appears to be shorter than that expected on the basis of the results of some other studies (Figurelli, 1958; Lundquist, 1961; Kaim and Klett, 1972).* Further evaluation of this approach by controlled studies will be needed to determine its efficacy. It would also seem to be important to evaluate the possible hazard of aspiration during sleeping, an issue that has been raised regarding sleep therapies for other conditions. A second concern is whether the possible benefits of this treatment are related to correcting a state of sleep deprivation, as the author suggests, or whether they are related to some other mechanism. Among other things, this study could be viewed as a therapy in which large doses of a cross-tolerant drug, already known to be of use in treatment of withdrawal, are used.

One experimental approach to the treatment of alcohol withdrawal has been the administration of NAD (nicotinamide adenine dinucleotide-nadide), a cofactor active in such reactions as the metabolism of ethanol by oxidation to acetaldehyde and, ultimately, acetic acid (Caldwell and Sever, 1974). Although initial results had suggested that NAD might be of benefit, a 10-day trial of 3 g daily was found to produce no difference from controls in measures of sleep or clinical tests (Smith, Johnson, and Burdick, 1971). Subsequently, it has become apparent that ethanol is metabolized by a nonoxidative pathway in several tissues, including the brain (Laposata and Lange, 1986), an observation that may lead to new ways of studying ethanol toxicity or dependence.

Another therapeutic approach has been the administration of 5-hydroxytryptophan (5-HTP), a precursor of serotonin (see Fig. 2-1).

---

*Actually, most studies give data on the duration of delirium tremens, without defining this state. As noted earlier, it is usually thought to include hallucinations, disorientation, and autonomic changes. The Bates paper apparently refers to the duration of hallucinations only, in patients with delirium tremens. Thus, it is somewhat difficult to compare these data with those of other studies.

Zarcone and Hoddes (1975), reasoning that ethanol may create an imbalance of serotonergic sleep mechanisms, gave 300 mg of 5-HTP for four nights to 12 alcoholics who had been abstinent for at least 23 days. There was no change in total amount of REM sleep, although the fragmentation of REM sleep periods, which was characteristic of alcoholics, greatly decreased. This supports the hypothesis that at least some of the sleep disturbances in alcoholics are related to abnormal serotonergic control mechanisms. Whether correction of these sleep disturbances by agents such as 5-HTP will change the clinical course of alcoholism is, of course, unknown.

Animal studies of ethanol have in many ways paralleled broader trends in neuroscience. There has been a great deal of attention paid to peptides, which is reflected in a report that neurotensin potentiates sedation (the loss of the righting reflex) by ethanol without affecting brain or blood concentration (Luttinger, Frye, and Bissette, 1982). Similar effects have been noted with bombesin and beta-endorphin (Luttinger et al., 1981). In contrast, thyrotropin-releasing hormone (TRH) may block various behavioral measures of sedation in mice (Mailman et al., 1980).

Following the interest in drug receptors, studies appeared showing the interaction of ethanol with the benzodiazepine receptor complex (Chapter 4). One implication is that drugs that block various components of the receptor complex might modify the effects of ethanol. Mendelson et al. (1985a), for instance, found that "cage convulsants," which bind at or near the chloride channel site, greatly reduce the duration of ethanol-induced loss of the righting reflex (Fig. 4-11). Indomethacin may decrease ethanol mortality, which supports the hypothesis mentioned earlier that alterations in the membrane-bound arachidonic acid cascade might mediate some of the pharmacological effects of ethanol (George, Elmer, and Collins, 1982).

ETHANOL AND HYPNOTICS

Ethanol and hypnotics are often found in the blood together for a variety of reasons. In addition to the purposeful mixing of the two in overdose situations, this may also occur inadvertently when a person receiving a long-acting hypnotic at night takes a drink the following evening. The complex pharmacological interactions of ethanol and benzodiazepines are reviewed by Mendelson (1980) and are discussed in Chapter 3. In summary, the results of studies of moderate doses of ethanol and benzodiazepines may indicate potentiation, no effect, or even antagonism, depending on the variable measured. In large doses, ethanol greatly potentiates the toxicity of benzodiazepines, which often leads to coma and death.

ETHANOL AND SLEEP APNEA

Ethanol is, of course, a respiratory suppressant. Although this is of little clinical significance when moderate amounts are consumed by healthy individuals, ethanol may greatly enhance respiratory impairment in patients with sleep apnea syndrome (Fig. 6-8). It is important, then, that such patients be cautioned not to take ethanol (Chapter 6).

SUMMARY

Ethanol potently affects sleep. This may be attributable to alterations in neuronal membranes, which, in turn, may alter the flux of ions including chloride and calcium. A variety of changes in biogenic amines have been found, but their relation to the known effects on sleep is not clear. Acutely, ethanol given to normal subjects decreases the percentage of REM sleep. Whether this occurs in only the first half of the night or all night may be dose related. Slow-wave sleep may increase in the first half of the night. "Dry" chronic alcoholics have disturbed sleep characterized by multiple awakenings, normal to mildly increased REM sleep, and decreased slow-wave sleep. These disturbances have been likened to the sleep of the elderly, and to subjects treated with reserpine. When alcoholics drink, the percentage of REM sleep decreases, whereas slow-wave sleep increases. The large increases in REM sleep that occur during ethanol withdrawal have been related by some authors to the development of hallucinations, and to the process of dependence itself. It is not clear whether sleep stage changes are related etiologically to these phenomena or whether they merely reflect them. Knowledge from sleep studies, however, has led to experimental approaches to treating alcoholism. Thyrotropin-releasing hormone, chloride channel blockers, and a prostaglandin synthetase inhibitor have ameliorated ethanol-induced sedation or toxicity in animals and conceivably could lead to new treatments in the future.

CHAPTER 9

Affective Disorders

The patients [with melancholia] are dull or stern, dejected or unreasonably torpid, without any manifest cause: such is the commencement of melancholy. And they also become peevish, dispirited, sleepless, and start up from a disturbed sleep.
—Aretaeus of Cappadocia (81-138 AD)
On the Causes and Symptoms of Chronic Disease

Sleep and depression are intimately related. The complaint of decreased sleep is very common, in almost 90% of endogenously depressed patients (Nelson and Charney, 1980), and improvement in sleep has often been considered to be one of the first signs of impending recovery (Mayer-Gross, Slater, and Roth, 1960). In sleep disorder centers, psychiatric illness (often depression) is the most common diagnosis made in patients complaining of insomnia (Table 9-1). Another intriguing association is that a variety of manipulations of sleep may effectively treat depressed patients. As a starting point, we will examine the phenomenology of sleep in depression, as well as sleep-related treatments and theoretical models that have arisen from them. In reviewing reports on the sleep of depressed patients, we will look at cross-sectional studies (in which actively ill patients are compared to controls) and longitudinal data on patients who are followed across time. Findings will be separated into descriptions of non-REM and REM sleep.

OBSERVATIONS OF PATIENTS

Symptomatic Depressed Patients Compared to Controls

Non-REM Variables

A number of studies have examined unmedicated depressed patients (Coble, Foster, and Kupfer, 1976; Foster *et al.*, 1976; Gresham,

TABLE 9-1. Disorders of Initiating and Maintaining Sleep in
5000 Patients in a Collaborative Study of 11 Sleep Disorder Centers

Diagnostic category	N	DIMS[a] (%)	Range/ center (%)	Total (%)
Psychiatric disorders	424	34.9	3.9–66.8	10.9
Psychophysiological disorders	186	15.3	1.0–32.9	4.8
Drug and ethanol dependency	151	12.4	2.9–25.2	3.9
Sleep-related myoclonus, restless leg syndrome	148	12.2	2.8–26.3	3.8
No insomnia abnormality	112	9.2	0.0–28.7	2.9
Sleep apnea syndromes	75	6.2	0.0–18.4	1.9
Other insomnia conditions	68	5.6	0.0–12.6	1.7
Medical, toxic, and environmental conditions	46	3.8	0.0–12.6	1.2
Childhood-onset insomnia	4	0.3	0.0–1.6	0.1
Total	1214	99.9	—	31.2

(From Coleman et al., 1982. Reprinted by permission.)
[a]DIMS, disorders of initiating and maintaining sleep.

Agnew, and Williams, 1965; Kupfer, 1976; Kupfer et al., 1978, 1979, 1980, 1985; Mendels and Hawkins, 1967a, 1968; Reynolds et al., 1980; Vogel et al., 1980; Kupfer and Foster, 1972; Jovanovic, 1977; Gillin et al., 1979b; Diaz-Guerrero, Gottlieb, and Knott, 1966; Jernajczyk, 1986). One fairly consistent finding was the fragmented nature of the sleep, as reflected in frequent brief awakenings, a high rate of stage changes, and low sleep efficiency. There is usually more stage 1 sleep and less slow-wave sleep. Although delta sleep declines across the lifetime in normal subjects (see Chapter 1), it is lower yet in depressed patients (Gillin et al., 1981). In general, total sleep time is reduced as a consequence of longer sleep latencies, increased intermittent waking time, and early morning awakenings. Groups in whom this is most clear include unipolar (Duncan, Pettigrew, and Gillin, 1979), older (Gillin et al., 1978), and more agitated (Kupfer, 1976) patients. There is some suggestion that a subgroup of depressives—perhaps 9%—may actually have longer sleep times (Michaelis and Hoffman, 1973), a finding also seen in questionnaire data (Nelson and Charney, 1980; Detre et al., 1972). In the latter study, hypersomnia was associated with weight gain, feeling worse in the morning, and more frequent hospitalization. Total sleep time of young depressives (i.e., under age 27) may be greater than controls when they are allowed to sleep ad libitum (Taub, Hawkins, and Van de Castle, 1978; Hawkins, Taub, and Van de Castle, 1985). A 24-hr study of six primary and secondary depressed patients also reported that their total sleep was greater than that of controls, but this was the result of increased sleep during the day (Schizimu *et al.*, 1979). In summary, then, cross-sectional studies of most depressed patients show fragmented, inefficient, and often shorter sleep. A minority of patients may suffer from hypersomnia.

Our discussion so far has centered on sleep changes in depression from studies in which sleep stages are interpreted by traditional criteria (Rechtschaffen and Kales, 1968). More recently, the sleep EEG has been examined, using frequency analysis procedures. Borbely *et al.* (1984) reported that in both unipolar patients and controls the power density in the delta (0.25–2.5 Hz) and total EEG (0.25–25 Hz) bands was highest in the first non-REM period and declined across subsequent periods. In the patients, the power was lower than in controls. As we will see later in the discussion of theoretical models of sleep in depression, these differences were not observed in a subsequent study of primarily bipolar depressed patients (Mendelson *et al.*, 1986g, 1987b).

REM Sleep Variables

An early view put forth by such investigators as Snyder (1969a) proposed that a lack of REM sleep led to depression. This was supported by clinical observations of early morning awakenings, the polygraphic finding that REM sleep tends to occur in largest amounts toward the morning (see Chapter 1), and experimental reports that REM sleep deprivation might lead to psychiatric disorders. As data became available, however, it appeared that in depression total REM sleep is usually normal or only slightly reduced; the most striking quality is its variability (Hawkins and Mendels, 1966). Later work cast doubt on the observation of psychiatric disturbance consequent to REM deprivation (Dement, 1969), and, thus, this particular view of the genesis of depression seems less likely.

REM Latency

A number of authors have suggested that the *timing*, in contrast to the total amount, of REM sleep is altered in depression. Since the 1960s, there have been many reports of short REM latency; that is, that REM sleep appears early relative to sleep onset (Green and Stajduher, 1966; Hartmann, 1968; Snyder, 1968; Hawkins *et al.*, 1967; Kupfer and Foster, 1972; Vogel *et al.*, 1980; Svendsen and Christensen, 1981; Mendlewicz *et al.*, 1984a; Kupfer *et al.*, 1985). REM latency decreases across the lifetime of normal subjects, but, in a manner analogous to delta sleep, it may be decreased more in depressives than in age-matched controls (Gillin et al., 1981). There are also reports that REM latencies are short in both hyposomniac and hypersomniac depressed patients (Kupfer et al., 1972) and that the degree of lengthening of REM latency after amitriptyline administration may predict a subsequent antidepressant response (Kupfer, Hanin, and Spiker, 1980b).

It was initially thought that the degree of shortening of REM latency in individual patients was related to the severity of symptoms (Spiker et al., 1978). Giles et al. (1986) also found that unipolar patients with a REM latency of less than 70 min were more severely depressed than those with latencies of more than 70 min. Zammit et al. (1986) reported that patients with either a short REM latency or nonsuppression of cortisol by dexamethasone tended not to respond to placebo. Ansseau et al. (1984a) and Shipley et al. (1986), however, did not find an association of REM latency with severity, and Mendlewicz et al. (1984a) actually found a positive correlation between the two.

Subsequent to the initial findings of short REM latency in depression, a number of studies questioned its sensitivity and specificity for depression. Normal REM latencies have been found in groups of unipolar (Hauri et al., 1974; Taub et al., 1978; Taub, 1982) and bipolar (Jovanovic, 1977; Jernajczyk, 1986; Thase et al., 1986; Mendelson et al., 1986g, 1987b) patients. REM latencies may also be normal in childhood depression (Mendlewicz et al., 1984b; Puig-Antich et al., 1982). Reports of adolescent depression have described short (Lahmeyer, Poznanski, and Bellur, 1983) and normal (Cashman et al., 1986) latencies.

The specificity of the short REM latency has also been questioned in a number of studies. Although it initially appeared that a short REM latency might distinguish primary from secondary depression, subsequent data indicate that it may be found in secondary depression as well (Lund and Berger, 1981). Short REM latency has also been reported in a number of other patient groups. These include narcolepsy (see Chapter 7), obsessive-compulsive disorder (Insel et al., 1982), depressed alcoholics (Spiker et al., 1977), divorcing women (Cartwright et al., 1980), anorexia nervosa (Neil, Merkanges, and Foster, 1980), hypomania and mania (Mendels and Hawkins, 1971a; Post et al., 1976a), subaffective dysthymia (Akiskal et al., 1980), schizophrenia (Jus et al., 1973), and primary alcoholism (Gillin et al., 1986). It may occur in normal subjects following sleep deprivation (Dement, 1960) and during temporal isolation (Czeisler et al., 1980; see Chapter 10). REM-onset sleep is also seen during multiple sleep latency tests in patients with sleep apnea (Walsh et al., 1982).

Interpretation of short REM latencies in depression or other conditions in which it has been reported is difficult because of the variability in the normal population. Mean REM latencies for groups of normal subjects have been as low as 63 (Mendelson *et al.*, 1986g, 1987b), 67 (Jernajczyk, 1986), and 70.4 min (Hiatt *et al.*, 1985). Kupfer *et al.* (1986) found the most common category of REM latencies among 52 younger and 23 older controls to be 53–71 min. These findings show how variable the normal REM latency may be, and hence how important it is to have carefully matched controls.

The issue of stability of the short REM latency was explored by Schulz *et al.* (1979), who reported on data from 90 polysomnograms taken from six patients during depression. Even within the usually accepted definition of a "short" REM latency there was a bimodal distribution, with one peak less than 10 min and the other peak greater than 60 min. Similarly, Coble, Kupfer, and Shaw (1981), in a study of 22 patients, found two peak incidences of REM onset, one at less than 10 min, the other between 40 and 60 min. If the very short REM latencies were excluded, then the remaining ones were relatively normally distributed between 10 and 90 min. Shipley *et al.* (1986), who recorded 62 patients for two nights, also found a bimodal distribution, with peaks at less than 10 min and between 40 and 49 min. A study of 92 depressed inpatients across four nights did not find a bimodal REM latency but rather a unimodal distribution with a peak frequency between 50 and 59 min (Ansseau *et al.*, 1984a). Kerkhofs *et al.* (1985) described relatively normal initial values that then tended to decrease across three nights of recordings in both major and minor depressive disorders. Ansseau *et al.* (1985) found that relatively even numbers of patients increased or decreased latencies across two nights of recording. Those with the greatest increase in REM latency from the first to the second night tended to have poorer clinical responses to tricyclics. Hopefully, as more longitudinal studies are performed, the likelihood of a given patient's having a short REM latency over several nights will be established. It might then be possible to define a positive test as one in which a patient has a certain number of short REM latencies during several nights' recordings, in much the same way as a diagnosis of narcolepsy is made by observing at least two REM-onset sleep episodes during five possible sleep periods (Chapter 7).

The relationship of the short REM latency to other potential biological markers of depression is still being evaluated. Perhaps the best known marker is nonsuppression of cortisol during the dexamethasone suppression test, or DST (Carroll, 1986). Several studies indicated that there is relatively little relation between the short REM latency and DST nonsuppression (Rush *et al.*, 1982, 1983; Ansseau *et al.*, 1984b). On the other hand, Mendlewicz *et al.* (1984a) reported that DST nonsuppressors had shorter REM latencies than DST suppressors. Shipley *et al.* (1986) found that nonpsychotic patients with REM latencies of less than 10 min tended to be nonsuppressors. Similarly, Zammit *et al.* (1986) found that in unipolar patients who did not respond to placebos, REM latencies were inversely correlated with postdexamethasone plasma cortisols at 4:00 PM. It remains to be seen, then, whether short REM latencies and the DST identify similar or unrelated populations of depressed patients.

In summary, many studies have described a short REM latency in depression, although a number of negative reports have also appeared. Studies of the short REM latency are complicated by issues of variability in the normal population, stability across successive nights, and occurrence in a wide range of psychiatric illnesses. The meaning of a short REM latency is not clear. As we will see later, the same observation can be interpreted several different ways—as evidence of a state of chronic REM deprivation, of a circadian rhythm phase advance of REM sleep (see Chapter 10), or of an increased cholinergic sensitivity.

Distribution of REM Sleep

In primary depression the distribution of REM sleep may be altered so that there is a greater proportion of REM in the first third of the night (Kupfer, Foster, and Detre, 1973; Gresham *et al.*, 1965). Instead of a progressive lengthening of REM periods across the night, as in normal subjects (Chapter 1), the length of successive REM periods remains roughly the same in unipolar depression. This difference is not seen in elderly primary (Gillin *et al.*, 1981) or bipolar depressed (Duncan *et al.*, 1981) patients. Indeed, even in unipolar depressed patients the number of minutes of actual REM in the first REM period is not significantly greater than in normal subjects (Duncan *et al.*, 1981), and the longer total length of the full REM period (including REM sleep and brief awakenings) presumably reflects less ''efficient'' REM.

REM Density

REM sleep may be more ''intense'' (an increase in REM density) in primary depressed patients (Gillin *et al.*, 1981; Mendlewicz *et al.*, 1984a; Kupfer *et al.*, 1985) and may differentiate psychotic from neurotic depressions (Snyder, 1969a; Kupfer and Foster, 1973; Kerkhofs *et al.*,

1985). Increased REM density is particularly evident in the first REM period (Schulz and Trojan, 1979), in contrast to normal subjects, in whom REM density (like REM period duration) increases across the night. It has also been suggested that the percentage of REM sleep in which eye movements occur may be positively correlated with the degree of depression found on the Beck Inventory, although the total number of eye movements (REM index) does not show this relationship (Hauri and Hawkins, 1971). Mendlewicz *et al.* (1984a), however, found that REM density could not be related to severity of depression. For the researcher studying sleep in depression, REM density has been both intriguing and disappointing: the former because increased REM density has been reported to persist even during remission (Schulz and Trojan, 1979; Sitaram *et al.*, 1982), the latter because increased REM density has not always been found even during illness (Gillin *et al.*, 1979b). One suspects that some of the differences between studies are the result of the relatively inexact way in which eye movements are quantified (frequently by assigning a value on a nine-point scale). A number of investigators are developing more precise measures of eye movement activity (e.g., Benson and Zarcone, 1981), which may clarify the situation.

Longitudinal Studies

Non-REM Sleep

As might be expected, as depression improves, total sleep time and amount of delta sleep increase (Lowy, Cleghorn, and McClure, 1971; Mendels and Hawkins, 1971a; Kupfer and Foster, 1973). Even in remission, however, sleep may not be fully normal. Delta sleep may be the slowest in returning (Hawkins *et al.*, 1967) and may remain lower than normal, while there may be longer sleep latencies and more awakenings (Hauri *et al.*, 1974).

REM Sleep

Some studies indicate relatively low amounts of REM sleep during acute illness with an increase as the patient improves (Gresham, Agnew, and Williams, 1965; Mendels and Hawkins, 1967b; Snyder, 1972a,b). Others have found normal percentage REM which increased further during electroconvulsive therapy (ECT) (Green and Stajduher, 1966), or elevated REM which declines toward normal upon improvement (Hartmann *et al.*, 1966). The variability of results casts doubt on the notion that actively ill patients have a prolonged decrease of REM sleep.

Just as non-REM sleep may remain altered during remission, there may also be changes in REM, and particularly, elevations of REM density (Sitaram *et al.*, 1982; Schulz and Trojan, 1979). Coble, Kupfer, and Shaw (1981) found little difference across five weeks in the percent of REM latencies of less than 20 min and greater than 60 min. There was, however, a negative correlation between clinical change on the Hamilton Rating Scale and percentage of REM latencies of less than 20 min.

SLEEP AND THE SWITCH PROCESS IN BIPOLAR PATIENTS

In bipolar patients, the switch process into mania is often preceded for one or two nights by decreased sleep (Bunney *et al.*, 1972). In the first few nights of mania, REM sleep may be decreased. Although the most common time to switch is between 7:00 AM and 3:00 PM, patients who change during sleep may have higher mania ratings and more insomnia in the first few days (Sitaram, Gillin, and Bunney, 1978). A study of one patient who switched at least four times during sleep indicated that the last recorded sleep was always REM (Gillin *et al.*, 1977). Changes in REM density may also distinguish nights before mania from nights before depression (Kupfer and Heninger, 1972).

THEORIES OF SLEEP IN DEPRESSION

These intriguing observations of sleep in depression have led to a number of theoretical explanations (Table 9-2). In a sense, the various

TABLE 9-2. Theories of Sleep in Depression

REM deprivation
Extended sleep, sleep satiety
Chronobiological (phase advance)
Altered function in the two-process model
  (inadequate buildup of process S)
Altered function in the Hobson–McCarley model
Neuropharmacological (increased cholinergic,
  decreased aminergic activity)

theories reflect the history of modern sleep research: When a new insight into sleep regulation occurs, its authors often attempt to apply it to the problem of depression. Another quality of these models is that many overlap and do not necessarily contradict one another. The neurochemical theory, based on heightened cholinergic activity, for example, is consistent with the altered cholinergic function of the Hobson–McCarley reciprocal interaction model.

REM Deprivation

As mentioned earlier, this hypothesis, put forth by Frederick Snyder, proposed that in the early stages of a depressive episode there is decreased total sleep and particularly decreased REM sleep (Snyder, 1968, 1969a). Insofar as REM sleep tends to occur late in nocturnal sleep, it was thought that the early morning awakening associated with depression would tend to reduce it selectively. Reflecting the interest at the time in studies that seemed to indicate that REM sleep deprivation led to psychiatric disturbances, it was thought that the mood disorder might result from the REM deprivation. In the recovery phase of depression, the amount of REM sleep was thought to increase. Although this model is derived from some well-known principles, such as the REM rebound phenomenon, few data support it. Coble et al. (1979), for instance, followed unmedicated patients for 35 days during which there was a general improvement in their depression, although complete recovery did not occur. During this time, REM latency and sleep efficiency remained low, while percentage REM and REM density decreased. Individual case reports of relapses from remission into depression (Cairns et al., 1980) or mania (Knowles, Waldron, and Cairns, 1979) indicated that sleep efficiency decreased only a few days before clinical illness appeared, leaving little time for significant sleep deprivation to occur. This is obviously a small data base, and hopefully more longitudinal studies will become available to clarify this.

Another difficulty with the REM deprivation hypothesis is that, as mentioned earlier, some depressed patients who become hypersomnic still show short REM latencies (Kupfer, Foster, and Detre, 19733; Kupfer et al., 1972). It is difficult to reconcile the REM deprivation theory with later observations that total, partial, or selective REM sleep deprivation may decrease depression. Finally, studies done subsequent to the propounding of this view have indicated that the association of REM deprivation with psychological disturbance is much more tenuous than it was once thought to be (Dement, 1969).

Extended Sleep and Sleep Satiety

Aserinsky (1969) and more recently Feinberg, Rein, and Floyd (1980) observed extended sleep (i.e., longer than 6–8 hr) in normal volunteers and noted both a high REM density and a tendency for successive REM periods to become progressively shorter. Both of these findings were also seen by Vogel et al. (1980), in endogenously depressed patients compared to insomniac controls; noting this similarity, they suggested that both situations share a common quality of REM sleep disinhibition. It was speculated that a circadian rhythm disturbance, such as a phase advance of the REM–non-REM cycle or a loss of rhythmicity, might account for this phenomenon. Gillin et al. (1984), aware of Aserinsky's concept that such measures as increased REM density might reflect "sleep satiety," and noting that in both conditions there is apparent difficulty initiating and maintaining sleep, proposed that depressed patients were in a continuous state of sleep satiety. If this were so, then depressed patients might be expected to show increased wakefulness during the day. A multiple sleep latency test (MSLT) study by Kupfer et al. (1980a) found this to be the case. Patients who slept least during the MSLT were also more likely to respond to tricyclic antidepressants.

The sleep satiety hypothesis is strengthened by reports of therapeutic benefits of total or partial sleep deprivation. It does not, however, account for observations on hypersomnic depressed patients. Another problem is that the studies (Aserinsky, 1969; Feinberg et al., 1980) did not control for the circadian differences when subjects had extended sleep.

Circadian View of Depression

There are, of course, many rhythmic aspects to depression. Among these are the daily cycle of mood, the marked regularity of illness and remission in "rapid cyclers," and seasonal depressions in some patients. It was only natural, then, that a number of investigators would come to examine depression as a consequence of disordered rhythms. Much of the work in this area centers around what has come to be known as the "REM phase advance hypothesis."

The REM Phase Advance Hypothesis

Wever (1979) proposed that there are at least two major oscillators, one that regulates REM sleep, temperature, and cortisol secretion, and another that controls the sleep–wake rhythm (Chapter 10). The REM phase advance hypothesis suggests that the circadian rhythm of REM sleep is phase-advanced relative to the sleep–wake rhythm (Papousek, 1975). Evidence for this view has come from several different types of studies. Weitzman et al. (1970a) described sleep in subjects who had undergone an acute 12-hr phase shift to a new bedtime of 10:00 AM. As Snyder pointed out in his discussion of this study, a number of aspects of their sleep—a short REM latency, increased REM in the first part of sleep, and increased wakefulness—resembled that found in depression. Plasma cortisol was elevated early in sleep. Other investigators examined cortisol and temperature rhythms in depression for evidence of a phase advance (Wehr, 1984; Wehr and Goodwin, 1983). Wehr, Muscattola, and Goodwin (1980) reported an advance of the temperature rhythm in depressed patients compared to controls. Wehr, Gillin, and Goodwin (1983) and Kripke et al. (1978) both described an advance of temperature acrophase and a shortening of REM latency relative to clock time in hypomania, although their findings during depression differed. Other studies have failed to find an advance of temperature (Pflug, Johnsson, and Ekse, 1981; Avery, Wildschiodtz, and Rafaelsen, 1982) but did note higher mean values. The latter appeared to be the result of a lesser decline in temperature during sleep in the depressed patients.

Studies of depressed patients have also described earlier cortisol minima relative to clock time (Fullerton et al., 1968a,b; Conroy, Hughes, and Mills, 1968; Yamashita et al., 1969). Linkowski et al. (1985) reported that the nadir of cortisol secretion occurred almost three hours earlier in unipolar, but not bipolar depressed patients, compared to controls. Once again, there may be an elevation of mean cortisol levels (Sachar et al., 1973a). There are also reports that cortisol secretion occurs earlier during active illness compared to remission (Doig et al., 1966; Yamashita et al., 1969) although this was not seen by Sachar et al. (1973a). Wehr, Muscattola, and Goodwin (1980) also reported that urinary 3-methoxy-4-hydroxyphenylglygol (MHPG) excretion occurs earlier in depressed patients compared to normal subjects. Other evidence for a phase advance comes from a clinical case study by Wehr et al. (1979), in which a patient was put to bed six hours earlier than usual, at 5:00 PM. On two of four trials, there was a brief clinical improvement and an advance of the time of the temperature maximum. In the two trials in which the patient did not improve, temperature rhythms were actually delayed. One interpretation of these observations is that clinical improvement occurred when a more normal relationship between sleep–waking times and REM sleep times was established. In another clinical study, depressed patients were allowed to nap at different times (Kupfer et al., 1980a). REM latency remained about the same from early evening to late afternoon, perhaps indicating a loss of rhythmicity of REM latency. The total amount of REM sleep was greater in morning naps, however, which suggested a more normal rhythm. Interpretation of the data is made more difficult by the number of subjects who slept very little (and, hence, contributed less to the sleep data), and who later turned out to have the best response to drug treatment.

One of the most intriguing aspects of the phase advance hypothesis is that it postulates a circadian rhythmic situation that can be at least partially induced by several experimental manipulations. These include east–west travel, living in an unentrained situation with an unusually long circadian day (e.g., 27 hr), undergoing an experimentally induced phase delay in sleep onset, and living under free-running conditions in temporal isolation. The latter situation has received the most attention in terms of its relevance to depression. A number of studies of normal volunteers in temporal isolation found that the period of the rest–activity cycle increases in duration to between 24 and 25 hr. Moreover, in many subjects, REM sleep, temperature, and cortisol rhythms become phase advanced relative to the sleep–wake cycle. Thus, they may have shorter REM latency and increased REM in the first part of sleep, although no increase in REM density was observed (Czeisler et al., 1980; Zimmerman et al., 1980). Data suggesting this altered phase relationship include a report by Dirlich et al. (1981) of a temporal isolation study of a unipolar patient with a 48-hr mood cycle. During isolation, the periodicity of mood persisted; the rest–activity cycle dropped to 19.5 hr, while the cortisol and temperature rhythm had a period of about 24 hr.

There have also been anecdotal accounts of depressive symptoms in volunteers undergoing temporal isolation. Lund (1974) found increased neuroticism and physical symptoms, which might be seen as exaggerations of natural patterns. Siffre (1975) described depressed feelings during six months of isolation. In one well-known incident, a volunteer committed suicide two weeks after a study that involved a 12-hr shift ended; there was some suggestion that he was to some degree internally desynchronized even before the study began (Rockwell et al., 1978). Knowles and MacLean (1985) presented data on the effects of delaying sleep in normal subjects. This manipulation, which might be expected to phase advance REM sleep relative to sleep onset, led to a short REM latency and depressive symptoms.

Several lines of evidence suggest that caution is in order regarding the phase advance hypothesis. As we have just described, the data on possible advances of temperature and cortisol rhythms include results from several negative studies. Some persons who consider themselves to be "morning types" may have relatively early temperature peaks without any evidence of an affective disorder (Horne and Ostberg, 1977). Several studies have found that patients who improved after various treatments continue to have short REM latencies or increased REM sleep (Green and Stajduhar, 1966; Mendels and Chernik, 1975; Vogel et al., 1980). Many subjects underwent temporal isolation without developing obvious depressive features. Indeed, Wever (1979) found that such subjective measures as a "contentment" scale and objective performance measures were actually *highest* during times of greatest internal desynchronization in temporal isolation and that there was no evidence that a depressed mood developed over the course of isolation. The observation that free-running subjects do not usually have increased phasic REM activity implies that this situation is not fully analogous to sleep in depression. Finally, as we will see later, sleep deprivation will effectively alleviate depression; it is controversial, however, whether it induces changes in body rhythms.

A related viewpoint, the *internal desynchronization hypothesis*, derives from studies of bipolar rapid cyclers (Kripke et al., 1978; Wehr et al., 1982). It postulates that, in this particular group, the sleep–wake rhythm and the REM–temperature–cortisol rhythm have different frequencies, so that they are continually going in and out of phase with each other (Wehr et al., 1982). The long periods without sleep that sometimes occur during the switch to mania are likened to the "long days"—often 36 hr or more—that often occur in normal subjects during temporal isolation. They are also similar in the sense of having short sleep latencies, enhanced total sleep time, and little change in REM density. The analogy is not perfect; normal volunteers do not usually develop manic symptoms after experiencing long days.

In summary, circadian rhythm studies have opened up new and exciting ways of looking at depression. It is probably valuable to view them in the context of circadian studies of diseases as a whole. In his classic studies, Richter (1965) described many illnesses—including infections, forms of arthritis, and agranulocytosis—that have clear rhythmic qualities. It is important to remember his caution that the presence of a rhythmic aspect does not necessarily mean that a dysrhythmia is the cause of the illness. One counterargument in the case of depression would be that certain manipulations of sleep and waking may actually be effective treatments, a topic to be discussed later.

Implications of the Two-Process Model

In Chapter 1, we outlined the two-process model of sleep regulation, which postulates a sleep-dependent process S and a circadian process C (Borbely, 1982b). Process S is thought to be reflected in the power density of the delta wave band (0.25–2.50 Hz), which increases during recovery following total sleep deprivation (Borbely *et al.*, 1981). Borbely *et al.* (1984) later examined power density in the delta band and the whole EEG spectrum (0.25–25 Hz) in unipolar depressed patients and controls. Power decreased across the first three non-REM periods in both groups; at each period, however, the depressives had lower values. One implication was that in depression there might be a deficit in the build-up of process S (Fig. 9-1). This concept was tested further in a group of 41 inpatient depressives and controls by Kupfer *et al.* (1984a,b), who used automated measures of both delta power and eye movements. The total delta waves positively correlated with time asleep in both groups, and the amount of delta sleep was less in depressed patients. The average delta wave count (delta waves per minute) over the whole night and in the first non-REM period also decreased in patients. (This may not have been seen in later non-REM

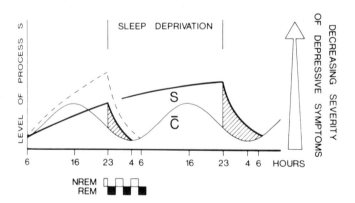

FIGURE 9-1. Sleep processes in a healthy subject (– – –) and in a depressive patient (———) plotted for a regular sleep-wake cycle and for sleep deprivation. The sleep periods of the depressive patient are indicated by shading. Because of the deficiency of process S, the sleep propensity and the amount of slow-wave sleep are reduced and the sleep period is shortened. The deficiency of process S leads to disinhibition of the REM sleep-controlling process in the first part of sleep. Consequently, the latency to the first REM sleep period is shortened and its duration increased (□, ■). Sleep deprivation normalizes not only the depressive sleep pattern but also induces a remission of depressive symptomatology (arrow, right ordinate). (From Borbely and Wirz-Justice, 1982. Reprinted by permission.)

periods because of the declining amplitude of delta waves, which might be below the amplitude criterion of 75–200 μV).

Another aspect of the two-process model suggests that the amount of phasic REM activity is inversely proportional to process S activity. Kupfer et al. (1984a) found that REM activity and density (activity per minute of REM sleep) were enhanced in depressives. Automated measures of number of rapid eye movements were highest in the first REM period compared to controls. Measures of the timing and duration of REM sleep were less clear. The short REM latency in depression might be viewed as resulting from disinhibition of REM sleep propensity when the process S is deficient. The data here indicated that the average delta count in the first cycle was positively correlated with REM latency. The length of the first REM period and the total delta count in the first period, however, were positively correlated, an observation less easily reconciled with the model. Other aspects of sleep in depression may also be encompassed by the model. If initiation of sleep is dependent on process S, then the long sleep latencies and frequent sleep interruptions in depression may also be seen as related to a decrease in process S.

The two-process principle has also been applied to depression by the use of computer models (Beersma, Daan, and Van den Hoofdakker, 1985). They found that two types of single variable changes could account for the known sleep alterations: either a deficient accumulation of process S or an increased amplitude in the random fluctuations of process C. (The latter could be the result of an oversensitivity to various internal and external stimuli.) These alternatives would predict very different findings in terms of both EEG power studies of sleep and the response to temporal isolation. A defect in process S accumulation, for instance, would predict power density values that were conceivably lower than those already reported. In the model with increased noise in process C, the prediction of increased sleep interruptions seemed to be borne out; observations of low EEG power density might be the result of the many interruptions that prevented the full expression of sleep EEG power. Under free-running conditions, the former proposed change would also predict a long sleep–wake cycle period on the order of 60 hr; the latter would predict short cycles of perhaps 13 hr.

Borbely (1987), reviewing some of the implications of the process S deficiency approach, pointed out a number of the complexities that must be considered. These include a large interindividual variation, as well as a changing rate of decay of process S across the night. It is also possible that a deficiency in process S in depression reflects both an "intrinsic" disorder and also such extrinsic factors as daytime napping.

In summary, the two-process model may be applied to depression. Before it is explored more fully, it may be well to examine the empirical data on which it rests. Mendelson *et al.* (1986g, 1987b), did not observe significant differences in either delta or whole EEG spectrum power between primarily bipolar depressed patients and controls (Fig. 9-2). Similarly, Van den Hoofdakker *et al.* (1985) found no significant disparity in delta power between depressive patients and controls, although the former had reduced slow-wave sleep, as read by conventional criteria. Further replication studies are clearly needed.

Reciprocal Interaction Model

As described in Chapter 1, Hobson, McCarley, and Wyzinski (1975) proposed that there is a reciprocal discharge pattern between noradrenergic cells of the gigantocellular tegmental field (FTG), which temporally corresponds to the REM–non-REM cycle. Although understanding of the anatomy of these systems is still evolving, functionally, they may be thought of as excitatory and inhibitory cell groups

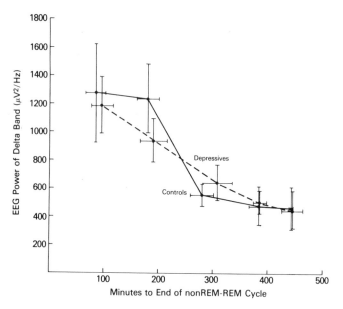

FIGURE 9-2. Power (EEG) in delta band (0.23–2.5 Hz) across sequential non-REM periods (as defined by Borbely *et al.*, 1984) in depressed patients (seven bipolar, one unipolar) and controls. (From Mendelson *et al.*, 1987b. Reprinted by permission.)

with respect to REM sleep. Vogel (1980) noted that when mathematical models of this relationship were manipulated, a combination could be found that might in principle produce sleep with a short REM latency and a long first REM period. These could be produced if there were a reduction in both generator and inhibitor strengths and in inhibitory level at cycle onset. Hobson, McCarley, and McKenna (1976) and Hobson (1983) also pointed out that a relative weakness of the aminergic inhibitory process might result in short REM latency, as well as increased REM percentage and density. Beersma, Daan, and Van den Hoofdakker (1984) also concluded that in this model a decrease in the initial value of the REM inhibitory process might account for the findings in terms of REM latency, accumulation of REM sleep, frequent awakenings, and other features. It is not clear, however, whether this might also be consistent with increased eye movement activity in depression. McCarley and Massaquoi (1985) described a limit cycle model of sleep in depression, based on decreased activity of aminergic REM-inhibitory cells in the reciprocal interaction model. It appears to account for the short REM latency, REM cycle period length, REM intensity, and REM episode duration when sleep is initiated at different times.

If there is a relatively weak REM inhibitory process, then the efficacy of REM deprivation treatment for depression (to be discussed later) would be due to preventing a fall in catecholaminergic activity. This might result in higher functional levels and relatively less cholinergic activity upon subsequent waking. Thus, REM deprivation might act like some tricyclic antidepressants, which enhance noradrenergic activity and have anticholinergic properties. Hobson (1983) also points out that such alterations in the model during depression would be consistent with theories that there is a functional decrease in catecholaminergic activity in depression (Schildkraut, 1967).

The reciprocal interaction model should also be seen in context with other systems in which an aminergic–cholinergic balance has been postulated. The best known is the nigrostriatal system, in which dopaminergic activity inhibits, and cholinergic activity enhances, parkinsonian tremor (Duvoisin, 1967). As we shall see, pharmacological studies of both sleep and depression have also been interpreted as showing a similar process.

Pharmacological Models

Several of the features of sleep in depression may be induced by various pharmacological agents. Hernandez-Peon et al. (1963) demonstrated that acetylcholine crystals placed in the limbic midbrain and forebrain induced sleep with an early REM period. A series of animal studies subsequently indicated a close relationship of cholinergic agonists and various qualities of REM sleep (see the review by Gillin, Sitaram, and Mendelson, 1982). In human subjects, both intravenous physostigmine (Sitaram *et al.*, 1977) and the cholinergic agonist arecoline (Sitaram *et al.*, 1978b) induced REM sleep when given during the first or second non-REM period in subjects pretreated with a peripheral cholinergic blocker. These effects were time dependent; physostigmine induced REM sleep more potently when given 35 min, compared to 5 min, after sleep onset. Similarly, the dose of physostigmine (0.5 mg) that induced REM sleep during the first non-REM period produced wakefulness when given during the second; a lower dose (0.25 mg), however, was followed by REM sleep when given 25 min after the first REM period. In contrast to the cholinergic system, drugs that inhibit biogenic amines may facilitate REM sleep (see Chapter 2). Thus reserpine, which depletes serotonin and catecholamines, and the alpha-adrenergic blocker thymoxamine may lead to short REM latencies (Oswald *et al.*, 1975).

Not surprisingly, these pharmacological manipulations of REM sleep have been applied to the problem of depression. Sitaram, Moore, and Gillin (1979) suggested that if muscarinic cholinergic hypersensitivity might be induced in humans, the consequent sleep would resemble that seen in depression. The muscarinic antagonist scopolamine was given every morning for three days on the assumption that by evening a hypersensitivity of muscarinic receptors would have been induced. The REM latency became shorter across the three days, REM density increased, and total sleep and sleep efficiency declined. The effects of arecoline in inducing REM sleep were enhanced, suggesting that there was, indeed, a state of muscarinic hypersensitivity. Applying this principle to affective disorder patients, arecoline has been reported to induce REM sleep more rapidly both during illness and remission, compared to normal volunteers and to nonaffective psychiatric patients (Jones *et al.*, 1985; Sitaram *et al.*, 1980, 1981, 1982). The latter authors also noted hypersensitivity response in anorexia nervosa patients with affective features and in some normal volunteers with positive family histories for depression. Nurnberger *et al.* (1983) reported that monozygotic twins may have high concordance for sensitivity to REM induction by arecoline. The hypersensitive arecoline response was also thought to be positively correlated with REM latency (Jones *et al.*, 1985).

Although the possibility of cholinergic hypersensitivity as a trait marker remains intriguing, at least one study indicates that this is more likely to be state-dependent (Berger et al., 1986). There has also been some difficulty in repeating the original finding, perhaps because of relatively weak test–retest reliability and other factors (Gillin et al., 1985). Even if an overactive cholinergic system were integral to depression, it also seems clear that it would only be one aspect of a complex mechanism. For instance, although physostigmine may induce some depressive symptoms in normal subjects (Risch et al., 1981), it clearly does not induce a full-blown syndrome.

Turning to the aminergic systems, reserpine as well as AMPT, which induces catecholamine synthesis, may produce depressivelike symptoms in man. Gillin et al. (1984) also found hypersomnia and short REM latency in volunteers given alpha-methyl-paratyrosine. Upon withdrawal decreased sleep and a hypomaniclike state occurred.

These pharmacological studies led Gillin et al. (1984) to conclude, as did the authors of the reciprocal interaction model (Hobson, 1983), that sleep in depression may result from an imbalance in a critical cholinergic–noradrenergic relationship. This is similar to the earlier proposal of Janowsky et al. (1972). The view, derived from the human pharmacological sleep studies to date, would add that muscarinic supersensitivity may be state-independent, whereas aminergic activity may be state-dependent. Certainly, replication of the findings of cholinergic supersensitivity would help substantiate this approach.

MANIPULATIONS OF SLEEP AS TREATMENTS FOR DEPRESSION

Perhaps the strongest argument for the case that sleep alterations in depression are not merely epiphenomena, but rather are central to the disease process, comes from the observation that some manipulations of sleep may effectively treat depression. The major forms of treatment, currently of interest, reviewed by Gillin (1983), include:

1. REM sleep deprivation
2. Total sleep deprivation
3. Partial sleep deprivation
4. Phase advance of sleep onset

In passing, it should be mentioned that the earliest manipulation of sleep as a treatment for psychiatric illness was drug-induced extended sleep. Described in 1901 by Wolf and later widely used after the studies of Klasi (1922), the treatment involved inducing continuous sleep with barbiturates for two to four weeks. Rationales for its use ranged from the biological to the psychodynamic, and, in general, responses were thought to have been better in schizophrenia than in affective disorders. Perhaps because of the dangers involved, as well as its questionable effectiveness, drug-induced extended sleep lost favor and is rarely, if ever, used.

REM Sleep Deprivation

As mentioned earlier, a popular view in the early 1960s was that REM sleep deprivation would produce psychological damage. By the late 1960s, however, a number of studies had questioned this view, and there were indications that REM deprivation actually had relatively little if any deleterious effects (Vogel, 1968). Indeed, Vogel et al. (1975a) pointed out a number of reasons indicating that REM deprivation might actually benefit depressive patients. They are as follows:

1. Antidepressant medications (tricyclics and MAO inhibitors) are more potent REM sleep inhibitors than are non-antidepressant drugs (Hishikawa et al., 1965; Hartmann, 1968b; Le Gassicke et al., 1965; Jouvet, 1967).
2. Electroconvulsive treatment may decrease REM sleep.
3. Reserpine, which may induce depressive symptoms in some persons, has been reported to increase REM sleep (Hartmann, 1966).
4. REM sleep deprivation in animals has been reported to make animals hypersexual, hyperactive, and hyperphagic (Dement, 1965), qualities that could be viewed as the opposite of a depressive symptomatology.

In a nonblind pilot study, Vogel (1975) deprived nine depressed patients of REM sleep. Five improved substantially and one slightly. Interestingly, those who improved had more evidence of REM pressure accumulation. (REM pressure is the tendency for REM sleep to occur during and after deprivation; one measure of REM pressure would be the amount of REM sleep on the recovery night.) These findings led to a blind crossover study of 34 endogenous and 18 reactive depressed patients (Vogel, 1975). In the active treatment, patients were awakened for 3 min whenever they entered REM sleep each night up to 30 awakenings or until the end of six consecutive nights, whichever came first. This process was repeated for several weeks. The control treatment consisted of awakenings during non-REM sleep to match the number of REM awakenings during one of the experimental nights. It was found that 17 of the 34 endogenously depressed patients, and one of the reactively depressed patients, recovered sufficiently to be discharged after these treatments. Eleven patients who had not improved from REM sleep deprivation received a course of imipramine; nine of these patients were treated for at least four weeks. Only one improved sufficiently to be discharged. Of the remaining ten patients who did not respond to imipramine, seven were given ECT and all but one had good responses. A review of the literature indicates that the rate of improvement after REM sleep deprivation is approximately the same as that for imipramine. The successful use of ECT seems to imply that among the endogenous patients there were at least two groups; that is, a group who improved with REM sleep deprivation and a second group that was largely unresponsive to imipramine but responsive to ECT.

In a later study, Vogel et al. (1980) compared REM sleep deprivation in 14 endogenous depressives and 14 nondepressed controls with chronic insomnia. Both groups had similar total sleep times and REM and delta sleep percentage during baseline conditions. The depressives had lower REM latency, higher eye movement activity, and greater variability in "early REM" percent and "late REM" percent. (Early REM percent refers to the duration of the first REM period multiplied by 100 and divided by total sleep time; late REM percent is an analogous calculation for all subsequent REM times after the first period.) During recovery, REM percentage was approximately the same in the two groups, but the distribution across the night differed; in the depressed patients, early REM percent was larger, and late REM percent smaller. Improvement did not correlate with any baseline sleep variables; it did correlate with recovery night late REM percent, increase in late REM percent, and increase in total REM percent.

The findings in the baseline sleep of depressives, the clinical response to REM sleep deprivation, and the particular pattern of REM sleep during the recovery night can be interpreted several different ways. As we shall see later, they can be described in terms of the reciprocal interaction model of sleep regulation as well as a (possibly resultant) circadian rhythm disturbance. As Vogel pointed out, antidepressant drugs are known to produce a variety of biochemical effects, primarily on biogenic amines; none of these pharmacological effects in isolation, however, ameliorate symptoms. REM sleep inhibition, however, is the one known action of antidepressants that, when duplicated, produces clinical improvements. Although not very practical as a clinical tool, the REM deprivation response is well documented, and any hypothesis of depression would have to take it into account.

Total Sleep Deprivation

After descriptions by Schulte (1971) and by Pflug and Tolle (1971a,b), many studies of total sleep deprivation have appeared (Fig. 9-3). Most involved a single night (e.g., Nasarallah and Coryell, 1982; Fahndrich, 1981; Gerner, 1979; Roy-Byrne *et al.*, 1984), although others have been done for two nights (e.g., Van den Burg and Van den Hoofdakker, 1975b; Knowles *et al.*, 1981). In general, the response occurred the next day or even during the deprivation itself, although some patients were reported to improve only after the night of recovery sleep (Loosen *et al.*, 1974; Wirz-Justice, Puringer, and Hole, 1976). This rapid response contrasts with that in REM sleep deprivation and phase advancing sleep, in which improvement may not occur for days or even weeks, respectively. Gillin (1983) calculated that 852 patients had been systematically treated by total sleep deprivation, with improvement in

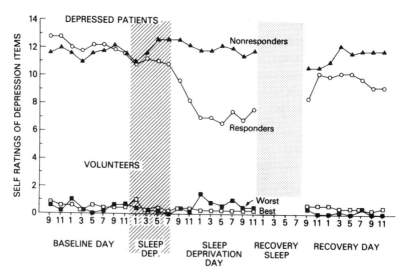

FIGURE 9-3. The effects of sleep deprivation on self-rated items of depression in depressed patients and normal volunteers. The marked improvement in mood observed in patient responders occurred in the early morning hours following sleep deprivation. Volunteers, including a subgroup who tolerated the procedure "best," showed little change in these depression items. (From Gerner, 1979. Reprinted by permission.)

57.9%. The best results were in the endogenously depressed patients, for whom the rate of improvement was 66.8%. Effectiveness may also depend on medication status and type of affective disorder. Wehr and Breitmeier (unpublished) and Wehr *et al.* (1982), for instance, found that in 14 hospitalized rapidly cycling bipolar patients, a single night of sleep deprivation was beneficial in 70% of those who were drug free but in only 15% of those on medication (usually lithium). Elsenga and Van den Hoofdakker (1983) found that sleep deprivation, in combination with clomipramine, induced a faster onset of improvement than the drug alone.

In general, the benefits of sleep deprivation have been reported to last only a few days; often exacerbations occur after the night of recovery sleep. Knowles *et al.* (1979) actually described a patient in whom symptoms would occur after brief naps. Pflug (1978) has presented data suggesting that sleep deprivation may shorten the total duration of the episode. Prophylactic value has been reported in a case report (Christadoulou *et al.*, 1978) and a series (Papadimitriou *et al.*, 1981), but this was not evident in three rapid cyclers (Wehr and Breitmeier, unpublished). In the latter study, patients became manic following the night of sleep deprivation, raising the possibility that the treatment may even help induce the switch.

Several studies have examined whether concentrations of neurotransmitter metabolites can predict response to sleep deprivation. There is some evidence that urinary and cerebrospinal fluid MHPG may be higher in responders than nonresponders; after sleep deprivation, it declined in responders and rose in nonresponders (Matussek *et al.*, 1974, 1977; Gerner *et al.*, 1979). Matussek *et al.* (1977) also found higher baseline urinary norepinephrine/epinephrine in responders, perhaps because they synthesize norepinephrine more rapidly. Baseline cerebrospinal fluid homovanillic acid (HVA) concentrations have been reported to be lower in responders (Gerner *et al.*, 1979).

In view of the many hypotheses of circadian disorders in depression, it seems reasonable to speculate that sleep deprivation might have beneficial effects by altering some rhythmic process. The data so far, however, are inconsistent. Gerner *et al.* (1979) found no difference between responders and nonresponders in baseline temperature curves. Responders showed no change after deprivation, although nonresponders had some flattening during and after deprivation. Pflug *et al.* (1981) reported that sleep deprivation lowered mean body temperature without obviously changing its timing, although the rhythmicity was extremely variable in depression. A preliminary rat study also seemed to indicate that 24-hr sleep deprivation does not alter the circadian rest–activity cycle (Borbely, 1982a), throwing further doubt on the possibility that this is the mechanism of action of sleep deprivation in depression. Czeisler *et al.* (1985), however, reported that two days of sleep deprivation in two normal volunteers resulted in a 4.5–6 hr phase advance and a 0.4–1.1 hr decrease in period of the rest–activity cycle (Fig. 9-4).

It is not clear whether sleep deprivation has a specific antidepressant effect or whether it leads to a nonspecific activation response to stress. In view of the finding that baseline cerebrospinal fluid HVA concentrations may be lower in responders, it should be noted that stress as well as stimulants may restore sensorimotor functions in rats with dopamine-depleting brain lesions (Marshall, Levitan, and Stricker, 1976). The observation of an increase in serum cortisol in responders relative to nonresponders seems consistent with a nonspecific stress response, although the decline in MHPG does not (Gerner *et al.*, 1979; Roy-Byrne, Uhde, and Post, 1984). The role of stress could be addressed better if sham treatments had been included in the studies. The difficulty, of course, is that it is hard to design a sham treatment for a study of total sleep deprivation. The question of specificity of the effect is also raised by reports that sleep deprivation may be beneficial in schizophrenia (Koranyi and Lehmann, 1960; Luby and Caldwell, 1967) or at least for postpsychotic depression in schizophrenics (Fahndrich, 1981). A further test of the possible nonspecific activating effects of sleep deprivation would be to examine sleep deprivation in normal subjects. Gerner *et al.* (1979) found less activation and more dysphoria in volunteers after total sleep deprivation;

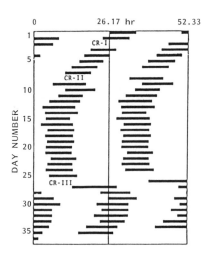

FIGURE 9-4. Rest–activity cycle in normal volunteers. Volunteers were trained to a 24-hr schedule during nights 1–10, except for being kept awake on the third (CR-I) and ninth (CR-II) nights. They then began following a self-selected routine; after 2½ weeks, they were kept up continuously for 50 hr (CR-III), and then returned to free-running. Note the phase advance shift of the rest–activity cycle and the change in the period of the synchronized run after CR-III. (From Czeisler *et al.*, 1985. Reprinted by permission.)

whether this would be true after partial sleep deprivation is not known.

Partial Sleep Deprivation

In studies of total sleep deprivation, patients often improved in the early morning hours. Pflug (1976) commented on a critical period at this time during which patients who would later respond complained particularly of poor mood and dysphoria. It seemed reasonable, then, to speculate that sleep deprivation during the latter half of the usual sleep time (late partial sleep deprivation or PSD-L) might be as beneficial as total sleep deprivation. Indeed, several studies have found PSD-L to be effective (Schilgen et al., 1976; Schilgen and Tolle, 1980: Philipp and Werner, 1979). Schilgen and Tolle (1980), for instance, awakened their 30 patients and kept them up after 1:30 AM; they found at least a modest improvement in 67%. Deprivation of sleep early at night (PSD-E) may have some benefits but apparently fewer than PSD-L. Goetze and Tolle (1981) studied 28 depressed patients who were allowed to sleep only from 1:30 AM until 7:00 AM and found at least a modest improvement in 13. The benefits, which often occurred only after four to eight days, were considered to be less than those seen after PSD-L or total sleep deprivation.

In terms of onset of response, PSD-L has often been reported to produce a response the next morning, or in some cases the following day. How long the benefits last is not clear, but they are thought to be measured in terms of days rather than weeks (Gillin, 1983). Partial sleep deprivation has also been reported to extend the duration of response to total sleep deprivation (Van Bemmel and Van den Hoofdakker, 1981).

Advance of the Sleep–Wake Cycle

One implication of the phase advance hypothesis is that restoration of the normal relationship between the two oscillators might treat the disorder. This could be achieved by phase advancing the sleep–wake rhythm. One might do this by having the patient go to bed relatively early. In effect, this is done incidentally as a part of PSD-L, in which the patient typically goes to bed at 8:00 or 9:00 PM; in PSD-L, however, the total time in bed is also reduced. Wehr et al. (1979) and Wehr and Wirz-Justice (1982) reported that moving the bedtime forward to 5:00 PM through 11:00 PM elicited an antidepressant response. Two out of six patients had partial improvement within a week and two entered remission. Sack et al. (1985) described four patients who were un-

responsive to antidepressants, in whom phase advance resulted in eu-
thymia for months and, in one case, for a year. Similarly, Souetre *et al.*
(1985) reported that four of five bipolar depressed patients significantly
improved during 18 days of phase advance treatment.

SUMMARY

The vast majority of depressed patients complain of poor sleep.
Polygraphically, their sleep tends to be shorter, with more interruptions and minimal slow-wave sleep. A number of studies have
reported short REM latencies, increased phasic activity, and a shift of
the distribution of REM sleep toward the first third of the night. The
short REM latency has been considered to be a possible biological
marker for depression. There have been a number of negative studies
as well, which may reflect the variability in both normal subjects and
depressed patients. Short REM latencies have also been seen in a variety of other psychiatric illnesses. A number of hypotheses have been
advanced with regard to sleep in depression. These include the notions
that depressed patients are in a chronic state of REM deprivation and
that they may be in a state analogous to sleep satiety. Circadian
rhythm studies have been taken to imply that in depression, the oscillator regulating REM sleep, cortisol secretion, and temperature may be
phase advanced relative to that controlling the sleep–wake cycle. A
related viewpoint, the internal desynchronization hypothesis, suggests
that in some patients these oscillators are in a continual process of going in and out of phase with each other. Both the two-process and the
reciprocal interaction models have been applied to depression. Pharmacological studies have suggested that sleep in affective disorder may
be the result of an imbalance of cholinergic and aminergic activity.

A number of manipulations of sleep may effectively ameliorate
symptoms of depression. These include total and partial sleep deprivation, REM sleep deprivation, and phase advancing the sleep–wake cycle. Total and partial sleep deprivation may induce relatively rapid
improvement, which may be short-lived. REM sleep deprivation has a
slower onset but may last longer. The phase advance treatment has
been studied less, but preliminary work suggested a relatively rapid
onset and raised the possibility of lasting benefits. The observation that
manipulation of sleep can treat depression suggests that the sleep disturbance of depression is not just a consequence of the disease but
rather an integral part of the process.

CHAPTER 10

Circadian Rhythms and Sleep

BACKGROUND

Part of our birthright as inhabitants of a spinning globe is continual exposure to rhythmical environmental changes and, in particular, the progression of day and night. It is no wonder that in the course of evolution organisms came to display rhythmic behaviors with an approximately 24-hr cycle. The ancient Greeks noted that various plants open their leaves by day and close them by night. The initial view of such rhythmic activities was that they were passive responses to changing stimuli, such as light and dark. By the eighteenth century, evidence began to accumulate suggesting that some rhythmic behaviors were *active* processes, which were manifestations of internal clocklike mechanisms. One of the earliest reports was made by Jean Jacques d'Ortous de Marian, who found that one particular plant would continue to open its leaves by day and close them by night, even in continuous darkness (Marchant, 1729). Perhaps more relevant to this discussion, de Marian went on to report that patients confined to bed would tend to keep a daily (circadian) rhythm of waking and sleep even when they did not know whether it was day or night. In the nineteenth-century, studies in environments without time cues (temporal isolation) began to lead to the conclusion that not only did organisms have active clocklike mechanisms but that they also might operate at rhythms that were slightly faster or slower than 24 hr (for a detailed review, see Moore-Ede, Sulzman, and Fuller, 1982). In 1962, temporal isolation studies by

Aschoff and Wever demonstrated the presence of endogenous rhythms in humans, including a rest–activity cycle of about 25 hr. An example of such a pattern in a later EEG-monitored study is seen in Figure 10-1. Under normal (entrained) circumstances, environmental cues (*zeitgebers*) reset body clocks so that they run in synchrony with day and night. In humans, these influences include social contacts and the timing of the sleep–wake cycle. Light is clearly the critical influence in animals; evidence is accumulating that this may be the case in humans as well (Czeisler *et al.*, 1986).

In addition to the many circadian processes—including rhythms of core temperature, cortisol secretion, and number of receptors for some neurotransmitters (Fig. 10-2)—there are many rhythmic activities with periods shorter or longer than a day. Some are measured in fractions of

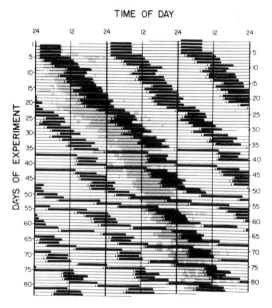

FIGURE 10-1. A sleep and low-temperature record of a subject who was released into a free-run in temporal isolation starting on the fifth day of the study: dark bars, EEG-defined sleep; stippled bars, core body temperature below mean established during first four days of the experiment (when subject was constrained to a 24-hr cycle with an 8-hr sleep period). The subject developed a sleep–wake cycle of about 25.1 hr and a temperature cycle of about 24.9 hr until day 35. After that, he became internally desynchronized with a sleep–wake cycle of 29.3 hr and a temperature cycle of 24.5 hr. The sleep–wake cycle began to have very variable durations at that time as well. (From Kronauer *et al.*, 1982. Reproduced by permission.)

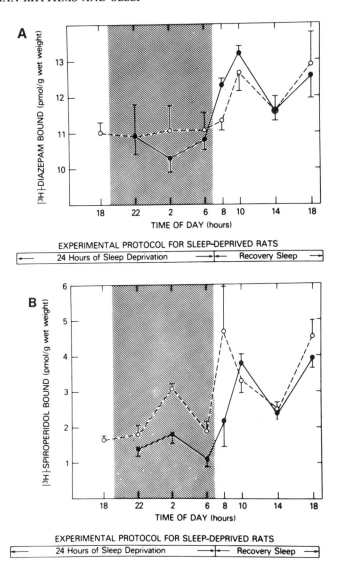

FIGURE 10-2. Neurotransmitter receptor binding during the last 13 hours of a 24-hr sleep deprivation protocol (○) and the first 12 hr of recovery sleep, together with non-sleep-deprived control groups (●) at the same time points in the dark and light phase. Measurements were made at 4-hr intervals. (A) Specific binding of [³H]diazepam to the benzodiazepine receptor and (B) specific binding of [³H]spiroperidol to the striatal dopamine receptor. Note that only minor changes in receptor rhythm resulted from sleep deprivation (induced by forced locomotion) and recovery sleep. (From Wirz-Justice *et al.*, 1981. Reprinted by permission.)

a second (i.e., the alpha rhythms of the electroencephalogram), seconds (i.e., respiration), minutes (the REM–non-REM cycle), months (the menstrual cycle), or years (estrous behavior, seasonal depressions). Further, there need not be just one clock in an organism; on the contrary, there are presumably many different clocks. This has led some authors to view various bodily functions as responses to a "clockshop." A large body of evidence indicates that this clockshop is centered in the suprachiasmatic nucleus (SCN) of the hypothalamus (Rietveld, 1985). This nucleus, perched above the optic chiasm, contains cells with intrinsic rhythmic properties. One major input into the SCN is the retinohypothalamic pathway, which provides information on light in the environment. In addition, there are approximately 20 known inputs from areas including the hypothalamus, thalamus, septum, and midbrain (including the raphe nuclei). Efferents go to a similar number of locations, often in the limbic system, regulating timing of rhythmic behaviors (Guldner, 1985). Among the efferent connections is an adrenergic path that, via the sympathetic chain, innervates the pineal gland and regulates melatonin secretion (see Chapter 3).

It is not entirely clear why organisms have such extensive rhythmical properties. In one sense, rhythmical qualities may be an almost inevitable consequence of any sophisticated regulatory system. In fact a major technological problem in building complex control systems is to *remove* the rhythmical qualities that seem to develop. Having an endogenous sense of time probably also has certain advantages. One which is often cited is that it allows an organism to anticipate important recurring events, for instance, to find shelter for the night before the onset of darkness. Another example of anticipation might be the progressive physiological stimulation in the hours before awakening, during which body temperature begins to climb and corticosteroid levels rise. This presumably creates the optimum situation for a mammal to begin the day (Moore-Ede and Sulzman, 1981). An inherent rhythm also makes it possible for an organism to develop several different states of behavior, which can occur at different times (Wehr and Goodwin, 1983; Moore-Ede and Sulzman, 1981). Oscillating systems may be particularly useful as control mechanisms; such systems may be particularly sensitive in distinguishing positive and negative deviations from the desired homeostatic goal (Oatley and Goodwin, 1971). Endogenous rhythms, however, may also lead to difficulties. Internal clock mechanisms may become misaligned with the outside world (external desynchronization); alternatively, two or more internal clocks may become misaligned with each other (internal desynchronization). The latter process is seen during temporal isolation experiments, in which the rhythm of body temperature takes on a different period from that of sleep and wakefulness. As we go on to discuss various disturbances of the rhythmical qualities of sleep, we will see examples of both situations.

In the years since de Marian first demonstrated cyclic rhythms in plants that have been isolated from day–night time cues, a variety of progressively more sophisticated studies were done on plants and small mammals under temporal isolation conditions. In 1962, Aschoff and Wever, in a study of six subjects in a Munich cellar, confirmed that humans, too, will operate on a non-24-hr rest–activity rhythm while free-running in temporal isolation. These initial studies did not, however, monitor sleep as measured by the polygraph. After initial EEG-monitored studies by Webb and Agnew (1972a,b) and Jouvet *et al.* (1974), a major long-term study of this type was carried out in a specially designed temporal isolation unit by Weitzman, Czeisler, and Moore-Ede (1979). Their findings in subjects who were studied for 25 to 105 days are generally representative of the sophisticated isolation studies from which subsequent theories of circadian regulation were derived. As in previous studies, they confirmed that free-running humans develop various cycles with periods approaching 25 hr. A number of subjects also spontaneously developed relatively long biological days of over 35 hr, often alternating with short days of 25 hr. Interestingly, the ratio of sleep time to total time remained about the same under free-running conditions, at about 0.30. REM sleep tended to occur much earlier in sleep, sometimes as soon as 10 min after sleep onset (see the discussion of short REM latency in Chapter 9). Slow-wave sleep retained its usual relationship to the early part of sleep (Chapter 1). During long sleep periods of over 12 hr, however, episodes of slow-wave sleep would reappear at about 14–16 hr. The relation of core body temperature to sleep onset was also altered. Under entrained conditions, the usual evening bedtime is during the descending temperatures following a late afternoon peak. In free-running conditions, however, the temperature rhythm advanced 6–8 hr relative to sleep onset; subjects tended to go to bed at the trough in the temperature cycle. There was often an additional drop in temperature after sleep onset, which was more obvious on those occasions when subjects went to sleep at times of higher temperatures. Plasma cortisol rhythm, like temperature, advanced 6–8 hr, increasing before sleep onset, with a second rise later. Growth hormone retained its usual secretory pattern during the first 2 hr of sleep (see Chapter 3), suggesting that there was relatively little direct circadian influence on its secretion.

The wealth of information from various temporal isolation studies, and of course, the long-standing observations of rhythms under entrained conditions, led a number of authors to speculate on the mechanisms of regulation of biological rhythms. This has resulted in a number of models. In evaluating the merits of various proposed models, it is well to remember that the ideal one would be able to account for all the observations just described.

MODELS OF SLEEP–WAKE REGULATION

In the 1960s, authors such as Wever (1964) and Aschoff (1964) suggested that a single oscillator controls the circadian cycle of motor activity, with inactivity resulting whenever its oscillation falls below a fixed point. Although this approach, as elaborated in a detailed model by Enright (1980), played a critical role in thinking in this field, it did not fully explain several observations. These include the wide range of frequencies of sleep phenomena, which vary from the circadian to the ultradian REM–non-REM cycle (Daan, Beersma, and Borbely, 1984). Other observations such as the phenomena of splitting and internal desynchronization led to the need for more flexible models. (*Splitting* refers to the tendency of a process, such as motor activity in small mammals, to split into two distinct portions when external timing cues are ambiguous.) One response to the need to explain these phenomena was the development of a model involving two pacemakers (Wever, 1975, 1979; Kronauer *et al.*, 1982). In this view, a dominant body pacemaker (X) regulates temperature, cortisol secretion, and REM sleep; a second, weaker pacemaker (Y) affects sleep versus waking (Fig. 10-3). The effect of X on Y is thought to be four times more potent than the effect of Y on X. Periodic time cues from the environment (Z) are seen as primarily affecting Y. Desynchronization during temporal isolation occurs when the intrinsic periods of X and Y become so different that the processes they regulate uncouple. In this view, an organism sleeps during one portion of the cycle of Y. This model allows for a wider variety of observed phenomena. It does, however, appear to require a pacemaker of extremely broad range, including a noncircadian period (Daan *et al.*, 1984). Those less inclined to this view have suggested that it is hard to relate these proposed pacemakers to any known physiology.

An alternative approach, presented by Borbely (1982), is based on the interaction of a homeostatic principle with a circadian principle (Daan *et al.*, 1984). The former, process S, is a sleep-regulating variable that accumulates during wakefulness and dissipates during sleep. (Fig. 9-1). It possibly corresponds to one of the hypnotoxins (see Chapter 2). One measurable manifestation of process S may be the power density in the delta waveband of the sleep EEG, which is thought to decline across successive non-REM periods of the night. Although originally it

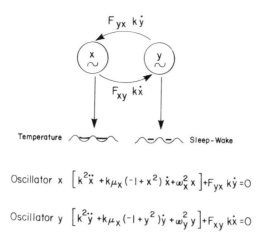

Oscillator x $\left[k^2 \ddot{x} + k\mu_x \left(-1 + x^2 \right) \dot{x} + \omega_x^2 x \right] + F_{yx} k\dot{y} = 0$

Oscillator y $\left[k^2 \ddot{y} + k\mu_x \left(-1 + y^2 \right) \dot{y} + \omega_y^2 y \right] + F_{xy} k\dot{x} = 0$

FIGURE 10-3. The two-pacemaker model of circadian regulation. See the text for a discussion. (From Kronauer *et al.*, 1982. Reproduced by permission.)

was thought to decline exponentially; later data suggested that a linear function is more appropriate; there is also some indication that the decay rate may first increase and then decrease during the night (Borbely, 1987). Evidence for its accumulation during waking comes from the observation of the increased power density of the EEG in sleep after sleep deprivation. A second principle, process C, is the circadian regulatory system, which may correspond physiologically to the suprachiasmatic nuclei. Thus in this model there is a single pacemaker that, under normal conditions, is entrained daily by external time cues. This circadian process imposes a rhythm on a variety of physiological activities and could conceivably synchronize other systems that have their own inherent rhythm (an example of the latter may be mammalian body temperature rhythms). Sleep onset would occur when the gradually rising process S intersects a threshold determined by process C ("point H"). After sleep onset, process S gradually declines, until it reaches another point determined by the circadian influence ("point L"), at which time awakening occurs.

After the original presentation of this model, it was necessary to refine it further to account for internal desynchronization. This was done by adding the assumption that during wakefulness the circadian threshold operates at a higher level than during sleep. One way to view this overall system is that process S may be the manifestation of a chemical substance, whereas points H and L represent the sensitivity of hypothetical receptors for S (Daan *et al.*, 1984). Other influences would also affect the timing of sleep and wakefulness. These might include changes in external conditions, such as ambient temperature, and conscious decisions, for example, whether to take a nap. In summary, various models have been developed to explain the rhythmical aspects of sleep. As time goes on, their utility will be determined by the ease with which they can be related to known anatomical and physiological systems and their ability to predict the outcome of experiments involving alterations of sleep schedules.

DISORDERS OF THE SLEEP–WAKE SCHEDULE

Transient Disturbance

Two types of transient disturbances are recognized in the ASDC nosology (1979): rapid time zone changes ("jet lag") and work shift changes in a conventional sleep–wake schedule.

Jet Lag

Jet lag includes the insomnia and excessive daytime sleepiness that occur after transmeridian flights. It is presumably the result of desynchronizaion between the endogenous sleep–wake rhythm and the rhythm imposed by the new environment. When flying west, a traveler finds himself phase-advanced relative to the new environment and, hence, would tend to go to bed earlier and arise earlier than those people who are accustomed to the local time. In readjusting, the traveler phase-delays his rhythms until they become synchronous with outside stimuli. A study by Kovacevic–Ristanovic et al. (1978) of subjects who flew from Brussels to Chicago indicated that initially there was less REM sleep and more stage 4 sleep in the second half of the night. The total amount of REM returned to normal by the tenth night. Sleep latency was initially reduced. Nicholson et al. (1986), describing sleep after westward trans-Atlantic flight, also reported increased slow-wave sleep and a decreased REM–non-REM sleep ratio. As might be expected, sleep was more disturbed in the second half of the night, as manifested by increased awake and stage 1 time. The disruptions of an acute phase-delay have been described in a laboratory setting by Seidel et al. (1984) and will be discussed in the pharmacology section later in the chapter.

When flying east, a traveler becomes acutely phase-delayed relative to the environment, tending to go to sleep later and getting up later than others. The readjustment would involve a phase-advance of his endogenous rhythms. There is some indication that it may be more difficult to adjust to eastward travel. It is possible that this is the result of the natural drift of the sleep–wake rhythm in the direction of the phase-delay. Klein *et al.* (1977) found that 22% of a group of eastward travelers required 14 to 18 days to readjust to a 6-hr shift in terms of psychomotor performance; none of the westbound travelers required more than six days. As Weitzman *et al.* (1981) pointed out, this suggests that some individuals may have relatively less ability to phase-advance, a topic discussed in the later section on the phase lag syndrome. There is also probably a limit to the ability of most individuals to acutely phase-advance, perhaps in the area of 6–8 hr. Mills, Minors, and Waterhouse (1978) found that when subjects were experimentally given sleep–wake periods that were phase-advanced by 8 hr, most subjects ultimately achieved this schedule by phase delaying themselves 16 hr.

It should be pointed out that travel can, of course, cause sleepiness for a variety of other reasons, which may include sleep loss and changes in diet. A vivid example of the latter is presented by Price and Holley (1982) in their description of the work conditions of the crew of Flight 182, which collided with a light plane over San Diego in September, 1978. Their schedule indicates that, cumulatively, they had had a deficit of 8 hr of sleep over the previous three days and that they were sometimes unable to find meals at the hours they had available for eating. In thinking about performance and sleepiness during and after trips, it is useful to separate these problems from the discomfort arising from desynchronization of endogenous rhythms with the environment, which can occur during transmeridian flights in the absence of any sleep loss. Another possible contribution is the effects of internal desynchronization, which in principle could be the result of different rhythms becoming entrained to the new environment at different rates.

There appears to be a great deal of individual difference in the ability to readjust to new time zones. Aschoff (1978) has suggested that individuals with the least amplitude of various rhythms can shift more easily, a notion supported by studies of Reinberg *et al.* (1978,a,b). Several authors have suggested that increasing the strength of environmental cues may help readjustment (Vernikos-Danellis and Winget, 1979). Many persons also take hypnotics in this situation, a topic that will be covered later in this chapter.

Work Shift Change

Perhaps 20% of workers in industrialized countries are engaged in shift work (Maurice, 1975). The clear benefits to society of providing production and services around the clock are tempered by the variety of stresses shift work places on the individual. Rotating shift workers tend to consult physicians, develop serious illness, and require hospitalization more frequently compared to fixed schedule workers (Khaleque and Rahman, 1982). We will only address one facet of this problem—the reciprocal relationship between altered work hours and altered sleep. Other areas include decrements in performance during shift work, as well as personal and domestic difficulties. In terms of the latter, Presser and Cain (1983) found that 30% of American dual-income nonfarm families have at least one spouse working on shifts. In 10% of these families, the other spouse worked entirely different shifts.

As Akerstedt (1984) pointed out, shift work is a general term for at least four types of schedules: "permanent night work, 3-shift work (regular alternation between thirds of the 24 hours), roster work (less regular and less strict 24 hour coverage) and irregular work hours." In the ASDC (1979) nosology, occasional, intermittent alterations of schedule are considered a transient work shift change in a conventional sleep–wake schedule. This is phenomenologically similar to jet lag. Once again, the endogenous rhythms of an individual are out of phase with the environment; the difference is that, in this case, it is the result of a sudden change in the schedule, rather than in the environment. In contrast, continuously rotating shift work is considered a persistent, frequently changing sleep–wake schedule (ASDC, 1979) and will be discussed in the next section.

Persistent Disturbance

Delayed Sleep Phase Syndrome ("Phase Lag Syndrome")

The phase lag syndrome may be the most common problem of the sleep–wake schedule in patients seen at sleep disorder centers (Fig. 10-4). Patients with this disorder have a characteristic history, the primary element of which is a chronic inability to fall asleep at conventional bedtimes. This will often have gone on for months or years. Typically, these patients can only sleep when they go to bed at 2:00–6:00 AM (Weitzman et al., 1981). Once sleep occurs, it is felt to be sound. Although the initial complaint is often insomnia, they have great difficulty awakening early in the morning and often seek medical help because of problems in reporting to work or to school on time. Often the cumulative sleep loss also results in a complaint of excessive daytime sleepiness. On weekends or vacation they will sleep for a normal sleep length (usually well into the morning) before awakening. In an effort to deal with this, they will often have taken hypnotics or alcohol,

Disorders of the Sleep-Wake Schedule (DOSWS)				
Diagnosis	N	% DOSWS	Range/Center, %	% Total
Delayed sleep phase syndrome	45	39.1	0-100	1.2
Irregular sleep-wake pattern	32	27.8	0-100	0.8
Not otherwise specified	13	11.3	0-50.0	0.3
Advanced sleep phase syndrome	10	8.7	0-40.0	0.3
Work shift, transient	6	5.2	0-37.5	0.2
Frequently changing SWS	5	4.3	0-50.0	0.1
Jet lag	2	1.7	0-50.0	0.0
Non-24-hr SWS syndrome	2	1.7	0-3.8	0.0
Total	115	99.8	. . .	2.9

FIGURE 10-4. Diagnoses among patients with disorders of the sleep–wake schedule. These data are taken from a multicenter study of 5000 patients. (From Coleman et al., 1982. Reproduced by permission.)

sometimes to the point of abuse. Hence the recognition of this syndrome may be complicated by superimposed alcohol or drug problems.

Patients with the phase lag syndrome often describe themselves as "night people," and usually have scores that confirm this on such tests as the Horne-Ostberg (1976). Speaking more anecdotally, this author finds that, if asked, they will often say that there have been periods in their lives when they were allowed to stay up late and sleep into the morning, during which they functioned well. This may have been in college, or when working an evening shift job. Again anecdotally, one has the impression that many drift into careers that allow them to work and sleep at unusual hours, for instance, as computer programmers who can come and go to a 24-hr computer facility as they choose.

The phase lag syndrome is thought to be the result of a sleep–wake cycle that is phase-delayed with respect to the usual *zeitgebers*. This represents movement in the direction of the "natural" activity rhythm of 25 hr, and hence may be the result of a partial failure of the normal entrainment mechanism. The end result is a delayed but stable relationship to the usual environmental cues of day and night.

This proposed pathophysiology of the phase lag syndrome may be expressed in terms of the phase–response curve (PRC). The PRC is a measure used primarily with plants and small animals so far, in which it is determined whether nonentrained subjects can be entrained by stimuli given at various periods. The range of periods over which a subject can be entrained is known as the range of entrainment (ROE). It has been postulated that patients with phase lag syndrome have a very narrow ROE, which may be primarily limited to periods equal or greater than 24 hr (Weitzman *et al.*, 1981). In theory, this could be the result either of a very low amplitude of response in the "advance" portion of the PRC, or of an unusually long normal endogenous period (Czeisler *et al.*, 1981a,b). Regardless of the mechanism, the consequence is a very poor ability to phase-advance each day, resulting in a delayed sleep–wake rhythm.

Czeisler *et al.* (1981a) proposed treating the phase lag syndrome with chronotherapy, in which patients go to bed three hours later each night. Eventually they move around the clock to more conventional bedtimes. Rearrangement of sleep by delaying, rather than advancing, takes advantage of the natural circadian drift. Czeisler *et al.* (1981a) presented data on five patients who were successfully treated in this manner, with an average follow-up of 260 days. Once on the new schedule, the patient needs to rigorously maintain it; the clinical impression is that staying up unusually late for a few nights will allow a phase delay to reoccur.

A final, tantalizing issue is whether the phase lag syndrome is associated with psychiatric illness. Weitzman *et al.* (1981) did not find this to be the case and also made the point that the frequently observed ruminations of the insomniac could be the consequence, rather than the cause, of poor sleep. This author has had the impression that many if not most of these patients have histories of depression or character disorder, and recommends that this issue be considered unsettled until further case series have been performed.

Non-24-Hr Sleep–Wake Syndrome

In this disorder the patient's inherent sleep rhythm is incrementally delayed each day relative to generally accepted sleep times. Clinically this is sometimes described as going to bed later and later each night; the patient will then often try to go to bed at a more usual bedtime and be unable to sleep for several hours. As in the phase lag syndrome, there is often an attempt to deal with this with drugs or alcohol, which may secondarily complicate the clinical picture. It is thought that this disorder results from the sleep–wake cycle operating at a period of more than 24 hr, often approaching 25 hr. This may result from a relatively complete inability to phase-advance each day in response to environmental cues. In a sense, it is the end of a continuum of ability to be synchronized by environmental cues: On one end is the normal situation, in which one is phase-advanced daily in response to *zeitgebers*; in the middle is phase lag syndrome, in which there is a partial response to *zeitgebers* so that there is a delayed but stable relation to the environment; at the far extreme is this syndrome, in which the sleep–wake cycle is not responsive to *zeitgebers* and is apparently free-running.

If the patient develops a life-style in which he goes to bed during his progressively cycling sleep times, the situation is usually very recognizable. Many patients try to maintain normal hours, and, hence complain of both insomnia and daytime sleepiness. One helpful part of the history is that every few weeks their sleep improves greatly, as their endogenous rhythm temporarily synchronizes with the environment. Not surprisingly, there is some suggestion that persons who are blind may be particularly vulnerable to developing this problem (Miles, Raynal, and Wilson, 1977).

Frequently Changing Sleep–Wake Schedule

In this disorder, the sleep schedule is repetitively altered as the result of such situations as frequent travel across time zones, permanently rotating shift work, or the unusual hours of a disco afficionado. The usual clinical picture is often a combination of insomnia as well as daytime sleepiness, even at times when there is a return to more conventional hours. Often the sufferer resorts to hypnotics or alcohol, which can superimpose difficulties on those already present. There may also be a "shift maladaption syndrome," including not only sleep difficulties but also gastrointestinal and cardiovascular pathology (Moore-Ede and Richardson, 1985).

Not surprisingly, a number of studies have documented that subjective distress is higher after shift work than after a regular day schedule. Tepas, Walsh, and Armstrong (1981), for instance, found that permanent night workers and rotating workers reported decreased total sleep and a higher incidence of sleep difficulty. The permanent night workers and rotators who complained of poor sleep had shorter reported total sleep than workers on the same schedule who did not experience discomfort. Among the permanent day and evening shift workers, there was no difference in reported sleep time between those who did and did not describe disturbed sleep.

Several studies have examined polygraphically monitored sleep during shift work (Foret and Lantin, 1972; Tilley *et al.*, 1982; Dahlgren, 1981; Torsvall, Akerstedt, and Gillberg, 1981; Foret and Benoit, 1978; Webb, 1983). The general findings have been similar, with decreased total sleep after the three successive shifts (Table 10-1; Fig. 10-5). In the Torsvall study, for example, total sleep time after the day shift was 8.0 hr, dropping to 4.3 hr after the night shift. During the day sleep after

TABLE 10-1. Sleep Studies of Shift Work[a]

References	TST	SWS	REM	RL	SL	Comparisons among types of workers
Foret and Lantin, 1972	↓ in AM	NC	↑ in AM	Not listed	Not listed	Engineers / Very irregular hours, comparison of three shifts
Torsvall et al., 1981	Dependent on bedtime; ↓ in AM	NC	↓ in AM	NC	↓ in day sleep	Engineers / Very irregular hours, comparison of three shifts in same group
Dahlgren, 1981	↓ in rotators	NC (SWS %)	↑ (%) in rotators	↓ in rotators	NC	Newspaper workers / Morning study in rotators vs. permanent night shift
Tilley et al., 1982	↓ in AM	↓ in day sleep	NC	Not listed	NC	Industrial workers / Weekly alternating three-shift system
Matsumato, Sasagawa, and Kawamori, 1978	↓ in AM	NC	NC	↓ in day sleep	NC	Nurses / Day sleep vs. night sleep
Foret and Benoit, 1978	↓ in AM	↓ in day sleep	NC	Not listed	Not listed	Research center workers / Day sleep vs. night sleep
Webb, 1983	Not listed	NC	NC	↓ in day sleep	↓ in day sleep	Nurses / Night shift vs. controls
Walsh, Tepas, and Moss, 1981	↓ in AM sleep	NC (↓% in day sleep)	→	→	→	Workers recruited through labor unions / Comparison of regular day, regular night, and rotating workers (studied at night); more complained of poor sleep

[a]Key: NC, no change; TST, total sleep time; SWS, slow-wave sleep; REM, rapid eye movement; RL, REM latency; SL, sleep latency.

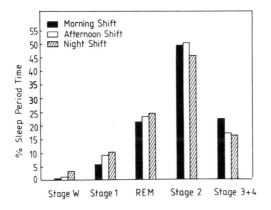

FIGURE 10-5. Sleep in 12 male shift workers operating on a weekly, rotating three-shift system. (From Tilley *et al.*, 1982. Reproduced by permission.)

the night shift, total slow–wave sleep was usually reported as unchanged or decreased, but the total minutes of REM tended to be reported as unchanged. In terms of sleep stage distribution, there was also a tendency for REM sleep and slow-wave sleep to become more even across the night. One reflection of this is the frequent finding of decreased REM latency.

Walsh, Tepas, and Moss (1981), who found that night workers had decreased total sleep, REM sleep, and shorter REM latency, commented that the changes were similar to those seen after chronic partial sleep deprivation (Mullaney *et al.*, 1977; Webb and Agnew, 1974). This suggests that night workers live in a chronic condition of partial sleep deprivation. Tune (1969a), however, observed that cumulative total sleep over the entire sleep cycle may not be reduced compared to that of day workers, presumably because of napping and longer sleep times on days off. It is possible that total cumulative sleep obtained in this manner may have a different physiological meaning than sleep that contains the same number of total hours of sleep but with more continuity.

One serious question from the point of view of public health is whether a career of shift work might leave a permanent imprint on a worker's sleep. There is so far little evidence to suggest this. Walsh, Tepas, and Moss (1981), who were admittedly studying workers who did not complain of sleep difficulty, found no difference in the sleep of rotators recorded at night compared to day workers. Similarly, Webb (1983) found little difference in the nighttime sleep of nurses with a history of nightwork compared to non-shift work women.

There has been a number of strategies for dealing with shift work. Tepas (1982) pointed out that these tend to be divided into two basic orientations: The "endogenous approach" seeks to change or maintain biological rhythms, implying that full adaptation with normal sleep is indeed possible; the "exogenous approach" is aimed at reducing deficits, suggesting that complete adaptation may not be feasible. Czeisler, Moore-Ede, and Coleman (1982), drawing upon principles from circadian rhythm research, devised a program for shift workers that was successfully applied at a potash plant in Utah. Before the schedule was rearranged, workers were changed weekly in a phase-advancing direction (night shift to swing shift to day shift). As part of the study, two groups of workers were placed on schedules in which they moved in the direction of phase delay, either weekly or every 21 days. In the latter group, complaints about the schedule dropped from 90% to 20%. There was an improvement in a measure of health, a decrease in job turnover, and increased productivity.

As Czeisler *et al.* (1982) have pointed out, other strategies for dealing with shift work in the past have included keeping workers in permanent shifts. The difficulty is usually one of finding personnel for the night shift, as well as the discomfort they experience when they keep more conventional hours on their days off. Another technique is a rapid rotation of shifts to avoid partial adaptation, although there is some evidence that this may still occur. Other strategies involve selecting workers with the greatest tolerance for rapidly changing schedules. An interesting approach was suggested by Kogi (1982), who showed that naps taken around midnight or the early morning hours helped reduce nighttime fatigue.

Irregular Sleep–Wake Pattern

This, too, is a problem of mixed insomnia and daytime sleepiness in a person in whom the structure of day and night becomes disorganized and variable. Typically, this pattern occurs in elderly persons living alone and in bedridden and institutionalized individuals for whom there are little or no social constraints on being awake at night or sleeping by day. The problem of irregular sleep–wake patterns is phenomenologically similar to that in "frequently changing sleep–wake schedule." In the latter, however, there is more of a sense that the individual knowingly and voluntarily allows the multiple changes in his sleep and waking pattern. One possible useful distinction which by history helps separate these conditions from the more psychologically oriented forms of insomnia (e.g., persistent psychophysiological insomnia; see Chapter 12) is that often in the latter the patient is unable to nap. Treatment consists of following the principles of sleep hygiene (Chapter 12), with emphasis on regular sleep hours.

PHARMACOLOGY

It has long been known that time of administration may change the pharmacological effects of a variety of drugs. For example, the degree of cataleptic response to haloperidol in rats (Campbell and Baldessarini, 1982) and the lethal effect of ethanol in mice (Haus and Halberg, 1959) vary at different times of day. Conversely, the effects of drugs on circadian processes have also been examined. Two major areas of interest have been the use of hypnotics after acute time zone shifts and the effects of drugs on fundamental circadian rhythms in animals.

Use of Hypnotics in Acute Phase Shifts

It may be useful to think of two different issues here. One is the effects of hypnotics in aiding sleep at the new bedtime. The other is whether the prior use of hypnotic alters wakefulness and performance at the new waking time. In one of the early studies in this area, Pollack, McGregor, and Weitzman (1975) gave 30 mg of flurazepam to normal volunteers who had undergone an acute sleep–wake cycle reversal. This treatment did indeed improve polygraphic measures of daytime sleep in subjects who had been kept awake all night, but they reported as much sleepiness the following evening as the controls. Allnut and O'Conner (1971) examined the effects of 5 mg of nitrazepam and 100 mg of secobarbital on subjects who went to bed at 8:00 PM and arose at 3:00 AM, which simulated the effect of traveling eastward. They described improved sleep on drug nights, although sleep on placebo nights was experienced as "average." During the daytime, performance as a whole was not improved, and it actually declined in the signal detection test. Seidel et al. (1984) observed normal volunteers who had undergone an acute phase delay of 12 hr and had then been given a placebo or one of two hypnotics. Under these conditions, subjects receiving the placebo had a marked reduction in total sleep and stage 2 and an increase in wake time at the end of the sleep period. This sleep loss was prevented by 30 mg of flurazepam or 0.5 mg of triazolam. Studies of the multiple sleep latency test (MSLT) at the new waking time (evening) showed enhanced sleepiness in placebo subjects, a marked increase in sleepiness in the flurazepam subjects, and no

312   CHAPTER TEN

change in the triazolam subjects. It should be noted that the marked sleepiness with flurazepam followed a period of relatively efficient sleep. Various performance measures worsened in the new waking period after placebo (vigilance reaction time) or flurazepam (vigilance visual tracking and digital symbol substitution), but remained the same or improved with triazolam administration. In contrast to these differences in objective performance tests, all groups had similar subjective responses, primarily sleepiness and mood disturbances. Bonnet *et al.* (1986) examined the effects of placebo and three doses of triazolam on volunteers who had undergone an acute 12-hr phase shift. During the night (the new ''subjective daytime''), MSLT scores showed enhanced wakefulness, and performance was improved on the Wilkinson vigilance test. In general, performance and alertness were best after a dose of 0.25 mg of triazolam. Nicholson *et al.* (1986) found that 0.25 mg of brotizolam improved some measures of sleep on the first night after westward trans-Atlantic flight. It was not possible to identify a drug effect on the second night, since sleep in the placebo condition returned to preflight values. After eastward flight, there was a modest improvement in waking time on the second, but not the first or the third, night.

In one of the few studies of a hypnotic given during persistent schedule shifts, Walsh, Muehlbach, and Schweitzer (1984) gave 0.5 mg of triazolam to 10 rotating shift workers during the first several mornings of the night shift. During the first two mornings, triazolam increased total sleep and sleep efficiency; for the subsequent two mornings, when no drug was given, there was no evidence of increased adaptation to the new schedule. No adaptation was seen in subjects given placebo for two days followed by two more days of recording. Hence, triazolam was observed to improve sleep when it was given under these conditions, but it did not seem to improve adaptation to a new schedule.

Circadian Rhythm Alteration by Drugs

Several compounds have been reported to alter circadian rhythmicity. Cahill and Ehret (1982), for instance, found that in the rat AMPT, which inhibits dopamine and norepinephrine synthesis (Chapter 2), shifted the acrophase of the temperature rhythm either earlier or later depending on the time of injection. Inhibition of norepinephrine synthesis in the early evening (when turnover was maximal) produced the greatest degree of phase advance, which suggests that this is the mechanism of action. In other rodent studies, various rhythmic processes were altered by pentobarbital and theophylline (Ehret, Potter, and Dobra, 1975), parachlorophenylalanine (Honma, Kenji, and Hiroshiga, 1979), dexamethasone (Horseman, Meinart, and Ehret, 1979), lithium (Kripke and Wyborney, 1980), clorgyline (Tamarkin et al., 1983), imipramine (Wirz-Justice et al., 1980a,b), and triazolam (Turek and Losee-Olson, 1986). Caffeine (Mayer and Scherer, 1975) and forskolin (Eskin and Takahashi, 1983) may alter rhythmicity in invertebrates, as may prednisone (Reindl et al., 1969) in humans.

In addition to directly altering rhythmicity, pharmacological agents may also affect the entraining effects of light. Ralph and Menaker (1985), for instance, found that in hamsters the GABA antagonist bicuculline may prevent phase delays normally induced by light pulses late in the subjective night, suggesting that the effects of light may be mediated by different pathways at different times.

Many of these observations may have relevance to human disorders. It has been speculated that alteration of circadian rhythms by antidepressants may be crucial to their therapeutic effects (Wirz-Justice et al., 1980b; see Chapter 9). Ehret, Groh, and Meinert (1980) used the possible clock-setting qualities of caffeine to devise schedules of eating and coffee consumption to potentially help treat jet lag. As mentioned earlier, an animal study found that the hypnotic triazolam (Chapter 3) may cause phase shifts that depend on time of administration (Turek and Losee-Olson, 1986). This might reasonably lead to human studies to determine if the judicious administration of hypnotics at specified hours would be useful for jet lag.

SUMMARY

Human physiology includes many rhythmic processes with periods that range from fractions of a second to years. The organization of many circadian rhythms is centered around the suprachiasmatic nucleus of the hypothalamus, which receives input from the retina and a variety of other sites throughout the central nervous system. A number of models have been designed to explain the rhythmic aspects of sleep and other behaviors. These include the one-oscillator, two-oscillator, and the two-process models. Several clinical sleep disorders can best be understood in terms of disrupted circadian rhythm processes. Transient disorders include jet lag and work shift change. Among persistent difficulties are the delayed sleep phase syndrome, non-24–hr sleep-wake syndrome, frequently changing sleep–wake schedule, and irregular sleep–wake pattern.

The interaction of drugs and circadian rhythms is a promising area of investigation. It has long been known that a number of agents have different effects when given at different times. Evidence is accumulating that short-acting benzodiazepines may be beneficial in clinical studies of acute phase shifts. In animal studies, a number of drugs alter circadian rhythms, and one hopes that these observations will lead to clinical applications.

CHAPTER 11

Nocturnal Myoclonus and the Restless Legs Syndrome

NOCTURNAL MYOCLONUS

Like sleep apnea, nocturnal myoclonus is a good example of abnormal processes appearing during sleep in the absence of obvious pathophysiology in the waking state. After the description by Sir Charles Symonds (1953) of patients who made kicking movements during sleep, case reports with polygraphic monitoring began to appear. By the 1970s, a syndrome of clonic leg movements as a cause of insomnia was recognized (Guilleminault et al., 1975a). These movements most typically involve dorsiflexion of the ankle, as well as fanning and dorsiflexion of the small toes and big toe; this may be followed by flexion of the knee and the hip (Smith, 1985). These events tend to occur in stage 2 sleep (Reimao, Lemmi, and Belluomini, 1984); they are detected on the anterior tibialis electromyogram (EMG), where they last 0.5–10 sec each, and appear at intervals of 20–40 sec (Fig. 11-1). These periodic leg movements (PLMs) are usually isolated movements of the lower limb and should be distinguished from movement arousals, in which anterior tibialis EMG activity is accompanied by the appearance of EMG activity or amplifier blocking artifacts on electrooculogram (EOG) or EEG channels (Rechtschaffen and Kales, 1968). It seems likely that the clinically significant movements are those that are followed by EEG evidence of arousal (alpha activity or a K complex). Presumably, these frequent interruptions of sleep continuity produce symptoms of insomnia or excessive daytime sleepiness.

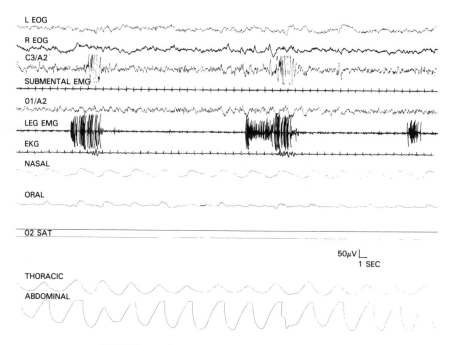

FIGURE 11-1. Recordings of periodic leg movements.

The ASDC (1979) nosology specifies that a formal diagnosis of nocturnal myoclonus requires three periods during the night, lasting from a few minutes to an hour or more, each containing at least 30 movements followed by partial arousal or awakening (ASDC, 1979). Alternative definitions have been listed by Kripke, Ancoli-Israel, and Okudaira (1982). One often seen is that there be more than five movements per hour. It has also been suggested that patients with this disorder segregate into those with relatively "solid" episodes of movements and those with a greater number of more "fragmented" episodes (Shafor *et al.*, 1986). Definitions of individual movement events also differ: Hartman and Scrima (1986), for instance, studied "arousals associated with muscle activity in the legs" that did not meet the formal standard criteria for repetitiveness or duration. When reading articles on the subject, it is important to determine whether the presence of EEG arousals following movements is required before the movements are counted, as those without EEG changes are often more frequent and possibly of less significance clinically.

Prevalence

Among patients seen in sleep disorder centers, nocturnal myoclonus and restless legs syndrome (RLS) may occur in 12.2% of patients complaining of insomnia and 3.5% of those with excessive daytime sleepiness (Coleman et al., 1982). Myoclonus is more prevalent in elderly patients complaining of sleep difficulties, where it has been found in 23% (Roehrs et al., 1983b) to 30% (Ancoli-Israel et al., 1981). A number of patients with narcolepsy are found to have significant numbers of periodic leg movements. The prevalence in the general population is uncertain. In a study of 100 persons with no sleep complaints, 5% were reported to have three periods of at least 30 movements accompanied by arousals (Bixler et al., 1982b). There is no known association with depression; in a study of 86 depressed inpatients, only one was found to have myoclonus (Reynolds et al., 1982).

Relation to Sleep Disturbance

Nocturnal myoclonus may present as insomnia or as excessive daytime sleepiness. There is some evidence that patients who complain of insomnia have more PLMs and sleep disruption (Saskin, Moldofsky, and Lue, 1985). In many cases, the patient will be unaware of the clonic movements but rather will describe sleep as disturbed and not restful.

The role of myoclonic movements in sleep disturbances has been the subject of some debate. As mentioned above, PLMs are found in normal volunteers, which has led some authors to question whether they do in fact induce a sense of poor sleep. Moreover, Coleman, Pollak, and Weitzman (1980) found that the prevalence of nocturnal myoclonus was no higher among insomniac patients than among those with syndromes of excessive daytime sleepiness or other sleep–wake disorders. This raised the possibility that in addition to being the cause of subjectively poor sleep, myoclonus may also be a nonspecific response to sleep disturbed by a variety of processes. However, the definition of nocturnal myoclonus used in this study was 40 movements, and it is not known if this same finding would be evident with stricter criteria. Hartman and Scrima (1986), who also used a less strict definition of movement events, did not find a higher prevalence of movements in sleep apneic patients, which argues against the notion that they represent a nonspecific response to sleep disruption.

Certain patient groups are also more likely to have PLMs. Leg movements during sleep are more common in narcoleptics than controls (Hartman and Scrima, 1986), and myoclonus may appear with uremia and other metabolic disorders. Leukemic children who had previously received both radiation and methotrexate may have more periodic leg movements than controls (Kotagal et al., 1985). Myoclonic movements may also appear during the sleep of newborns and infants (in whom a Babinski sign may normally be present) and then disappear in the first few months of life (Blennow, 1985). The physiology under-lying such movements (either spontaneous or under these pathological conditions) is unknown. Smith (1985) has commented on the similarity of these movements to the Babinski sign (which may occur normally during non-REM sleep) and suggests that they are the result of a loss of supraspinal inhibition of movement.

Drugs Associated with Myoclonus

Nocturnal myoclonus may appear during anticonvulsant and hyp-notic withdrawal. There is some evidence that tricyclic antidepressants may cause or exacerbate myoclonic movements, although Coleman (1979) did not find their use more common than other classes of medi-cation in a review of 53 patients. One case history suggested that lithium may induce nocturnal myoclonus and restless legs syndrome (Heiman and Christie, 1986). Several cases of myoclonus, hyper-reflexia, and diaphoresis have been reported in depressed patients in whom L-tryptophan was given in combination with phenelzine (Levy, Bucher, and Votolato, 1985). Ethanol may not alter the number of movements, but doses above 0.4 g/kg may decrease the number of as-sociated arousals (Scrima et al., 1986).

Differential Diagnosis

A number of other conditions leading to abnormal motor activity in bed should be kept in mind (Bamford, Snider, and Beutler, 1983). Noc-turnal myoclonus, in which clinical EEGs have shown no evidence of spiking, should be distinguished from myoclonic and other types of seizures occurring during sleep. In partial complex seizures, spiking ac-tivity is often brought out during drowsiness and sleep. If the patient awakens, the history will be similar to that for episodes during waking, including an aura, confusion, and possible automatic behavior. Gener-alized seizures are often heard by other family members; the patient may also awaken later with headache, injury to the tongue, or evi-dence of soiling. Paraplegic patients may develop flexor spasms, espe-cially at night. Cramps or painful contractions of the calves may occur on the night following exercise. This is often a normal condition but may also appear in spinal cord disease, hypothyroidism, hypocalcemia, and other conditions. Movements that are the result of basal ganglia disorders usually disappear during sleep, but if patients awaken and then have movements the history may resemble that of nocturnal myoclonus. Hypnogogic myoclonic jerks may also appear in parkinsonian patients started on L-DOPA (see Chapter 2). Palatal myoclonus was originally thought to occur in sleep as well as wakefulness, but later evidence suggests that it tends to disappear during sleep (Montagna, Cirignotta, and Lugaresi, 1983). Nocturnal myoclonus should be distinguished from hypnic jerks, a normal phenomenon of generalized movements that may occur at sleep onset. There is also a syndrome of brief (<150 msec) myoclonic movements in non-REM sleep, which may be seen in patients with sleep-related respiratory disorders, narcolepsy, and other disorders (Broughton, Tolentino, and Krelina, 1985).

Treatment

A variety of agents, including some hypnotics, muscle relaxants, and 5-hydroxytryptophan, have been given with little benefit (Dement, Holman, and Guilleminault, 1976). Perhaps the most widely recognized treatment is clonazepam (0.5–1.5 mg), although results have been variable. Only a few of 15 patients in a study at Stanford University reported clear benefits (Coleman, 1982). Coleman (1979) found that polygraphic measures improved in only one of three patients. Oshtory and Vijayan (1980), however, described successful treatment of two cases. Mitler et al. (1986b) found that 1 mg of clonazepam improved sleep without reducing the number of myoclonic movements.

The most common side effect of clonazepam is sleepiness. In those patients with concurrent myoclonus and sleep apnea, the possibility that clonazepam may exacerbate the disordered breathing events must be considered (see Chapter 6). It seems good practice to administer clonazepam initially to such patients under observation in the laboratory.

Some clinicians have the impression that short-acting benzodiazepines may be of benefit in nocturnal myoclonus; the only systematic data available are for 30 mg of temazepam, which was as effective as clonazepam (Mitler et al., 1986b). Baclofen (20–40 mg) has been reported to decrease such signs of arousal as alpha activity and K complexes in myoclonus. During non-REM sleep, it may increase the number of movements but decrease their amplitude (Fig. 11-2; Guilleminault and

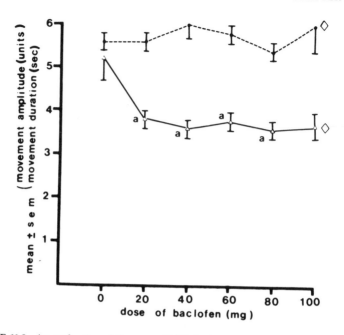

FIGURE 11-2. An evaluation of the mean EMG discharge obtained by monitoring the anterior tibialis muscle using surface electrodes. Duration (●) and amplitude (△) of the discharge were plotted separately. A diamond indicates that no statistical analysis was performed because the number of patients (three) receiving this size dose (100 mg) of baclofen was too small. Baclofen has an effect on the amplitude but not the duration of the discharge. a, A muscle discharge with an amplitude significantly less than at baseline (0); (From Guilleminault and Flagg, 1984. Reprinted by permission.)

Flagg, 1984). Nocturnal myoclonus appears to be exacerbated by anxiety, and it seems wise to look for ways to decrease stress in the patient's life.

RESTLESS LEGS SYNDROME

Clinical Features

Although described as early as the seventeenth century, modern interest in the restless legs syndrome comes from the work of Eckbom (1945). In this intriguing condition, patients report a dysesthesia of the legs, sometimes described as a creepy or prickly sensation, which occurs at rest (Frankel, Patten, and Gillin, 1974). It is relieved by movement. Since the sensation comes on when lying down at bedtime, it often results in difficulty going to sleep. Symptoms may become worse after sleep loss, or during pregnancy, and may actually get better with fever. It often occurs in uremia and may appear in 5 to 20% of dialysis patients (Read, Feest, and Nassim, 1981). As many as 15% of surgical outpatients may have the restless legs syndrome (Braude and Barnes, 1982). Prevalence is thought to increase with advancing age, although one case series found the dominant group among 174 patients to be middle-aged females (Telstad *et al.*, 1984). In the latter study, symptoms were worse among patients with lower hemoglobin concentrations, although the mean of the group was normal. Restless legs syndrome may also appear in iron deficiency anemia (Ekbom, 1975) and vitamin B12 deficiency (Lugaresi *et al.*, 1968b). In general, about one-third of patients may have a positive family history.

Nocturnal myoclonus patients occasionally have the restless leg syndrome; however, many or most patients with RLS also have myoclonic movements during sleep (e.g., Ambrosetto *et al.*, 1965). Aside from the frequently concurrent evidence of myoclonus, there are no definitive polygraphic findings in restless legs syndrome. Often, increased anterior tibialis EMG activity is seen before sleep onset.

Treatment

Opioids such as oxycodone are frequently used to treat the restless legs syndrome (Trzepacz, Violette, and Sateia, 1984), and it has been speculated that underactivity of the opioid system may be involved in its pathogenesis (Sandyk and Gillman, 1986). Trials with diazepam (Morgan, 1967) and clonazepam (Montagna *et al.*, 1984; Read *et al.*, 1981) have been favorable, and it has been suggested that alprazolam might be useful (Bee, 1985). In a large Norwegian study, both placebo and carbamazepine led to an improvement, but carbamazepine was significantly more effective than placebo (Telstad *et al.*, 1984).

The differential diagnosis for RLS should include leg cramps associated with iron or calcium deficiencies and drug-induced akathisia. Patients with fibrositis syndrome have musculoskeletal pain and areas of tenderness which are not relieved by movement. They often have alpha intrusions into non-REM sleep and myoclonus on polysomnography (Moldofsky *et al.*, 1984). Increased motor activity because of anxiety should also be considered. This is sometimes difficult, since many patients with RLS develop emotional complications, including anxiety and depressive symptomatology. These need to be addressed in any treatment plan.

SUMMARY

Nocturnal myoclonus is characterized by repetitive movements of the legs, including dorsiflexion of the ankle and toes and flexion of the knee and hip. These movements are accompanied by brief EEG arousals. Clinically, nocturnal myoclonus may result in either insomnia or excessive sleepiness. Often the patient is unaware of movements during sleep, and the neurological examination while awake is normal. Some periodic leg movements may appear in asymptomatic persons; it is not understood how they differ from those who experience poor sleep. The observation of frequent periodic leg movements in other conditions such as narcolepsy has led some researchers to argue that, in addition to causing a sleep disorder, myoclonic movements may be a consequence of other sleep disturbances. Such movements may also be induced or exacerbated by withdrawal of anticonvulsants or hypnotics and, possibly, by administration of tricyclic antidepressants or lithium. Treatment with clonazepam and short-acting benzodiazepines may be of some benefit.

Restless legs syndrome is a dysesthesia of the legs that occurs at rest and is relieved by movement. Its incidence increases in uremia and in iron or vitamin B12 deficiency anemias. Many restless leg syndrome patients also have nocturnal myoclonus. There are no definitive polygraphic signs, aside from possibly increased anterior tibialis EMG activity before sleep onset. Some relief may come from the use of oxycodone, benzodiazepines, and possibly carbamazepine.

CHAPTER 12

Chronic Insomnia

Approximately one-third of all Americans report difficulty falling asleep or maintaining sleep, and perhaps one-half of these unhappy persons consider this to be a major problem in their lives (Mellinger and Balter, 1983). The general approach of this book has been to emphasize that the complaint of chronic poor sleep is often the expression of underlying pathophysiology (e.g., sleep apnea or nocturnal myoclonus) of which the patient is often unaware. In other cases, psychiatric disorders such as depressive illness are evident. In both of these conditions, a specific treatment is often available: for example, CPAP for sleep apnea or a tricyclic antidepressant for an affective disorder. In addition to these situations perhaps one-quarter of all patients seen for insomnia in sleep disorder centers have difficulties that are currently described primarily in psychological terms: persistent psychophysiological DIMS (disorder of initiating and maintaining sleep, or insomnia) and subjective DIMS complaint without objective findings (Coleman *et al.*, 1982). In this chapter, we will describe these conditions and present some tantalizing findings that suggest their etiology. The use of hypnotics to treat insomnia has been discussed in Chapter 3; here we will present some nonpharmacological approaches.

PERSISTENT PSYCHOPHYSIOLOGICAL DIMS

In this disorder, the act of trying to go to sleep, or the setting in which it occurs, induces a conditioned arousal response. The classic history of such a patient—which is rarely evident at the first interview—

is that at some time in the past he experienced a traumatic event in his personal or professional life that might be expected to have briefly disturbed sleep. Instead of dwelling on the trauma, however, he focused attention on the resultant sleep difficulty. Eventually, the concern about the original upset is healed, but worry about being able to sleep has taken on a life of its own, which perpetuates the sleep disturbance. Often the bedroom itself can trigger anxiety about sleeping. Thus in response to questioning the patient will say that he sleeps better away from home. Similarly, he will report that he can easily fall asleep when he is not trying to—when watching television, for example—but is unable to sleep when he later goes to bed. The history is often confused by the previous use of hypnotics. In some ways, persistent psychophysiological DIMS is the equivalent among sleep disorders of the conditioned negative reactions seen in many fields of medicine. Patients who have been successfully treated with chemotherapy for Hodgkin's disease, for example, may develop nausea and other symptoms years later when going to their physician or when they are reminded of their previous illness (Cella, Pratt, and Holland, 1986).

In the laboratory, the patient with persistent psychophysiological DIMS often sleeps well—perhaps because he is away from home, perhaps because he is so sure that he will not sleep in this strange environment that he does not try. Whether he sleeps well or not, however, the subjective report of sleep the next morning will be in general agreement with the polygraphic findings.

SUBJECTIVE DIMS WITHOUT OBJECTIVE FINDINGS

The patient with this disorder complains of poor sleep; when studied in the laboratory the record is relatively normal or only mildly disturbed, yet the patient will insist that he slept very little and had a poor night. There is no major psychiatric diagnosis evident and one does not get a sense of hypochondriasis in the rest of his life. The patient may have used hypnotics extensively, and—as in all illnesses—some aspects of negative conditioning may secondarily occur. The cause of this disparity between subjective distress and objective findings is not clear. Some have suggested that it is the result of excessive mental activity during sleep, a poor sense of the passing of time, or a deficit in the ability to recognize one's state of consciousness. Alternatively, it may be that objective abnormalities are present but are too subtle to be seen in sleep studies as they are currently performed. Whatever its cause, this is the equivalent in sleep disorders of a problem seen in many areas of medicine. One is reminded, for instance, of patients who complain of dyspnea, but in whom complete pulmonary examinations and function tests are normal.

OTHER FORMS OF CHRONIC INSOMNIA

Although this chapter is oriented to a detailed discussion of persistent psychophysiological DIMS and subjective DIMS without objective findings, it is important to be aware of several other conditions associated with chronic poor sleep. Just as insomnia may be a complaint in major depressive disorder (Chapter 9) and schizophrenia, it may also appear in persons with excessive anxiety, obsessive-compulsive disorder, and personality disorders. In the Association of Sleep Disorder Centers nosology (1979), such persons are considered to have *DIMS with symptom and personality disorders*. In these conditions, the severity of the sleep disturbance often has a temporal association to the severity of the psychiatric symptomatology. In *childhood onset DIMS* there is a history of initial or maintenance insomnia going back to childhood. There is a lack of history of conditioning factors which can be found in persistent psychological DIMS, and there is no evidence of the psychopathology found in DIMS with symptom and personality disorders. Unlike the latter two conditions, poor sleep persists relatively unchanged during periods of high or low stress or anxiety.

All of the forms of insomnia we have discussed are chronic problems, and should be distinguished from *transient and situational DIMS*, which is related to an emotional situation or loss or unfamiliar sleep environment. By definition, such sleep disturbances last less than three weeks. Persons with chronic insomnia also should be distinguished from *natural short sleepers*, individuals whose total sleep is less than 75% of that which is typical for their age (see Chapter 1). The polysomnogram on natural short sleepers shows a normal sleep latency, few interruptions of sleep, and normal amounts of slow-wave sleep, although there may be less REM sleep. These persons apparently have less need for sleep than most of the population. Unlike insomniacs, they do not complain of daytime disturbances such as fatigue, irritability, or lack of concentration. Because they have often been led to believe that they should sleep more, they may have had unsuccessful attempts at longer sleep times. The "treatment" primarily is to explain that they are at one end of the continuum of normal need for sleep.

QUALITIES ASSOCIATED WITH INSOMNIA

In a number of studies, the complaint of insomnia is a special manifestation of personality or life-style qualities that are present 24 hr a day. One of the difficulties in interpretation, however, is that such studies were often done on "insomniacs" or "poor sleepers" without further diagnostic specificity. With this caveat in mind, however, they are still instructive in that they suggest some common qualities in patients with chronic poor sleep in whom obvious pathophysiology is not present.

Minnesota Multiphasic Personality Inventory (MMPI) tests have been performed on insomniacs for many years. Monroe (1967), in one of the earliest studies, examined volunteers classified as good and poor sleepers, although the latter had not specifically sought help for their difficulties. The poor sleepers were found to have higher scores on a variety of scales including F, depression, hypochondriasis, masculinity-femininity, paranoia, psychasthenia, schizophrenia, and social introversion. Studies in Los Angeles and Hershey found that 80 to 85% of insomniacs had an elevated score on at least one scale (Kales *et al.*, 1976b); a study in Durham found elevations in 63% (Edinger, Stout, and Hoelscher, 1986). Zorick *et al.* (1984a) reported that patients with persistent psychophysiological insomnia tended to have 2.1 elevations, while those with subjective DIMS without objective findings had a mean of 2.8 elevations.

It has often been noted that the three most common scale elevations are on depression, hysteria, and psychasthenia, but other studies reported increases across a broad range of seven scales (Kales *et al.*, 1978). Roth, Kramer, and Lutz (1976b) found the highest scores in the "neurotic triad" of depression, hypochondriasis, and hysteria and Coursey, Buchsbaum, and Frankel (1975) reported similar changes, as well as elevations of psychasthenia. Mendelson *et al.* (1984c) and Mendelson *et al.* (1986d) examined two groups of 10 insomniacs, and found that no group means on any scale were greater than 70 (the generally accepted threshold for pathology). Insomniacs, however, significantly differed from matched controls on several scales. In the former study, the insomniacs had higher values on the F, D, and SI scales and lower values on the K scale. This suggests a greater sense of distress, depression, and social introversion and less defensiveness about responses. In the latter study, insomniacs rated higher on the hysteria and psychopathic deviance scales (Fig. 12-1). Levin, Bertelson, and Lacks (1984) found that sleep-onset insomniacs had higher scores than normal subjects on a wide range of scales including hypochondriasis, depression, hysteria, psychopathic deviance, and psychasthenia. Interestingly, patients with more severe insomnia had higher scores on the paranoia scale than controls or more mild insomniacs. In a later study, Bertelson and Masch (1986) found that sleep-onset insomniacs

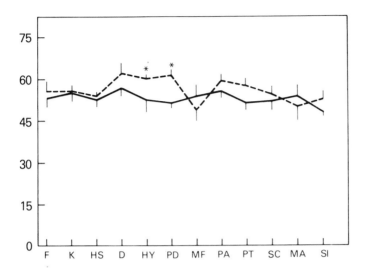

FIGURE 12-1. Mean MMPI scores for 10 insomniacs (– – –) and controls (———).
*Groups differ by $p<0.05$. (From Mendelson *et al.*, 1986. Reprinted by permission.)

had more psychopathology, as manifested by a greater number of elevated scales, than sleep-maintenance insomniacs. Thus, MMPI studies tend to indicate differences from normal, often involving the depression, hysteria, hypochondriasis, and psychasthenia scales, although without a clearly convincing pattern. With time, statistical clustering procedures (e.g., Edinger, Stout, and Hoelscher, 1986) may help clarify these findings.

Efforts to look for DSM-III-R diagnoses and personality traits have also been inconclusive. Tan *et al.* (1984) found that 92 of 100 patients complaining of insomnia had one or more axis I diagnoses. They concluded that the patients tended to internalize difficulties centered around anxiety, depression, obsessive-compulsiveness, phobias, and excessive somatic concerns. Marchini *et al.* (1983) examined qualities of life-style in good and poor sleepers. The poor sleepers seemed less busy and were less involved in their work and with other people. They tended to be more concerned about their immediate physical environment and to have more passive forms of entertainment. Obviously, insomniacs are a heterogeneous group, which makes these studies harder to interpret. It is also possible, of course, that the MMPI or personality qualities found in insomniacs are the result, rather than the cause, of poor sleep. As these problems continue to be explored, though, many investigators are left with a sense that certain personality and life-style qualities are somehow associated with chronic insomnia.

DAYTIME SLEEPINESS

It seems reasonable to suppose that the subjectively disturbed nocturnal sleep of insomnia might lead to daytime sleepiness. This has been examined using the multiple sleep latency test (MSLT), a measure of the tendency to go to sleep as assessed during four or five 20-min nap periods (see Chapter 7). Most studies have indicated, though, that both young and elderly insomniacs are no more sleepy than controls during the MSLT (Mendelson et al., 1984c, 1986d; Dement, Seidel, and Carskadon, 1982, 1984; Fig. 12-2). The lack of objective sleepiness in insomniacs might be interpreted several different ways. It might suggest that the actual sleep deficit of insomniacs is not as great as their subjective distress seems to indicate. If the discomfort of patients with "subjective DIMS without objective findings" is relatively greater than the polygraphically defined degree of sleep disturbance, it might not be surprising that they are not excessively sleepy by day. Alterna-

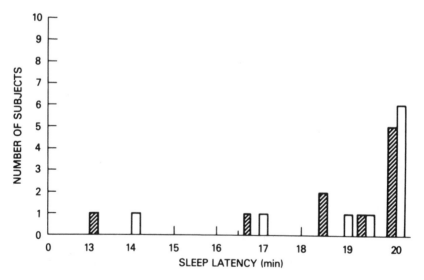

FIGURE 12-2. Mean sleep latency during multiple sleep latency test for 10 insomniacs (■) and controls (□). (From Mendelson et al., 1984c. Reprinted by permission.)

tively, the MSLT data suggest that insomniacs have trouble sleeping at any time, whether day or night.

Interruptions of nocturnal sleep may have different effects on daytime sleepiness in insomniacs, compared to normals or persons with sleep apnea or myoclonus. Stepanski et al. (1984) found that in normal subjects the number of arousals at night had little relationship to daytime sleepiness as measured by the MSLT. In sleep apnea and myoclonus, arousals correlated positively with sleepiness, as might be expected. In insomniacs, however, the number of arousals were negatively correlated with sleepiness.

DAYTIME PERFORMANCE

The ability of insomniacs to go about their daily waking lives is still poorly understood. Just as there is no difference in objectively measured sleepiness, it also appears there is no significant difference in amounts of motor activity when awake (Thoresen et al., 1981a). Church and Johnson (1979) found that poor sleepers did as well as control subjects on the 4-Choice Reaction Task and the Digit Symbol Substitution Task. Bonnet (1984) also found insomniacs and controls similar in baseline reaction time. Mendelson, Garnett, and Linnoila (1984d) found no difference in a wide variety of measures, including reaction time, continuous performance, and continuous tracking. There have, however, been reports of some deficits. Linnoila, Erwin, and Logue (1980), examining a group of insomniacs who had not been characterized by polysomnography, reported greater variability in performance measures over time and decrements in tracking and reaction time. Mendelson, Garnett, and Linnoila (1984d) noted that insomniacs had a greater degree of movement on the Romberg test. Sugarman, Stern, and Walsh (1984) found that patients with subjective insomnia had more misses on an auditory vigilance task than those with objectively disturbed sleep or normal controls. There are, then, several negative studies, and the few positive findings indicate that any of the deficits are subtle and inconsistent.

SLEEP STUDIES OF INSOMNIACS

The degree of alteration of objective sleep measures in insomniacs is also unclear. There have been many studies over the years, the earlier ones documented in detail by the Institute of Medicine (1979a).

Interpretation is difficult, however, because most studies were done on the basis of clinical history and without the benefit of polysomnography to rule out such illnesses as sleep apnea. The tendency has been to find small but significant evidence of sleep disturbance. Gillin *et al.* (1979), for instance, found that insomniacs differed from controls by having less total and delta sleep, lower sleep efficiency, and longer sleep latency. In studies in which polygraphic screening has been performed and age-matched normal controls are used, the differences become more subtle. Mendelson *et al.* (1984c) found that 10 insomniacs differed significantly from controls only in having more intermittent waking time and lower sleep efficiency (Table 12-1). In a later study, insomniacs differed from controls only in having more early morning awakening time, although there was a trend toward shorter sleep and lower sleep efficiency (Mendelson *et al.*, 1986d). In a study of 10 patients with persistent psychophysiological insomnia who were polygraphically screened, Reynolds *et al.* (1984a) reported that sleep efficiency was 81.5% and total sleep was 359.8 min. Although there was no normal comparison group, both values were only slightly lower than controls in the three previously mentioned studies. Carskadon *et al.* (1976) found the mean total sleep time in 122 insomniacs screened for apnea and myoclonus to be 375 min, and only 27 averaged less than 5.5 hr a night. The implication seems to be that, as with daytime performance, insomniacs have some deficits in polygraphically measured sleep but that these are relatively small. It is possible, of course, that electrophysiological disturbances are very much present but are too subtle, or of a different nature, than those that can be detected by current polygraphic techniques. It is easy to be left with the feeling, though, that the degree of distress experienced by insomniacs in these studies is out of proportion to the objectively measured sleep disturbance. This view has led to studies of the relation of subjective sleep reports to polygraphic measures.

THE SUBJECTIVE EXPERIENCE OF INSOMNIACS

One of the most complete studies of subjective reports of insomniacs was carried out by Carskadon *et al.* (1976), who examined 122 patients who had been screened to rule out sleep apnea and nocturnal myoclonus. The insomniacs overestimated the amount of time it took them to fall asleep and underestimated total sleep time. In view of the many MMPI studies showing elevations on the hypochondriasis scale, it might have been speculated that they tend to exaggerate all their

TABLE 12-1. Sleep Parameters in Chronic Insomniacs and Controls[a]

Sleep parameters	Insomniacs (n = 10)		Controls (n = 10)		t test
	Mean	SD	Mean	SD	
Total sleep (min)	364.70	103.02	389.82	34.55	NS
Sleep latency	46.27	40.08	25.90	11.79	NS
REM latency	86.67	40.04	84.45	19.85	NS
Total REM (min)	94.65	36.18	97.22	17.99	NS
Intermittent waking time	47.87	24.00	25.85	19.04	$p < 0.05$
Total recording time	467.45	123.77	450.87	36.85	NS
Sleep efficiency (%)	77.60	11.62	86.34	4.36	$p < 0.05$
REM (%)	24.89	4.48	24.92	3.63	NS
REM density	1.39	0.43	1.38	0.33	NS
REM index	121.40	71.91	102.70	26.56	NS
Non-REM	270.05	70.69	292.57	28.22	NS
Stage 1 (min)	17.45	11.25	11.45	9.95	NS
Stage 1 (%)	4.48	2.95	2.86	2.44	NS
Stage 2 (min)	195.47	62.17	220.65	33.48	NS
Stage 2 (%)	53.34	7.32	56.29	5.16	NS
Stage 3 (min)	21.05	9.64	24.17	10.58	NS
Stage 3 (%)	6.16	2.68	6.31	2.73	NS
Stage 4 (min)	36.07	21.61	36.30	16.44	NS
Stage 4 (%)	11.08	7.79	9.57	4.27	NS
Delta (min)	57.12	18.43	60.45	16.20	NS
Delta (%)	17.26	7.32	15.90	4.22	NS
EMA[b] (min)	12.25	13.74	9.30	11.55	NS

(From Mendelson et al., 1984c. Reprinted by permission.)
[a]All values except percentages refer to mean ± SD minutes.
[b]Early morning awakening time.

sleep disturbances. This was not the case, however, as they actually underestimated the number of awakenings during the night.

One explanation of the inaccuracy of insomniacs in reporting total sleep and sleep latency might be that they somehow misperceive their own state of consciousness. Several reports indicate that this might be the case. In a classic study, Rechtschaffen (1968) awakened 16 good and 16 poor sleepers 10 min after the first sleep spindle and asked them what they had been experiencing. Out of 22 such forced awakenings, six poor sleepers but only one good sleeper reported that they had already been awake. Similar results were found in two insomniacs studied by Engle-Friedman, Baker, and Bootzin (1985). Mendelson *et al*. (1984c) did not find this phenomenon when insomniacs were abruptly awakened by a loud (80 dB) tone but did observe it when a gradually louder tone was employed as part of an arousal threshold study (Mendelson *et al*., 1986d). In the latter case, insomniacs reported that they had been awake more often than controls at forced awakenings 5 min after the lights were turned out, 10 min after sleep onset, 5 min after the beginning of the first REM period, and during movement time. Although the insomniacs went back to sleep as quickly as the controls, and had the same amount of polygraphically defined sleep between the forced awakenings, they reported that they had been asleep only half as long. These findings suggest that insomniacs may suffer from some form of impairment in recognizing or remembering their state of consciousness.

Since many insomniacs get relief—in the short-term—from hypnotics, one might ask if these agents alter their perception of state of consciousness. Mendelson *et al*. (1987g) gave 10 chronic insomniacs 30 mg of flurazepam and placebo, and then awakened them 10 min after the first sleep spindle to ask if they believed that they had been awake or asleep. It was found that on flurazepam nights patients tended to be less likely to report that they had been awake, compared to placebo nights. Thus even when the EEG sleep stage is held constant, flurazepam tended to alter the insomniac's beliefs about their sleep. This raises the interesting possibility that in addition to enhancing polygraphically defined sleep, hypnotics may achieve therapeutic effects by altering perceptual or cognitive processes.

IS POOR SLEEP THE SAME AS "LIGHT" SLEEP?

Another possibility is that insomniacs experience discomfort because they are unusually sensitive to environmental stimuli during sleep. In order to examine this, Mendelson *et al*. (1986d) tested the auditory arousal threshold of insomniacs and controls. The procedure was carried out on two different nights, once using an electronic tone and once using a tape recording of a person calling out the subject's name. As seen in Figures 12-3 and 12-4, there were significant differences in arousal threshold at different sleep stages, and thresholds to the recording of the subject's name were lower than to the electronic tone. In both conditions, however, arousal thresholds for insomniacs and controls did not differ significantly. We mentioned earlier that in a study of experimental awakenings, insomniacs went back to sleep as

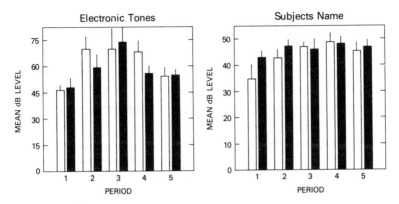

FIGURE 12-3. Arousal thresholds to an electronic tone and to a tape recording of the subject's name in 10 insomniacs and controls. An analysis of variance showed significant differences between sleep stages in both cases ($p < 0.05$) but no differences between the two groups or group × sleep stage interaction effects. It should be noted that three subjects in each group did not awaken 10 min after sleep onset, even when the equipment was set at the highest possible volume (100 dB). They were arbitrarily assigned a value of 100 dB. □, Controls; ■, insomniacs; 1, 5 min after lights out; 2, 10 min after sleep onset; 3, 5 min after stage 4 onset; 4, 5 min after first REM onset; 5, during MT. (From Mendelson *et al.*, 1986d. Reprinted by permission.)

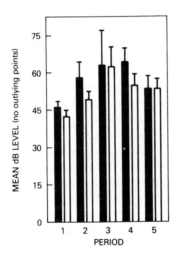

FIGURE 12-4. Subjects are from the same study as that of Figure 12-3, except that those subjects who did not awaken in response to electronic tones at 10 min after sleep onset have been eliminated. An analysis of variance showed a significant effect for sleep stage ($p < 0.05$), with highest arousal thresholds for stage 4 and REM (in both cases $p < 0.01$ compared to "5 min after lights out"). □, Controls; ■, insomniacs; 1, 5 min after lights out; 2, 10 min after sleep onset; 3, 5 min after stage 4 onset; 4, 5 min after first REM onset; 5, after MT. (From Mendelson *et al.*, 1986. Reprinted by permission.)

easily as controls. The arousal threshold data suggest that they are not more susceptible than controls to being awakened by external stimuli. This suggests that the poor sleep they experience is different from "light" sleep.

INSOMNIACS' PERCEPTION OF HABITUAL SLEEP

Another curious quality about insomniacs is the disparity between their belief about their habitual sleep and their perception about the current night. Mendelson et al. (1984c, 1986d) gave questionnaires to two groups of 10 insomniacs and matched controls regarding their typical sleep and daytime functioning. As might be expected, they differed significantly on a variety of questions dealing with whether they felt refreshed upon awakening and tired during the day and how they characterized their sleep. In contrast to their major differences in reporting habitual sleep, insomniacs and controls differed very little in their descriptions in the laboratory about the previous night. Out of an extensive battery of questions, they differed significantly only in that the insomniacs described less fatigue before going to bed (Mendelson et al., 1984c) and shorter total sleep time (Mendelson et al., 1986d). Similarly, although insomniacs and controls described their habitual daytime status very differently, their reports on how they felt at any given moment were quite similar. On the Stanford Sleepiness Scale, 100-mm line scales of alertness, fatigue and other measures, and on a Mood Rating Scale, there were virtually no differences between how insomniacs and controls rated themselves as to their current feelings (Table 12-2). Out of these many measures, the only significant contrast was that on the second baseline day, in one of the two studies, the controls reported a better sense of well-being (Mendelson et al., 1986d). We have already suggested that insomniacs may have some difficulty recognizing their own state of consciousness. The apparent discrepancy between how they describe their habitual sleep and daytime lives compared to how they perceive themselves at any given moment suggests that insomniacs may have some deficit in their ability to remember or to generalize from their current experience of wakefulness and sleep.

As these studies illustrate, the problem of insomnia is complex, and the few insights available are largely derived from subjective reports. Consequently, it has been difficult to design and evaluate treatments, and the amorphousness of the problem has led to much of the controversy about the efficacy of various approaches. Pharmacological treatment has been described in Chapter 3. We will present here the major nonpharmacological techniques.

TABLE 12-2. Self-Assessment of Daytime Mood and
Function in Insomniacs and Controls

Scale	p value
Mood rating	
Euphoria	0.04 (time effect)
Activation	0.001 (time effect)
Depression	NS
Dysphoria	NS
Physical symptoms	NS
Sleepiness	NS
Self-rating	
Reason clearly	0.04 (time effect)
Process information quickly	0.005 (time effect)
Ability to concentrate	0.01 (time effect)
Accurate decisions	0.005 (time effect)
Level of motor activity	NS
General mood state	NS
Asleep–alert	NS
Calm–anxious	NS
Tired–energetic	NS

(From Mendelson *et al.*, 1984c. Reprinted by permission.)
Note that in some cases, there were time-of-day effects, but no significant
differences between insomniacs and controls were observed.

TREATMENT OF INSOMNIA

Nonpharmacological Techniques

The great variety of nonpharmacological approaches testifies to our
uncertainty regarding the efficacy of any particular one. Some authors
have stressed the importance of psychotherapy for insomnia (Kales,
Kales, and Humphrey, 1975b; Berlin, 1985), viewing insomnia as a
complaint masking more profound intrapsychic conflicts. There have
been few or no systematic studies showing any benefits of long-term dy-
namically oriented psychotherapy for chronic insomnia. On the other
hand, there have been a variety of studies of behavioral approaches,
which are described in detail in several reviews (Mendelson, 1980; Borkovec, 1982; Nicassio *et al.*, 1985; Bootzin and Engle-Friedman, 1987).
Many of these are designed to achieve one or more of three major goals:
(1) replacing excessive arousal with relaxation; (2) reducing ruminations
or fears and concerns about sleep; and (3) minimizing problems that
result from habits or undesirable environmental cues.

Dealing with Excessive Arousal

Several methods have been employed to induce relaxation at bed-time. The classic *progressive relaxation* procedure of Jacobson (1938), which involves the systematic tensing and relaxing of individual muscle groups, has been reported to reduce insomnia (Jacobson, 1964) and has been widely used. *Biofeedback* based on the EMG (Budzynski, 1973) or to enhance theta or "sensorimotor rhythm" (SMR) activity (Hauri and Cohen, 1977) has been thought to be of benefit. *Autogenic training* (Nicassio and Bootzin, 1974) and meditation have also been employed. Freedman *et al.* (1978) reported a multicenter study comparing patients receiving biofeedback (EMG and EMG plus theta), relaxation procedures (progressive relaxation and autogenic training), and control procedures (electrosleep and exercise). There were no significant differences in outcome, suggesting perhaps that these procedures do not benefit groups of patients as a whole but may help selected individuals. In a subsequent study, Hauri (1981) found that neither EMG nor SMR biofeedback benefited psychophysiological insomniacs as a group. The amount of feedback learning correlated positively with improved sleep in the SMR but not the EMG group. In a 1982 study, Hauri *et al.* reported that both theta and SMR biofeedback benefited psychophysiological insomniacs as evaluated by home sleep logs. Using measures from the sleep laboratory, tense and anxious insomniacs benefited only from theta feedback; those who were relaxed at intake were helped only by SMR.

Behavioral self-management (Coates and Thoresen, 1977; Thoresen *et al.*, 1981b) emphasizes the need not only to master specific techniques such as progressive relaxation, but also to acquire skills in solving daytime problems associated with poor sleep. The importance of a sense of mastery in working out daily problems is stressed. A patient who traditionally brings home a great deal of office work, for instance, might learn both a relaxation procedure as well as time management skills to help him finish his work at the office and then have more free time in the evening. Studies that have included follow-ups as long as 6 to 36 months have had favorable results (Kirmil-Gray *et al.*, 1978; Thoresen *et al.*, 1978).

Reducing Ruminations or Fears and Concerns

In *systematic desensitization* the patient lists situations that are associated with poor sleep, arranged in ascending order of severity. He then is asked to picture these situations and couple them with the peaceful feeling derived from one of the relaxation procedures. Individual case

studies have indicated that this is useful. One group study that compared relaxation procedures alone, relaxation plus desensitization, a
quasi-desensitization procedure, and an untreated group found significant improvement in the two active treatment groups (Steinmark and
Borkovec, 1974). Since relaxation alone was roughly as effective as
relaxation plus desensitization, however, the benefit of desensitization
per se was called into question.

Paradoxical techniques have also been used to treat insomnia
(Rudestam, 1980). In one case, a patient was asked what chore he liked
least (Haley, 1963). When he replied that scrubbing floors was most
distasteful, the therapist suggested that he should do this whenever he
could not sleep. The patient rapidly learned to sleep. Alternatively, the
therapist can instruct the patient to try not to sleep. The patient may be
assigned a task and told to resist sleeping. In principle, this prevents
the self-defeating pattern that results from trying too hard to go to
sleep.

Cognitive focusing (Rudestam, 1980) may be used to prevent ruminations that prevent sleep. The concern is that when a patient awakens
during the night, he cannot return to sleep because he begins to have
repeated thoughts incompatible with sleep, to the effect of "Now I'm
in for it; I'll never get back to sleep." In this technique, the patient is
taught to repeat reassuring thoughts, and then to focus on a pleasant
image in order to avoid such ruminating.

Modifying Effects of Habits or Environmental Cues

As in systematic desensitization, the stimulus control technique is
derived from operant conditioning principles. Falling asleep is considered the instrumental act performed to induce sleep, which is the rein-
forcer (Bootzin, 1977). The object is to remove from the bedroom any
stimuli that induce behaviors incompatible with falling asleep, such as
worrying or watching television. Hence the patient is instructed to re-
serve the bedroom only for sleep or sex. If he finds himself engaged in
any other activity (including lying in bed unable to sleep) he is instructed to leave the bedroom and not return until he feels ready to
sleep (Table 12-3). Several studies have shown some benefit from this
approach (Bootzin, 1972, 1973, 1977; Haynes, Price, and Simons, 1975).
Puder et al. (1983) found that a four-week course of stimulus control
treatment significantly improved subjective measures of sleep in 16
older adults with sleep-onset insomnia and that benefits were maintained at a six-week follow-up. Bootzin and Engle-Friedman (1986)
compared this approach with progressive relaxation and with only

TABLE 12-3. Stimulus Control Instructions

1. Lie down intending to go to sleep *only* when you are sleepy.
2. Do not use your bed for anything except sleep; that is, do not read, watch television, eat, or worry in bed. Sexual activity is the only exception to this rule. On such occasions, the instructions are to be followed afterward when you intend to go to sleep.
3. If you find yourself unable to fall asleep, get up and go into another room. Stay up as long as you wish and then return to the bedroom to sleep. Although we do not want you to watch the clock, we want you to get out of bed if you do not fall asleep immediately. Remember the goal is to associate your bed with falling asleep *quickly!* If you are in bed more than about 10 minutes without falling asleep and have not gotten up, you are not following this instruction.
4. If you still cannot fall asleep, repeat Step 3. Do this as often as is necessary throughout the night.
5. Set your alarm and get up at the same time every morning, irrespective of how much sleep you got during the night. This will help your body acquire a consistent sleep rhythm.
6. Do not nap during the day.

(From Bootzin and Nicassio, 1978. Reprinted by permission.)

providing sleep hygiene information and support to 53 older insomniacs. All three techniques resulted in significant improvement in the short term. After two years, there were few differences between the three groups, although the stimulus control patients reported the most improvement in sleep latency and felt that their sleep was least affected by life events.

In *sleep restriction therapy* (Spielman, Saskin, and Thorpy, 1983, 1987) the patient keeps a sleep log, from which his estimated total sleep time is derived. He is then instructed to limit his total time in bed to what had previously been his total estimated sleep time. When sleep appears to be 90% efficient for five nights at this new and shorter time in bed, he is allowed to stay in bed progressively longer. The effort, then, is to make sleep more efficient by consolidating it. This approach may be of more benefit in patients who complain of severely disturbed sleep (Spielman, Saskin, and Thorpy, 1984). The implication is that excessive time in bed is an element that helps perpetuate insomnia, even though it may not be the original cause. At a 35-week follow-up, clear benefits in terms of total sleep, sleep efficiency, and wake time were still evident (Spielman, Saskin, and Thorpy, 1987).

General Features of Behavioral Therapies

One of the striking qualities of these behavioral therapies is that their similarities are greater than their differences. Although details of implementation vary, one senses that the broader methods and goals have several common features. These include:

1. Documentation: In behavioral treatments, keeping a log of the target behavior both before and during treatment is a key element. In addition to its obvious use—to establish a baseline from which to judge treatment—keeping a log may also have additional functions. It quantitates the behavior, which somehow makes it less mysterious to the patient. The ability to quantitate something gives a sense of being more able to control it. There are many instances in the treatment of a variety of disorders—from impulsiveness in hyperactive children to compulsive rituals—in which behaviors improve when the patient begins to keep track of them systematically.

2. Self-management: The spirit of many of these treatments is that the therapist is not there to fix a problem for the patient. Rather, the therapist is a consultant who provides him with a set of tools to use, during and after therapy, to deal with life difficulties.

3. Developing an active stance: When treating an insomniac, one is often struck by the passive manner in which the problem is formulated. The patient often speaks as if he is the passive victim of an affliction that, for unknown reasons, has been visited upon him. Most behavior therapies induce a feeling that the patient is more in charge of his feelings and ability to sleep than he might have imagined. As he develops skill in inducing a relaxed feeling during progressive relaxation, or when focusing on a tense situation during systematic desensitization, there is often a growing realization by the patient that he can bring on peaceful or anxious feelings by his own volition. They do not just happen to him.

4. Seeing sleep in the broader context of one's life: Insomniacs often describe their nighttime disturbance as if it occurs in isolation, unconnected to their daytime lives. This is particularly evident in systematic desensitization, when one is trying to establish a list of events associated with poor sleep. Most insomniacs will insist that their poor sleep just "happens out of the blue," and are often intrigued with the new knowledge they gain as they begin to see its associations with life events. Hauri (1986) has suggested that the therapist approach this in the same manner that is used with a pain patient: one does not argue whether he is feeling pain, but rather inquires whether some days might be better and some worse. When the patient agrees that this is the case, the therapist suggests that they try to determine what makes some days different from others. The behavioral self-management approach recognizes this as well, emphasizing learning skills that solve problems in the patient's daytime life as well as mastering relaxation procedures.

Sleep Hygiene

In addition to specific behavior therapies, it also seems beneficial to give the patient some specific guidelines about sleep, which have come to be known as "sleep hygiene." These include:

1. Keep regular hours of sleep time: Consistency in time of going to bed and arising is useful to insomniacs. It is important to avoid a life-style in which one becomes progressively more sleep-deprived during the week and then attempts to catch up during the weekend. Thus, weekend sleep hours should not differ greatly from those during week-days. Bedtimes should be predictable. It may be useful to incorporate a certain amount of ritual around going to bed, with a relatively constant sequence of putting on pajamas, washing, brushing teeth, and so forth. These events may then become cues to the behavior of going to sleep.

2. Avoid naps: Although naps may have some importance in some sleep disorders—notably narcolepsy—they should be avoided in insomnia. As with the injunction to keep regular hours for bedtime, the goal here is to confine sleep to a particular part of the 24-hr day.

3. Avoid stimulants and drugs that disturb sleep: Coffee and other caffeine-containing beverages must be eliminated from the diet. Alcohol may shorten sleep latency, but it induces wakefulness during the night, and hence, should be avoided. Patients who smoke should be encouraged to quit. It should be determined whether the patient is taking any medications that tend to disrupt sleep. These include beta-blockers, thyroid hormone, steroids, and cancer chemotherapy agents.

4. Exercise: Although there is some disagreement as to whether exercise has some more specific action or merely affects sleep by increasing core temperature, it appears likely that moderate exercise does aid sleep in physically fit persons. One should exercise in the late afternoon or early evening, since exercising late in the evening may disturb sleep.

5. Be aware of the role of eating on sleep: Heavy meals late at night may disturb sleep. Some persons, however, find that a glass of milk or a warm beverage seems to aid sleep.

6. Sleep in the right setting: The bedroom should be conducive to sleep. The patient should feel safe and comfortable. There should be no reminders of work or other stresses—for instance, no desk where he pays bills or does work from the office. The temperature should be right for the individual; in general, slightly cool may be best.

7. Don't lie in bed awake: If the patient finds himself experiencing the exquisite torture of lying in bed unable to sleep, he should get up and go into another room, and not return to bed until he feels ready to

sleep. Most persons, on hearing this advice, express worry about how they will function the next day if they have gotten up during the night. They should be reassured that the goal here is to help the long-term situation, and that a few nights of getting up occasionally will not interfere greatly with their ability to get work done.

8. Plan time in the evening to relax: Many persons slip into a lifestyle in which they come home from work late, have dinner at a late hour, and then are faced with going to bed in order to get up early for work. This "loss of the evening" seems to make it harder to go to sleep. The patient should address the way he plans and organizes the 24 hours in order to allow time to relax during the evening.

A Program for Patients

Once the major physiological disturbances of sleep have been ruled out, patients with chronic insomnia may benefit from a relatively short-term course of education in sleep hygiene and behaviorally oriented therapy. It should be emphasized that this advice is based as much on clinical experience as scientific endeavor, and that much more testing is needed before it is fully accepted. One major question is how to deal with the patient's requests for hypnotics. Certainly, the first thing to do is to point out that nightly use of hypnotics in chronic insomnia is likely to be unsuccessful. Occasional use may be of some benefit. Interestingly enough, there have been virtually no careful clinical studies of occasional administration. When short-term behavioral therapy is proposed, it is sometimes useful to respond to a request for hypnotics from a skeptical patient with a prescription for occasional use. In effect, one says to the patient: "Try this with me. While we are doing therapy you can feel assured that you will never go for more than four nights without a good night's sleep." Then begin therapy, emphasizing that the patient has an active role in his disturbance and is not merely its passive victim.

SUMMARY

Among patients with chronic sleep complaints is a fascinating group in whom no evidence of psychiatric disorders or of sleep apnea, nocturnal myoclonus, chronobiological disturbance, or other major pathophysiology of sleep can be found. Among these chronic insomniacs are those in whom a conditioned arousal response inhibits sleep ("persistent psychophysiological DIMS") and those in whom the degree of distress seems very disproportionate to the relatively minor objective sleep disturbance ("subjective DIMS without objective findings"). Their MMPI studies have tended to indicate a high incidence of elevated scores on various scales, particularly depression, hysteria, hypochondriasis, and psychasthenia. Although insomniacs describe great discomfort during the day, performance tests have found few if any consistent deficits, and MSLT testing has generally not shown increased sleepiness. During the night, after forced awakenings, subjective insomniacs go back to sleep as quickly as controls. As a group, they are not more easily aroused by auditory stimuli than controls, which suggests that their subjectively poor sleep is not necessarily "light" sleep. Their reports appear to exaggerate some, but not all, of the polygraphically observed sleep disturbances. After some forms of forced awakenings, they are more likely than controls to say that they had been awake during polygraphically defined sleep. A number of hypotheses have been advanced to explain these observations. One possibility is that subjective insomniacs suffer from a disability in recognizing their own state of consciousness and in remembering and generalizing from their experiences.

A number of nonpharmacological approaches may be used to treat chronic insomnia. Many carry the spirit of self-management, in which the therapist does not "fix" the patient's problem, but instead helps him acquire useful skills that can be used during and after therapy. Other themes that often emerge are documentation of behavior, as well as helping the patient to develop an active stance and to see the sleep disturbance in the broader context of his life.

Bibliography

Abrams, R. L., Grumbach, M. M., and Kaplan S. L., 1971, The effect of administration of human growth hormone on the plasma growth hormone, cortisol, glucose, and free fatty acid response to insulin: Evidence for growth hormone autoregulation, *J. Clin. Invest.* **50:**940–950.

Adamson, J., and Burdick, J. A., 1973, Sleep of dry alcoholics, *Arch. Gen. Psychiatry* **28:**146–149.

Adinoff, B., Majchrowicz, E., Martin, P., and Linnoila, M., 1986, The benzodiazepine antagonist Ro 15-1788 does not antagonize the ethanol withdrawal syndrome, *Biol. Psychiatry* **21:**643–649.

Adrien, J., 1978, Ontogenesis of some sleep regulation: Early postnatal impairment of the monoaminergic system, *Prog. Brain Res.* **48:**393–405.

Aghajanian, G. K., 1981, Studies on adrenergic receptors in the dorsal raphe nucleus, *Psychopharmacol. Bull.* **17:**21.

Aghajanian, G. K., Rosecrans, J. A., and Sheard, M. H., 1967, Serotonin: Release in the forebrain by stimulation of midbrain raphe, *Science* **156:**402–403.

Agnew, H. W., and Webb, W. B., 1971, Sleep latencies in human subjects: Age, prior wakefulness, and reliability, *Psychonomic Sci.* **24:**253–254.

Agnew, H. W., Webb, W. B., and Williams, R. L., 1964, The effects of stage four sleep deprivation, *Electroencephalogr. Clin. Neurophysiol.* **27:**68–70.

Aguirre, M. Broughton, R., and Stuss, D., 1985, Does memory impairment exist in narcolepsy–cataplexy? *J. Clin. Exp. Neuropsychol.* **7:**14–24.

Akerstedt, T., 1984, Work schedules and sleep, *Experientia* **40:**417–422.

Akerstedt, T., Gillberg, M., and Wetterberg, L., 1982, The circadian covariation of fatigue and urinary melatonin, *Biol. Psychiatry* **17:**547–554.

Akimoto, H., Honda, Y., and Takahashi, Y. 1960, Pharmacotherapy in narcolepsy, *Dis. Nerv. Syst.* **21:**704–706.

Akindale, M. O., Evans, J. I., and Oswald, I., 1970, Monoamine oxidase inhibitors, sleep and mood, *Electroencephalogr. Clin. Neurophysiol.* **29:**47–56.

Akiskal, H. S., Rosenthal, T. L., Haigel, R. F., Lemni, H., Rosenthal, R. H., and Scott-Strauss, A. 1980, Characterological depressions: Clinical and sleep EEG findings separating "subaffective dysthymics" from "character spectrum disorders," *Arch. Gen. Psychiatry* **37:**777–783.

Albertson, T., Bowyer, J., and Paule, M., 1982, Modification of the anticonvulsant efficacy of diazepam by RO-15-1788 in the kindled amygdaloid seizure model, *Life Sci.* **31:**1597–1601.

Alford, F. P., Baker, H. W., Burger, H. G., de Kretser, D. M., Hudson, B., Johns, M. W., and Masteron, J. P., 1973a, Temporal patterns of integrated plasma hormone levels during sleep and wakefulness. II. Follicle-stimulating hormone, luteinizing hormone, testosterone and estradiol, *J. Clin. Endocrinol. Metab.* **37:**848–854.

Alford, F. P., Baker, H. W., Burger, H. G., de Kretser, D. M., Hudson, B., Johns, M. W., and Masterson, J. P., 1973b, Temporal patterns of integrated plasma hormone levels during sleep and wakefulness. I. Thyroid-stimulating hormone, growth hormone and cortisol, *J. Clin. Endocrinol. Metab.* **37:**841–847.

Allen, R. P., Wagman, A., Faillace, L. A., and McIntosh M., 1971, Electroencephalographic (EEG) sleep recovery following prolonged alcohol intoxication in alcoholics, *J. Nerv. Ment. Dis.* **153:**424–433.

Allgulander, C., 1978, Dependence on sedative and hypnotic drugs—a comparative clinical and social study, *Acta Psychiatr. Scand. Suppl.* **270:**1–102.

Allnut, M. F., and O'Connor, P. J., 1971, Comparison of the electroencephalographic, behavioral and subjective correlates of natural and drug-induced sleep at atypical hours, *Aerosp. Med.* **42:**1006–1010.

Ambrosetto, C., Lugaresi, E., Coccagna, G., and Tasinart, C. A., 1965, Clinical and polygraphic remarks in the syndrome of restless legs, *Riv. Patol. Nerv.* **86:**245–252.

Amira, S. A., Johnson, T. S., and Logowitz, N. B., 1985, Diagnosis of narcolepsy using the multiple sleep latency test: Analysis of current laboratory criteria, *Sleep* **8:**325–331.

Amsterdam, J. D., Schweitzer, E., and Winokur, A., 1987, Multiple hormonal responses to insulin-induced hypoglycemia in depressed patients and normal volunteers, *Am. J. Psychiatry* **144:**170–175.

Ancoli-Israel, S., Kripke, D. F., Mason, W., and Messin, S., 1981, Sleep apnea and nocturnal myoclonus in a senior population, *Sleep* **4:**349–358.

Anonymous, 1889, Minutes from the Clinical Society of London, *Br. Med. J.* (Feb. 16):358.

Ansseau, M., Kupfer, D. J., Reynolds, III, C. F., and McEachran, A. B., 1984a, REM latency distribution in major depression: Clinical characteristics associated with sleep onset REM periods, *Biol. Psychiatry* **19:**1651–1666.

Ansseau, M., Scheyvaerts, M., Doumont, A., Poirrier, R., Legros, J., and Franck, G., 1984b, Concurrent use of REM latency, dexamethasone suppression, clonidine, and apomorphine tests as biological markers of endogenous depression: A pilot study, *Psychiatry Res.* **12:**261–272.

Ansseau, M., Kupfer, D. J., Reynolds, C. F., and Coble, P. A., 1985, "Paradoxical" shortening of REM latency on first recording night in major depressive disorder: Clinical and polysomnographic correlates, *Biol. Psychiatry* **20:**135–145.

Anton-Tay, F., Diaz, J. L., and Fernandez-Guardiola, A., 1971, On the effect melatonin upon the human brain. Its possible therapeutic implications, *Life Sci.* **10:**841–850.

Arendt, J., Borbely, A. A., Franey, C., and Wright, J., 1984, The effects of chronic small doses of melatonin given in the late afternoon on fatigue in man: A preliminary study, *Neurosci. Lett.* **45:**317–321.

Aschoff, J., 1964, Die tagesperiodik Licht- und dunkelaktiver Tiere, *Rev. Suisse Zool.* **71:**528–558.

Aschoff, J., 1978, Features of circadian rhythms relevant for the design of shift work schedules, *Ergonomics* **21:**739–754.

Aschoff, J., and Wever R., 1962, Spontanperiodik des Menchen bei Ausschluss aller Zeitgeber, *Naturwissenschaften* **49:**337–342.

Aschoff, J., Fatranska, M., Giedke, H., Doerr, P., Stamm, D., and Wisser, H., 1971, Human circadian rhythms in continuous darkness: Entrainment by social cues, *Science* 171:213–215.

Aserinsky, E., 1969, The maximal capacity for sleep: Rapid eye movement and density as an index of sleep satiety, *Biol. Psychiatry* 1:147–159.

Aserinsky, E., and Kleitman, N., 1953, Regularly occurring periods of eye motility and concomitant phenomena during sleep, *Science* 118:273–274.

Askenasy, J. J., and Yahr, M. D., 1985, Reversal of sleep disturbance in Parkinson's disease by antiparkinsonian therapy: A preliminary study, *Neurology* 35:527–532.

Association of Sleep Disorder Centers, 1979, Diagnostic classification of sleep and arousal disorders, *Sleep* 2:1–137.

Autret, A., Minz, T., Beillevaire, T., Degos, C., and Cathala, H. P., 1977, Clinical and polygraphic effects of *d*.1 5 HTP on narcolepsy–cataplexy, *Biomedicine* 27:200–203.

Avery, D. H., Wildschiodtz, G., and Rafaelsen, O. J., 1982, Nocturnal temperature in affective illness, *J. Affect. Disord.* 4:61–71.

Axelrod, J., 1974, The pineal gland: A neurochemical transducer, *Science* 184:1341–1348.

Azukizawa, M., Pekary, A. E., Hershman, J. M., and Parker, D. C., 1976, Plasma thyrotropin, thyroxine, and triiodothyronine relationships in man, *J. Clin. Endocrinol. Metab.* 43:533.

Badia, P., Harsh, J., Balkin, T., Cantrell, P., Klempert, A., O'Rourke, D., and Schoen, L., 1984, Behavioral control of respiration in sleep, *Psychophysiology* 21:494–500.

Baekeland, F., 1967, Pentobarbital and dextroamphetamine sulfate: Effects on the sleep cycle in man, *Psychopharmacologia* 11:388–396.

Baekeland, F., and Lundwall, L., 1971, Effects of methyldopa on sleep patterns in man, *Electroencephalogr. Clin. Neurophysiol.* 31:269–273.

Baghdoyan, H. A., McCarley, R. W., and Hobson, J. A., 1985, Cholinergic manipulation of brainstem reticular systems: Effects on desynchronized sleep, in: *Sleep: Neurotransmitters and Neuromodulators* (A. Wauquier, ed.), Raven Press, New York, pp. 15–27.

Baghdoyan, H. A., Rodrigo-Angulo, M. L., McCarley, R. W., and Hobson, J. A., 1987, A neuroanatomical gradient in the pontine tegmentum for the cholinoceptive induction of desynchronized sleep signs, *Brain Res.* 414:245–261.

Bailey, E., Jenner, F. A., and Wheeler, M. J., 1971, Renal function during the stages of sleep, *J. Physiol. (Lond.)* 218:40–42.

Bailie, G. R., Calder, I. T., Kesson, C. M., and Lawson, D. H., 1980, A comparison of temazepam with nitrazepam and with placebo as a hypnotic in medical patients in hospital, *J. Clin. Hosp. Pharm.* 5:311–317.

Baker, T. L., Foutz, A. S., McNerney, V., Mitler, M. M., and Dement, W. C., 1982, Canine model of narcolepsy: Genetic and developmental determinants, *Exp. Neurol.* 75:729–742.

Baker, T. L., Guilleminault, C., Nino-Murcia, G., and Dement, W. C., 1986, Comparative polysomnographic study of narcolepsy and idiopathic central nervous system hypersomnia, *Sleep* 9:232–242.

Ball, T., 1796, *An Inaugural Dissertation on the Causes and Effects of Sleep*, Budd and Bartram, Philadelphia, PA, p. 8.

Bamford, C. R., Snider, S. R., and Beutler, L., 1983, Nocturnal movements, *Ariz. Med.* (May):327–329.

Baraitser, M., and Parkes, J. D., 1978, Genetic study of narcoleptic syndrome, *J. Med. Gen.* 15:254–259.

Barker, J. L., and Ransom, B. R., 1978a, Amino acid pharmacology of mammalian central neurones grown in tissue culture, *J. Physiol.* **280**:331–354.

Barker, J. L., and Ransom, B. R., 1978b, Pentobarbitone pharmacology of mammalian central neurones grown in tissue culture, *J. Physiol.* **280**:355–372.

Barreca, R., Franceschini, R., Messina, V., Bottaro, L., and Rolandi, E., 1985, 24-Hour Othyroid-stimulating hormone secretory pattern in elderly men, *Gerontology* **31**:119–123.

Bartholini, G., Keller, H., Pieri L., and Pletscher, A., 1973, The effect of diazepam on the turnover of cerebral dopamine, in: *The Benzodiazepines* (S. Garattini, E. Mussini, and L. O. Pandall, eds.), Raven Press, New York, pp. 235–240.

Basile, A. S., and Skolnick, P., 1986, Subcellular localization of "peripheral-type" binding sites for benzodiazepines in the rat brain, *J. Neurochem.* **46**:305–308.

Bates, R. C., 1972, Delirium tremens and sleep deprivation, *Mich. Med.* **71**:941–944.

Batini, C., Moruzzi, G., Palestine, M., Rossi, G. F., and Zanchetti, A., 1958, Persistent patterns of wakefulness in the pretrigeminal midpontine preparation, *Science* **128**:30–32.

Batini, C., Magni, F., Paelstini, M., Rossi, G. F., and Zanchetti, A., 1959, Neural mechanisms underlying the enduring EEG and behavioral activation in the midpontine pretrigeminal cat, *Arch. Ital. Biol.* **97**:13–25.

Beary, M. D., Lacey, J. H., Crutchfield, M. B., and Bhat, A. V., 1984, Psychosocial stress, insomnia and temazepam: A sleep laboratory evaluation in a "general practice" sample, *Psychopharmacology* **83**:17–19.

Beck, W., and Stubbe, P., 1984, Pulsatile secretion of luteinizing hormone and sleep-related gonadotropin rhythms in girls with premature thelarche, *Eur. J. Pediatr.* **141**:168–170.

Bee, D. M., 1985, Restless legs and nocturnal myoclonus, *JAMA* **254**:361.

Beersma, D. G. M., Daan, S., and Van den Hoofdakker, R., 1985, The timing of sleep in depression: Theoretical considerations, *Psychiatry Res.* **16**:253–262.

Bell, C. C., Dixie–Bell, D. D., and Thompson, B., 1986, Further studies on the prevalence of isolated sleep paralysis in black subjects, *J. Natl. Med. Assoc.* **78**:649–659.

Bell, E., and Govindan, S., 1986, Obstructive sleep apnea and nocturnal myoclonus: KDS-1 state inventories, *Sleep Res.* **15**:87.

Benavides, T., Quarteronet D., Imbault, F., Malgouris, C., Uzan, A., Renault, C., and Dubroeucg, M. C., 1983, Labeling of "peripheral-type" benzodiazepine bindings sites in the rat brain by using (^{3}H) PK 11195; an isoquinoline carboxamide derivative: Kinetic studies and autoradiographic localization, *J. Neurochem.* **41**:1744–1750.

Benson, K. L., and Zarcone, V. P., 1981, A comparison of REM sleep eye movement measures as indicators of depression, *Sleep Res.* **10**:169.

Benson, K. L., and Zarcone, Jr., V. P., 1985, Testing the REM sleep phasic event intrusion hypothesis of schizophrenia, *Psychiatry Res.* **15**:163–173.

Benson, K. L., Berger, P. A., and Zarcone, V. P., 1981, The relationship of REM sleep to urinary and CSF MHPG in depressive disorder: A re-examination, *Sleep Res.* **10**:168.

Benson, K. L., Zarcone, U. P., Faull, K., Barnes, D. L. B., Barchas, J. D., and Berger, P. A., 1982, The relationship of the CSF serotonin metabolite 5-HIAA on REM sleep eye movement activity in psychiatric patients, *Sleep Res.* **11**:117.

Berger, H., 1929, Uber das Elektroencephalogramm des Menschen, *Arch. Psychiatr. Nervenkr.* **87**:527–570.

Berger, H., 1938, Das Elektroencephalogramm des Menschen, *Nova Acta Leopoldina* **6**:173–309.

Berger, R. J., 1961, Tonus of extrinsic laryngeal muscles during sleep and dreaming, *Science* **134**:840.

Berger, R. J., 1969, Physiological characteristics of sleep, in: *Sleep: Physiology and Pathology* (A. Kales, ed.), Lippincott, Philadelphia, PA, pp. 66–79.

Bergonzi, P., Chiurulla, C., Cianchett, C., and Tempesta, E., 1974, Clinical pharmacology as an approach to the study of biochemical sleep mechanisms: The action of L-DOPA, *Confin. Neurol.* **36:**5–22.

Berlin, R. M., 1985, Psychotherapeutic treatment of chronic insomnia, *Am. J. Psychother.* **39:**68–74.

Berlin, R. M., and Conell, L. J., 1983, Withdrawal symptoms after long-term treatment with therapeutic doses of flurazepam: A case report, *Am. J. Psychiatry* **140:**488–489.

Berman, K. F., Mendelson, W. B., Skolnick, P., Paul, S. M., and Wyatt, R. J., 1982, Effects of an adenosine agonist, L-phenylisopropyladenosine (L-PIA) on sleep and spontaneous motor activity in the rat, *Sleep Res.* **11:**54.

Bernard, P., Bergen, K., Sobiski, R., and Robson, R., 1981, An orally effective benzodiazepine antagonist, *Pharmacologist* **23:**201.

Berry, D. T., Webb, W. B., Block, A. J., Bauer, R. M., and Switzer, D. A., 1986, Nocturnal hypoxia and neuropsychological variables, *J. Clin. Exp. Neuropsychol.* **8:**229–238.

Berry, R. B., and Block, A. J., 1984, Positive nasal airway pressure eliminates snoring as well as obstructive apnea, *Chest* **85:**15–20.

Berson, S. A., and Yalow, R. S., 1968, Radioimmunoassay of ACTH in plasma, *J. Clin. Invest.* **47:**2725–2751.

Bert, J., 1972, Action de la P-chlorophenylalanine sur le sommeil du *babouin papio*, *Electroencephalogr. Clin. Neurophysiol.* **33:**99–103.

Bertelson, A. D., and Masch, J. K., 1986, MMPI characteristics among different types of insomnia, *Sleep Res.* **15:**90.

Berthon-Jones, M., and Sullivan, C. E., 1984, Ventilation and arousal responses to hypercapnia in normal sleeping humans, *J. Appl. Physiol.* **57:**59–67.

Betts, T. A., and Birtle, J., 1982, Effect of two hypnotic drugs on actual driving performance next morning, *Br. Med. J.* **285:**852.

Beutler, L. E., Ware, C., Karacan, I., and Thornby, J. I., 1981, Differentiating psychological characteristics of patients with sleep apnea and narcolepsy, *Sleep* **4:**39–47.

Billiard, M., and Seignalet, J., 1985, Letter, *Lancet* **1:**226–227.

Billiard, M., Seignalet, J., Besset, A., and Cadilhac, J., 1986a, HLA-DR2 and narcolepsy, *Sleep* **9:**149–152.

Billiard, M., Quera Salva, M., De Koninck, J., Besset, A., Touchon, J., and Cadilhac, J., 1986b, Daytime sleep characteristics and their relationships with night in the narcoleptic patient, *Sleep* **9:**167–174.

Binnie, G. A., 1983, Psychotropic drugs and accidents in a general practice, *Br. Med. J.* **287:**1349–1350.

Binns, E., 1852, *The Anatomy of Sleep or the Art of Procuring Sound and Refreshing Slumber at Will*, John Churchill, London.

Birkeland, A. J., 1982, Plasma melatonin levels and nocturnal transitions between sleep and wakefulness, *Neuroendocrinology* **34:**126–131.

Bivens, C. H., Lebovitz, H. E., and Feldman, J. M., 1973, Inhibition of hypoglycemia-induced growth hormone secretion by the serotonin antagonists cyproheptadine and methysergide, *N. Engl. J. Med.* **289:**236–239.

Bixler, E. O., Santen, R. J., Kales, A., Soldatos, C. R., and Scharf M. B., 1977, Inverse effects of thioridazine (Mellaril) on serum prolactin and testosterone concentrations in normal men, in: *The Testis in Normal and Infertile Men* (P. Troen and H. R. Nankin, ed.), Raven Press, New York, pp. 403–408.

Bixler, E. O., Soldatos, C. R., Scarone, S., Martin, E. D., Kales, A., and Charney, D. S.,

1978, Similarities of nocturnal myoclonic activity in insomniac patients and normal subjects, *Sleep Res.* **7:**213.

Bixler, E. O., Kales, A., and Soldatos, C. R., 1979, Sleep disorders encountered in medical practice, *Behav. Med.* **1:**13–21.

Bixler, E. O., Kales, A., Soldato, C. R., Vela-Bueno, A., Jacoby, J. A., and Scarone, S., 1982a, Sleep apneic activity in a normal population, *Res. Comm. Chem. Pathol. Pharmacol.* **36:**141–152.

Bixler, E. O., Kales, A., Vela-Bueno, A., Jacoby, J. A., Scarone, S., and Soldatos, C. R., 1982b, Nocturnal myoclonus and nocturnal myoclonic activity in a normal population, *Res. Comm. Chem. Pathol. Pharmacol.* **36:**129–139.

Blackard, W. G., and Heidingsfelder, S. A., 1968, Adrenergic receptor control mechanisms for growth hormone secretion, *J. Clin. Invest.* **47:**1407–1414.

Blennow, G., 1985, Benign infantile nocturnal myoclonus, *Acta Pediatr. Scand.* **74:**505–507.

Bliwise, D. L., Carey, E., and Dement, W. C., 1983, Nightly variations in sleep-related respiratory disturbance in older adults, *Exp. Aging Res.* **9:**77–81.

Bliwise, D., Carskadon, M., Carey, E., and Dement, W., 1984, Longitudinal development of sleep-related respiratory disturbance in adult humans, *J. Gerontol.* **39:**290–293.

Block, A. J., Boysen, P. G., Wynne, J. W., and Hunt, L. A., 1979, Sleep apnea, hypopnea and oxygen desaturation in normal subjects. A strong predominance, *N. Engl. J. Med.* **300:**513–517.

Block, A. J., Wynne, J. W., and Boysen, P. G., 1980, Sleep-disordered breathing and nocturnal oxygen desaturation in postmenopausal women, *Am. J. Med.* **69:**75–79.

Block, A. J., Wynne, J. W., Boysen, P. G., Lindsey, A., Martin, C., and Canter, B., 1981, Menopause, medroxyprogesterone and breathing during sleep, *Am. J. Med.* **70:**506–510.

Block, A. J., Dolly, R. F., and Slayton, P.C., 1984, Does flurazepam ingestion affect breathing and oxygenation during sleep in patients with chronic obstructive lung disease? *Am. Rev. Respir. Dis.* **129:**230–233.

Blois, R., Feinberg, I., Gaillard, J. M., Kupfer, D. J., and Webb, W. B., 1983, Sleep in normal and pathological aging, *Experientia* **39:**551–558.

Blum, K., Merritt, J. H., Wallace, J. E., Owen, R., Hahn, J. W., and Geller, I., 1972, Effects of catecholamine synthesis inhibition on ethanol narcosis in mice, *Curr. Ther. Res.* **14:**324–329.

Bodenheimer, W. S., Winter, J. S. D., and Faiman, C., 1973, Diurnal rhythms of serum gonadotropins, testosterone, estradiol and cortisol in blind men, *J. Clin. Endocrinol. Metab.* **37:**472–475.

Boehme, R. E., Baker, T. L., Mefford, J. D., Dement, W. C., and Ciaranello, R. D., 1984, Narcolepsy: Cholinergic receptor changes in an animal model, *Life Sci.* **34:** 1825–1828.

Bolger, G. T., Weissman, B. A., Lueddens, H., Basile, A. S., Mantione, C. R., Barrett, J. E., and Witkin, J. M., 1985, Late evolutionary appearance of "peripheral-type" binding sites for benzodiazepines, *Brain Res.* **338:**366–370.

Bonnet, M. H., 1984, The restoration of performance following sleep deprivation in geriatric normal and insomniac subjects, *Sleep Res.* **13:**188.

Bonnet, M. H., Mitler, M., Gillin, J. C., Mendelson, W. B., Dexter, J., Kripke, D., and James, S. P., 1986, Triazolam, sleep satiation, and nocturnal work shift sleepiness and performance, *Sleep Res.* **15:**28.

Bonvallet, M., Dell, P., and Hiebel, G., 1954, Tonus sympathique et activite electrique corticale, *Electroencephr. Clin. Neurophysiol.* **6:**119–144.

Bootzin, R. R., 1972, Stimulus control treatment for insomnia, *Proc, Am. Psychol. Assn.* pp. 395–396, Honolulu, Hawaii.

Bootzin, R. R., 1974, Stimulus control of insomnia, paper presented at the meeting of the Am. Psyc. Assn. Chicago, 1974

Bootzin, R. R., 1977, Effects of self-control procedures for insomnia, in: *Behavioral Self-Management* (R. B. Stuart, ed.), Bruner/Mazel, New York, pp. 175–196.

Bootzin, R. R., 1985, Insomnia, in: *Behavioral Therapy* (M. Hersen and C. G. Last, eds.), Springer, New York, pp. 132–143.

Bootzin, R. R., 1985, Nonpharmacological treatments of insomnia, Proceedings, IVth World Congress of Biological Psychiatry, Philadelphia.

Bootzin, R. R., and Engle-Friedman, M., 1981, The assessment of insomnia, *Behav. Assess.* 3:107–126.

Bootzin, R. R., and Engle-Friedman, M., 1987, Sleep disturbances, in: *Handbook of Clinical Gerontology* (B. A. Edelstein and L. L. Carstensen, eds.) Pergamon Press, New York, in press.

Bootzin, R. R., and Nicassio, P. M., 1978, Behavioral treatments for insomnia, *Prog. Behav. Mod.* 6:1–45.

Borbely, A. A., 1982a, Sleep regulation: Circadian rhythm and homeostasis, in: *Current Topics in Neuroendocrinology* (D. Ganten and D. Pfaff, eds.), Springer-Verlag, Berlin, pp. 83–103.

Borbely, A. A., 1982b, A two-process model of sleep regulation. I. Physiological basis and outline, *Hum. Neurobiol.* 1:195–204.

Borbely, A. A., 1986, Endogenous sleep-substances and sleep regulation, *J. Neural Trans.* 21S:243–254.

Borbely, A. A., and Wirz-Justice, A., 1982, Sleep, sleep deprivation and depression, *Hum. Neurobiol.* 1:205–210.

Borbely, A. A., Baumann, F., Brandeis, D., Strauch, I., and Lehmann, D., 1981, Sleep deprivation: Effect on sleep stages and EEG power density in man, *Electroenceph. Clin. Neurophys.* 51:483–493.

Borbely, A. A., Neuhaus, H. U., and Tobler, I., 1981, Effect of p-chlorophenylalanine and tryptophan on sleep, EEG, and motor activity in the rat, *Behav. Brain Res.* 2:1–22.

Borbely, A. A., Tobler, I., Loepfe, M., Kupfer, D. J., Ulrich, R. F., Grochocinski, U., Doman, J., 1984, All-night spectral analysis of the sleep EEG in untreated depressives and normal controls, *Psychiatry Res.* 12:27–33.

Bordeleau, J. M., Charland, P., and Tetreault L., 1970, Hypnotic properties of nitrazepam (Mogadon). A comparative study of chlordiazepoxide, diazepam, nitrazepam, secobarbital and placebo in psychiatric patients, *Dis. Nerv. Syst.* 31:318–323.

Borkovec, T. D., 1982, Insomnia, *J. Consult. Clin. Psychol.* 50:880–895.

Bornstein, S. K., 1982, Respiratory monitoring during sleep: Polysomnography, in: *Sleeping and Waking Disorders: Indications and Techniques* (C. Guilleminault, ed.), Addison-Wesley, Menlo Park, CA, pp. 183–212.

Bowersox, S. S., Kilduff, T. S., Kaitin, K. I., Dement, W. C., and Ciaranello, R. D., 1986, Brain benzodiazepine receptor characteristics in canine narcolepsy, *Sleep* 9:111–115.

Bowes, G., 1984, Arousal responses to chemical stimuli during sleep, *J. Develop. Physiol.* 6:207–213.

Bowling, G., and Richards, N. G., 1961, Diagnosis and treatment of the narcolepsy syndrome: Analysis of seventy-five case records, *Cleve. Clin. Quart.* 28:38–45.

Boyar, R., Finkelstein, J., Roffwarg, H., Kapen, S., Weitzman, E., and Hellman, I., 1972a, Synchronization of augmented luteinizing hormone secretion with sleep during puberty, *N. Engl. J. Med.* 287:582–586.

Boyar, R., Perlow, M., Hellman, L., Kapen, S., and Weitzman, E., 1972b, Twenty-four hour pattern of luteinizing hormone secretion in normal men with sleep stage recording, *Clin. Endocrinol. Metab.* **35**:73–81.

Boyar, R. M., Finkelstein, J. W., David, R., Roffwarg, H., Kapen, S., Weitzman, E. D., and Hellman, L., 1973, Twenty-four hour patterns of plasma luteinizing hormone and follicle-stimulating hormone in sexual precocity, *N. Engl. J. Med.* **289**:282–286.

Boyar, R. M., Rosenfeld, R. S., Kapan, S., Finkelstein, J. W., Roffwarg, H. P., Weitzman, E. D., and Hellman, L., 1974, Human puberty: Simultaneous augmented secretion of luteinizing hormone and testosterone during sleep, *J. Clin. Invest.* **54**:609–618.

Boyar, R. M., Finkelstein, J. W., Kapen, S., and Hellman, L., 1975, Twenty-four hour prolactin (PRL) secretory patterns during pregnancy, *J. Clin. Endocrinol. Metab.*, **40**:1117–1120.

Boyd, A. E., Lobovitz, H. E., and Pfeiffer, J. B., 1970, Stimulation of human growth hormone secretion by L-DOPA, *New Engl. J. Med.* **283**:1425–1429.

Braestrup, C., and Squires, R. F., 1978, Brain specific benzodiazepine receptors, *Br. J. Psychiatry* **133**:249–260.

Braestrup, C., Nielsen, M., and Olsen, F., 1980, Urinary and brain beta-carboline-3-carboxylates as potent inhibitors of brain benzodiazepine receptors, *Proc. Natl. Acad. Sci. USA* **77**:2288–2292.

Braestrup, C., Schmiechen, R., Nielsen, M., and Petersen, E. N., 1982, Benzodiazepine receptor ligands, receptor occupancy, pharmacological effect and GABA receptor coupling, in: *Pharmacology of Benzodiazepines* (E. Usdin, P. Skolnick, J. Tallmann, D. Greenblatt, and S. Paul, eds.), pp. 71–85.

Bramwell, B. C., 1909, Excessive sleepiness, *Clin. Stud. Edinb.* **8**:276–277.

Branchey, L., Branchey, M., and Nadler, R. D., 1971a, The influence of sex hormones on brain activity in male and female rats, in: *Influence of Hormones on the Nervous System* (D. H. Ford, ed.), Karger, Basel, pp. 334–340.

Branchey, L., Branchey, M., and Nadler, R. D., 1973, Effects of sex hormones on sleep patterns of male rats gonadectomized in adulthood and in the neonatal period, *Physiol. Behav.* **11**:609–611.

Branchey, M., and Kissin, B., 1970, The effects of alpha-methyl-paratyrosine on sleep and arousal in the rat, *Psychonom. Sci.* **19**:281–282.

Branchey, M., Branchey, L., and Nadler, R. D., 1971b, Effects of estrogen and progesterone on sleep patterns of female rats, *Physiol. Behav.* **6**:743–746.

Branchey, M. H., Begleiter, H., and Kissin B., 1970, The effects of various doses of alcohol on sleep in the rat, *Comm. Behav. Biol.* **5**:75–79.

Brandenberger, G., Follenius, M., Muzet, A., Ehrhart, J., and Schieber, J. P., 1985, Ultradian oscillations in plasma renin activity: Their relationships to meals and sleep stages, *J. Clin. Endocrinol. Metab.* **61**:280–284.

Brannan, J. O., and Jewett, R. E., 1969, Effects of selected phenothiazines on REM sleep in schizophrenics, *Arch. Gen. Psychiatry* **21**:284–290.

Braude, W., and Barnes, T., 1982, Clonazepam: Effective treatment for restless legs syndrome in uraemia, *Br. Med. Jr.* **284**:510.

Brazier, M. A. B., 1973, *The Electrical Activity of the Nervous System*, Pittman Publishing Corp., New York, pp. 240–292.

Brebbia, D. R., and Altshuler, K. Z., 1965, Oxygen consumption rate and electroencephalographic stage of sleep, *Science* **150**:1621–1623.

Breese, G. R., Colt, J. M., Cooper, B. R., Prange, A. J., and Lipton, M. A., 1974, Antagonism of ethanol narcosis by thytotropin-releasing hormone, *Life Sci.* **14**:1053–1063.

Bremer, F., 1935, Cerveau isolé et physiologie du sommeil, *Compt Rend. Soc. Biol. (Paris)* **118**:1235–1241.

Bremer, F., 1974, Historical development in ideas on sleep, in: *Basic Sleep Mechanisms* (O. Getre-Quadens and J. D. Schlag, eds.), Academic Press, New York, pp. 3–11.

Bricolo, A., Turella, G., Mazza, C. A., Buffatti, P., and Grosslercher, J. C., 1970, Modification del sonno nocturno in parkinsoniani trattati con L-DOPA, *Sist. Nerv.* **2:**181–190.

Bridges, P. K., and Jones, M. T., 1966, The diurnal rhythm of plasma cortisol concentration in depression, *Br. J. Psychiatry* **112:**1257–1261.

Brillon, D., Nabil, N., and Jacobs, L. S., 1986, Cholinergic but not serotonergic mediation of exercise-induced growth hormone secretion, *Endocrinol. Res.* **12:**137–146.

Broadbent, W. H., 1877, Cheyne-Stokes respiration in cerebral hemorrhage, *Lancet* **1:**307–309.

Brod, J., 1973, *The Kidney*, Butterworth and Company, London.

Brodie, H. K. H., Murphy, D. L., Goodwin, F. K., and Bunney, W. E., 1971. Catecholamines and mania: The effect of alpha-methyl-para-tyrosine on manic behavior and catecholamine metabolism, *Clin. Pharmacol. Exp. Ther.* **12:**218–224.

Broughton, R., 1982a, Human consciousness and sleep/waking rhythms: A review and some neurophysiological considerations, *J. Clin. Neuropsychol.* **4:**193–218.

Broughton, R., 1982b, Performance and evoked potential measures of various states of daytime sleepiness, *Sleep* **5:**135–146.

Broughton, R., and Mamelak, M., 1975, Gamma-hydroxy-butrate in the treatment of compound narcolepsy, *Sleep Res.* **4:**211.

Broughton, R., and Mamelak, M., 1980, Effects of nocturnal gamma-hydroxybutyrate on sleep/waking patterns in narcolepsy–cataplexy, *J. Canadien D Sci. Neurol.* **7:**23–31.

Broughton, R., Ghanem, Q., Hishikawa, Y., Sugita, Y., Nevsimalova, A., and Roth, B., 1981, Life effects of narcolepsy in 180 patients from North America, Asia, and Europe compared to matched controls, *Canada J. Neurol. Sci.* **8:**299–304.

Broughton, R., Low, R., Valley, V., Da Costa, B., and Liddiard, S., 1982, Auditory-evoked potentials compared to performance measures and EEG in assessing excessive daytime sleepiness in narcolepsy–cataplexy, *Electroencephalogr. Clin. Neurophysiol.* **54:**579–582.

Broughton, R., Ghanem, Q., Hishikawa, Y., Sugita, Y., Nevsimalova, A., and Roth, B., 1983, Life effects of narcolepsy: Relationships to geographic origin (North American, Asian or European) and to other patient and illness variables, *Canadian J. Neurol. Sci.* **10:**100–105.

Broughton, R., Tolentino, M. A., and Krelina, M., 1985, Excessive fragmentary myoclonus in NREM sleep: A report of 38 cases, *Electroencephalr. Clin. Neurophys.* **61:**123–133.

Broughton, R., Valley, V., Aguirre, M., Roberts, J., Suwalski, W., and Dunham, W., 1986, Excessive daytime sleepiness and the pathophysiology of narcolepsy–cataplexy: A laboratory perspective, *Sleep* **9:**205–215.

Broughton, R. J., 1968, Sleep disorders: Disorders of arousal? *Science* **159:**1070–1078.

Broughton, R. J., Guberman, A., and Roberts, J., 1984, Comparison of the psychosocial effects of epilepsy and narcolepsy/cataplexy: A controlled study, *Epilepsy* **25:**423–433.

Brouilette, R., Hanson, D., David, R., Klemka, L., Szatkowski, A., Ferubach, S., and Hunt, C., 1984, A diagnostic approach to suspected sleep apnea in children, *J. Pediatr.* **105:**10–14.

Browman, C. P., Gujavarty, K. S., Yolles, S. F., and Mitler, M. M., 1986, Forty-eight-hour polysomnographic evaluation of narcolepsy, *Sleep* **9:**183–188.

Brown, C. C., Horrom, N. J., and Wagman, A. M. I., 1979, Effects of L-tryptophan on sleep onset insomniacs, *Waking Sleeping* **3:**101–108.

Brown, G. M., and Reichlin, S., 1972, Psychologic and neural regulation of growth hormone secretion, *Psychosom. Med.* **34:**45–61.

Brownell, L. G., West, P., Sweatman, P., Acres, J. C., and Kryger, M. H., 1982, Protriptyline in obstructive sleep apnea: A double-blind trial, *New Engl. J. Med.* **307:**1037–1042.

Bruhova, S., and Roth, B., 1972, Heredo-familial aspects of narcolepsy and hypersomnia, *Arch. Suiesse, Neurol, Neurochir. Psychiat.* **110:**45–54.

Bryan, G. T., 1971, The role of urinary tryptophan metabolites in the etiology of bladder cancer, *J. Clin. Nutr.* **24:**841–847.

Buchsbaum, M. S., Coursey, R. D., and Murphy, D. L., 1976, The biochemical high-risk paradigm: Behavioral and familial correlates of low platelet monoamine oxidase activity, *Science* **194:**133.

Buckman, M. T., MacLean, C., Peake, G. T., Rhodes, J. M., and Srivastava, L. S., 1980, Absence of prolactin hypersecretion during sleep in men with gynecomastia, *Horm. Metab. Res.* **12:**344–345.

Budzynski, T. H., 1973, Biofeedback procedures in the clinic, *Semin. Psychiatry* **5:**537–547.

Budzynski, T. H., Stoyva, J., and Adler, C., 1970, Feedback-induced relaxation: Application to tension headache, *J. Behav. Ther. Exp. Psychiatry* **1:**205–211.

Bunney, B. S., and DeRiemer, S. A., 1982, Effects of clonidine on dopaminergic neuron activity in the substantia nigra: Possible indirect medication by noradrenergic regulation of the serotonergic raphe system, *Adv. Neurol.* **35:**99–104.

Bunney, W. E., Jr., Goodwin, F. K., Murphy, D. L., House, K. M., and Gordon, E. K., 1972, The switch process in manic-depressive illness. II. Relationship to catecholamines, REM sleep, and drugs, *Arch. Gen. Psychiatry* **27:**304–309.

Bunney, W. E., Kopanda, R. T., and Murphy D. L., 1977, Sleep and behavioral changes possibly reflecting central receptor hypersensitivity following catecholamine synthesis in man, *Acta Psychiat. Scand.* **56:**189–203.

Burday, S. Z., Fine, F. H., and Schalch, D. S., 1968, Growth hormone secretion in response to arginine infusion in normal and diabetic subjects: Relationship to blood glucose levels, *J. Lab. Clin. Med.* **71:**879–911.

Burwell, C. S., Robin, E. D., Whaley, R. D., and Bickelman, A. G., 1956, Extreme obesity associated with alveolar hypoventilation: A pickwickian syndrome, *Am. J. Med.* **21:**811–818.

Cabranes, J. A., Vela, A., Timoneda, F., Meyers, C. A., Coy, D. H., and Schally, A. V., 1984, Selective inhibition of sleep-related growth hormone release by phe-4-somatostatin, *Res. Comm. Chem. Pathol. Pharmacol.* **45:**421–430.

Cadieux, R. J., Kales, A., Santen, R. J., Bixler, E. O., and Gordon, R., 1982, Endoscopic findings in sleep apnea associated with acromegaly, *J. Clin. Endocrinol. Metab.* **55:**18–22.

Cahiff, A. L., and Ehret, C. F., 1982, Alpha-methyl-*p*-tyrosine shifts circadian temperature rhythms, *Am. J. Physiol.* **243:**R218–222.

Caine, E. D., Mendelson, W. B., and Loriaux, D. L., 1979, Neuroendocrine effects of haloperidol in an adolescent with Gilles de la Tourette's disease and delayed onset of puberty, *J. Nerv. Ment. Dis.* **167:**504–507.

Cairns, J., Waldron, J., MacLean, A. W., and Knowles, J. B., 1980, Sleep and depression: A case study of EEG sleep prior to relapse, *Am. J. Psychiatry* **25:**259–263.

Caldwell, J., and Sever, P. S., 1974, The biochemical pharmacology of abused drugs. II. Alcohol and barbiturates, *Clin. Pharmacol. Ther.* **16:**737–749.

Camjanovich, R. P., and MacInnes, J. W., 1973, Factors involved in ethanol narcosis: Analysis of mice of three inbred strains, *Life Sci.* **13:**55–65.

Campbell, A., and Baldessarini, R. J., 1982, Circadian changes in behavioral effects of haloperidol in rats, *Psychopharmacology (Berlin)* **77:**150–155.

Campbell, I. C., Wirz-Justice, A., Krauchi, K., McKernan, R. M., and Durcan, M. J., 1985,

Circadian studies of neurotransmitter receptors, in: *Circadian Rhythms in the Central Nervous System* (P. H. Redfern, I. C. Campbell, J. A. Davies, and K. F. Martin, eds.), VCH, Deerfield, FL, pp. 95–110.

Carlini, E. A., 1983, REM sleep deprivation and dopamine in the CNS, *Rev. Pure Appl. Pharmacol. Sci.* **4**:1–25.

Carlson, G. A., and Goodwin, F. K., 1973, The stages of mania, *Arch Gen. Psychiatry* **28**:221–228.

Carlson, H. E., Gillin, J. C., Gorden, P., and Snyder, F., 1972, Absence of sleep-related growth hormone peaks in aged normal subjects and in acromegaly, *J. Clin. Endocrinol. Metab.* **34**:1102–1105.

Carlsson, A., Corrodi, H., Fuxe, K., and Hokfelt, T., 1969, Effects of some antidepressant drugs on the depletion of intraneuronal brain catecholamine stores, *Eur. J. Pharmacol.* **5**:367–373.

Carmichael, F. J., and Israel, Y., 1975, Effect of ethanol on neurotransmitter release by rat brain cortical slices, *J. Pharmacol. Exp.* **193**:824–834.

Caroffs, S. N., and Winokur, A., 1984, Hormonal response to thyrotropin-releasing hormone following rest–activity reversal in normal men, *Biol. Psychiatry* **19**:1015–1025.

Caron, P. J., Nieman, L. K., Rose, S. R., and Nisula, B. C., 1986, Deficient nocturnal surge of thyrotropin in central hypothyroidism, *J. Clin. Endocrinol. Metab.* **62**:960–970.

Carroll, B. J., 1986, Informed use of the dexamethasone suppression test, *Clin. Psychiatr. (Suppl.)* **47**:10–12.

Carskadon, M. A., and Dement, W. C., 1975, Sleep studies on a 90-minute day, *Electroencephalogr. Clin. Neurophysiol.* **39**:145–155.

Carskadon, M. A., and Dement, W. C., 1981, Respiration during sleep in the aged human, *J. Gerontol.* **36**:420–423.

Carskadon, M. A., Dement, W. C., Mitler, M. M., Guilleminault, C., Zarcone, V. P., and Spiegel, R., 1976, Self-reports versus sleep laboratory findings in 122 drug-free subjects with complaints of chronic insomnia, *Am. J. Psychiatry* **133**:1382–1383.

Carskadon, M. A., Van Den Hoed, J., and Dement, W. C., 1980, Sleep and daytime sleepiness in the elderly, *J. Geriatr. Psychiatry* **13**:135–151.

Carskadon, M. A., Harvey, K., and Dement, W. C., 1981, Multiple sleep latency tests during the development of narcolepsy, *W. J. Med.* **135**:414–418.

Carskadon, M. A., Seidel, W. F., Greenblatt, D. J., and Dement, W. C., 1982, Daytime carryover of triazolam and flurazepam in elderly insomniacs, *Sleep* **5**:361–371.

Cartwright, R. D., 1984, Effect of sleep position on sleep apnea severity, *Sleep* **7**:110–114.

Cartwright, R. D., Monroe, L. J., and Palmer, C., 1967, Individual differences in response to REM deprivation, *Arch. Gen. Psychiatry* **16**:297–303.

Cartwright, R. D., Lloyd, S., Paul, L., and Stephenson, K., 1980, Pressure to dream during a major life crisis, *Sleep Res.* **9**:131.

Casanueva, F. F., Villanueva, L., Cabranes, J. A., Cabezas-Cerrato, J., and Fernandez-Cruza, A., 1984, Cholinergic medication of growth hormone secretion elicited by arginine, clonidine, and physical exercise in man, *J. Clin. Endocrinol. Metab.* **59**:526–530.

Cashman, M. A., Coble, P., McCann, B. S., Taska, L., Reynolds, C. F., and Kupfer, D. J., 1986, Sleep markers for major depressive disorder in adolescent patients, *Sleep Res.* **15**:91.

Canton, R., 1889, Case of narcolepsy, *Clin. Soc. Trans.* **22**:133–137.

Cavagnini, F., and Peracchi, M., 1971, Effect of reserpine on growth hormone response to insulin hypoglycemia and to arginine infusion in normal subjects and hyperthyroid patients, *J. Endocrinol.* **51**:651–656.

Cazzullo, C. L., Penati, G., Bozzi, A., and Mangoni, A., 1969, Sleep patterns in depressed patients treated with a MAO inhibitor: Correlation between EEG and metabolites of tryptophan, in: *The Present Status of Psychotrophic Drugs* (A. Cerletti and F. J. Bove, eds.), pp. 199–203.

Cella, D. F., Pratt, A., and Holland, J. C., 1986, Persistent anticipatory nausea, vomiting, and anxiety in cured Hodgkin's disease patients after completion of chemotherapy, *Am. J. Psychiatry* **143**:5.

Ceresa, F., Angeli, A., Boccuzzi, G., and Molino, G., 1969, Once-a-day neurally stimulated and basal ACTH secretion phases in man and their response to corticoid inhibition, *J. Clin. Endocrinol.* **29**:1074–1082.

Cerone, G., Murri, L., Rossi, B., and Fraioli, F., 1975, Gonadotropin secretion during sleep in chronic schizophrenic patients. Presented at the International Second Sleep Research Congress, Edinburgh, June 30–July 4, 1975

Chan, A. W. K., 1984, Effects of combined alcohol and benzodiazepine: A review, *Drug Alcohol Depend.* **13**:315–341.

Chan, A. W. K., Scanley, D. L., Leong, F. W., and Casbeer, D., 1982, Dissociation of tolerance and physical dependence after ethanol chlordiazepoxide intake, *Pharmacol. Biochem. Behav.* **17**:1239–1244.

Chandler, L. J., Leslie, S.W., Chweh, A. Y., and Swinyard, E. A., 1984, Correlation of benzodiazepine hypnotic potency with inhibition of voltage-dependent calcium uptake into mouse whole brain synaptosomes, *Soc. Neurosci.* (Abstr 125.20) **10**:420.

Chappel, S. C., 1985, Neuroendocrine regulation of luteinizing hormone and FSH: A review, *Life Sci.* **36**:97–103.

Charness, M. E., Gordon, A. S., and Diamond, I., 1983, Ethanol modulation of opiate receptors in cultured neural cells, *Science* **222**:1246–1248.

Chaudhary, B. A., Chaudhary, T. K., Kolbeck, R. C., Harmon, J. D., and Speir, W. A., 1986, Therapeutic effect of posture in sleep apnea, *S. Med. J.* **79**:1061–1063.

Chen, C. N., 1980, The use of clomipramine as an REM sleep suppressant in narcolepsy, *Postgrad. Med. J.* **56**:86–89.

Cherniack, N. S., 1981, Respiratory dysrhythmias during sleep, *Semin. Med. Beth Israel Hosp., Boston* **305**:325–330.

Cherniack, N. S., Longobardo, G. S., Gothe, B., and Weiner, D., 1980, Interactive effects of central and obstructive apnea, *Adv. Physiol. Sci.* **10**:553–560.

Chernik, D. A., Ramsey, T. A., and Mendels, J., 1973, Effect of parachlorophenylalanine on the sleep of a methadone addict, *Br. J. Psychiatry* **122**:191–199.

Chihara, K., Kato, Y., Marda, Y., Oligo, S., and Imura, H., 1976a, Suppressive effect of L-dopa on human-prolactin release during sleep, *Acta Endocrinol. (KBH)* **81**:19–27.

Chihara, K., Kato, Y., Maeda, K., Matsukura, S., and Imura, H., 1976b, Suppression by cyproheptadine of human growth hormone and cortisol secretion during sleep, *J. Clin. Invest.* **57**:1393–1402.

Chihara K., Kato Y., Maeda Y., Ohgo S., and Imura, H., 1976c, Suppressive effect of L-DOPA on human prolactin release during sleep, *Acta Endocrinol. (Copenhagen)* **81**:19–27.

Chihara, K., Kato, Y., Abe, H., Furumoto, M., Maeda, K., and Imura, H., 1977a, Sleep-related growth hormone release following 2-bromo-alpha-ergocriptine treatment in acromegalic patients, *J. Clin. Endocrinol. Metab.* **44**:78–85.

Chihara, K., Kato, Y., Maeda, K., Abe, H., and Furumoto, M., 1977b, Effects of thyrotropin-releasing hormone on sleep and sleep-related growth hormone release in normal subjects, *J. Clin. Endocrinol. Metab.* **44**:1094–1100.

Chihara, K., Arimara, A., and Schally, A. V., 1979, Immunoreactive somatostatin in rat hypophyseal portal blood: Effects of anesthetics, *Endocrinology* **104**:1434–1441.

Child, K. J., Currie, J. P., Davis, B., Dodds, M. G., Pearce, D. R., and Twissell, D. J., 1971, The pharmacological properties in animals of CT 1341, a new steroid anaesthetic agent, *Br. J. Anaes.* **43**:2–13.

Chin, J. H., and Goldstein, D. B., 1977, Effects of low concentrations of ethanol on the fluidity of spin-labeled erythrocyte and brain membranes, *Mol. Pharmacol.* **13**:435–441.

Chokroverty, S., 1986, Sleep apnea in narcolepsy, *Sleep* **9**:250–253.

Christodoulou, G. N., Milliaras, D. E., Lykouras, E. P., Papadimitriou, G. N., and Stafanis, C. N., 1978, Possible prophylactic effect of sleep deprivation, *Am. J. Psychiatry* **135**:375–376.

Church, M. W., and Johnson, L. C., 1979, Mood and performance of poor sleepers during repeated use of flurazepam, *Psychopharmacology* **61**:309–316.

Cianchetti, C., Masala, C., Magoni, A., and Gessa, G. L., 1980, Suppression of REM and delta sleep by apomorphine in man: A dopamine mimetic effect, *Psychopharmacology*, **67**:61–65.

Clarenbach, P., Birmanns, B., and Jaursch-Hancke, C., n. d., The effect of ritanserin on sleep and hormones in man (personal communication).

Clarenbach, P., Del Pozo, E., Brownell, J., Heredia, E., Spiegel, R., and Cramer, H., 1980, Characterization of ergot and non-ergot serotonin antagonists by prolactin and growth hormone profiles during wakefulness and sleep, *Brain Res.* **202**:357–363.

Clark, P. B. S., 1987, Recent progress in identifying nicotinic cholinoceptors in mammalian brain, *Trends Pharmacol. Sci.* **8**:32–35.

Clark, R. W., Schmidt, H. S., and Malarkey, W. B., 1979a, Disordered growth hormone and prolactin secretion in primary disorders of sleep, *Neurology* **29**:855–861.

Clark, R. W., Schmidt, H. A., Schaal, S. F., Boudoulas, H., and Schuller, D. E., 1979b, Sleep apnea: Treatment with protriptyline, *Neurology* **29**:1287–1292.

Clemens, J. A., Shaar, C. J., Smalstig, E. D., Tandy, W. A., and Roush, M. E., 1972, Preoptic area multiple unit activity and LH release during the sleep cycle of the rat, *Endocrinology* **91**:621–625.

Clemes, S., and Dement, W., 1967, The effect of REM sleep deprivation on psychological functioning, *J. Nerv. Ment. Dis.* **144**:485–491.

Clift, A. D., 1975, Prediction of the dependence-prone patient: A general practice investigation, in: *Sleep Disturbance and Hypnotic Drug Dependence* (A. D. Clift, ed.), Excerpta Medica, Amsterdam, pp. 107–153.

Coates, T. J., and Thoresen, C. E., 1977, *How to Sleep Better: A Drug Free Program for Overcoming Insomnia*, Prentice-Hall, Englewood Cliffs, NJ, pp. 1-324.

Coble, P., Foster, F. G., and Kupfer, D. J., 1976, Electroencephalographic sleep diagnosis of primary depression, *Arch. Gen. Psychiatry* **33**:1124–1127.

Coble, P. A., Kupfer, D. J., Spiker, D. G., Neil, J. F., and McPartland, R. J., 1979, EEG sleep in primary depression: A longitudinal placebo study, *J. Affective Disord.* **1**:131–138.

Coble, P. A., Kupfer, D. J., and Shaw, D. H., 1981, Distribution of REM latency in depression, *Biol. Psychiatry* **16**:453–466.

Coccagna, C., Montovani, M., Berti-Ceroni, G., Pazzaglea, P., Petrella, A., and Lugarese, E., 1970, Sindrome ipersonniche-ipoventilatore, *Ment. Med.* **61**:1073–1084.

Coccagna, C., Mantouani, M., Brignani, F., Parchi, C., and Lugaresi, E., 1972, Continuous recording of insomnia with periodic breathing, *Bull. Physiopathol. Resp.* **8**:1217–1227.

Coccagna, C., Cirignotta, F., Zucconi, M., Gerardi, R., Medori, R., and Lugaresi, E., 1984, A polygraphic study of one case of primary alveolar hypoventilation (Ondine's curse), *Bull. Eur. Physiopathol. Respir.* **20**:157–161.

Coccagna, G., Martinelli, P., and Lugaresi, E., 1982, Sleep and alveolar hypoventilation in myotonic dystrophy, *Acta Neurol. Belg.* **82:**185–194.

Coculescu, M., Serbanescu, A., and Temeli, E., 1979, Influence of arginine vasotocin administration on nocturnal sleep of human subjects, *Waking and Sleeping* **3:**273–277.

Cohen, D., Cohen, O., Marcadet, A., Massart, C., Lathrop, M., Deschamps, I., and Dausset, J., 1984, Class II HLA-DC beta-chain DNA restriction fragments differentiate among HLA-DR2 individuals in insulin-dependent diabetes and multiple sclerosis, *Proc. Natl. Acad. Sci. USA* **81:**1774–1778.

Cohen, H., Thomas, J., and Dement, W. C., 1970, Sleep styles, REM deprivation, and electroconvulsive threshold in the cat, *Brain Res.* **19:**317–321.

Cohen, H. B., Dement, W. C., and Barchas, J. D., 1973, Effects of chlorpromazine on sleep in cats pretreated with para-chlorophenylalanine, *Brain Res.* **53:**363–371.

Cohen, S., 1970,Benzodiazepin withdrawal, *Drug Abuse Alcoholism Newslett. (Vista Hill Found.)* **16:**1–4.

Coleman, R. M., 1979, Periodic nocturnal myoclonus in disorders of sleep and wakefulness, Ph.D. thesis, Yeshiva University, University Microfilms, Ann Arbor, MI.

Coleman, R. M., 1982, in: *Sleeping and Waking Disorders: Indications and Techniques* (R. Guilleminault, ed.), pp. 265–295.

Coleman, R. M., Pollak, C. P., and Weitzman, E. D., 1980, Periodic movements in sleep (nocturnal myoclonus): Relation to sleep disorders, *Ann. Neurol.* **8:**416–421.

Coleman, R. M., Roffwarg, H. P., Kennedy, S. J., Guilleminault, C., Cinque, J., Cohn, M. A., and Dement, W. C., 1982, Sleep-wake disorders based on a polysomnographic diagnosis: A national cooperative study, *JAMA* **247:**997–1003.

Colvin, C.L., and Tankanow, R.M., 1985, Pimozide: Use in Tourette's syndrome, *Drug Intell. Clin. Pharm.* **19:**421–424.

Colvin, G. B., Whitmoyer, D. I., and Sawyer, C. H., 1969, Circadian sleep–wakefulness patterns in rats after ovariectomy and treatment with estrogen, *Exp. Neurol.* **25:**616–625.

Conroy, R. T. W. L., Hughes, B. D., and Mills, J. N., 1968, Circadian rhythm of plasma II-hydroxycorticosteroids in psychiatric patients, *Br. Med. J.* **3:**405–407.

Coppen, A., 1967, The biochemistry of affective disorders, *Br. J. Psychiatry* **113:**1213–1264.

Coppola, J. A., 1971, Brain catecholamines and gonadotropin secretion, in: *Frontiers in Neuroendocrinology* (L. Martini and W. F. Ganong, eds.), Oxford University Press, New York, pp. 129–143.

Corda, M. G., Blaker, W. D., Mendelson, W. B., Guidotta, A., and Costa, E., 1983, Beta-carbolines enhance shock-induced suppression of drinking in rats, *Proc. Natl. Acad. Sci. USA* **80:**2072–2076.

Cordingly, G. J., Dean, B. C., and Harris, R. I., 1984, A double-blind comparison of two benzodiazepine hypnotics, flunitrazepam and triazolam, in general practice, *Curr. Med. Res. Opin.* **8:**714–719.

Corsini, G. U., Piccardi, M. P., DelZompo, M., and Gessa, G. L., 1977, Changes in CSF tryptophan and 5-HIAA induced by amino acids mixtures in man, *Proc. Int. Soc. Neurochem.* **6:**563.

Costa, E., Guidotti, A., and Mao, C. C., 1975, Evidence for involvement of GABA in the action of benzodiazepines: Studies on rat cerebellum, *Adv. Biochem. Psychopharmacol.* **14:**113–130.

Costa, E., Corda, M. G., Wise, B., Konkel, D., and Guidotti A., 1982, Benzodiazepines and GABA interactions: Role of GABA-modulin, *in: Pharmacology of Benzodiazepines* (E. Usdin, P. Skolnick, J. F. Tallman, D. Greenblatt, and S. F. Paul, eds.), Macmillan, London, pp. 111–120.

Coulter, J. D., Lester, B. K., and Williams, H. L., 1971, Reserpine and sleep, *Psychophar-macologia* 19:134–147.

Coursey, R. D., 1975, Personality measures and evoked responses in chronic insomniacs, *J. Abnorm. Psychol.* 84:339–349.

Coursey, R. D., Buchsbaum, M., and Frankel, B. L., 1975, Personality measures and evoked responses in chronic insomniacs, *J. Abnorm. Psychol.* 84:239–249.

Coutifaris, C., and Chappel, S. C., 1983, Involvement of hypothalamic luteinizing hormone-releasing hormone in the regulation of the estrous follicle-stimulating hormone surge in the female golden hamster, *Endocrinology* 113:563–568.

Cramer, H., Rudolph, J., Consbruch, U., and Kendel, K., 1974, On the effects of melatonin on sleep and behavior in man, *Adv. Biochem. Psychopharmacol.* 11:187–191.

Crawley, J. N., Marangos, P. J., Paul, S. M., Skolnick, P., and Goodwin, F. K., 1981, Interaction between purine and benzodiazepine: Inosine reverses diazepam-induced stimulation of mouse exploratory behavior, *Science* 211:725–727.

Crawley, J. N., Rojas-Ramirez, J. A., and Mendelson, W. B., 1982, The role of central and peripheral cholecystokinin in mediating appetitive behaviors, *Peptides* 3:535–538.

Crosignani, P. G., Lombroso, G. C., Mattei, A., Caccamo, A., and Trojsi, L., 1979, Effect of three serotonin antagonists on plasma prolactin response to suckling in puerperal women, *J. Clin. Endocrinol. Metab.* 48:335–337.

Crossland, J., and Slater P., 1968, The effects of some drugs on the "free" and "bound" acetylcholine content of a rat brain, *Br. J. Pharmacol.* 33:42.

Crowley, T. J., Pegram, G. V., and Smith, D. E., 1969, The biogenic amines and sleep in the monkey Primate electrophysiology particularly related to sleep. No. 5761, Aeromedical Research Laboratory, Dept. ART TR-69-3, Rep. 163. GPO, Holloman Air Force Base New Mexico.

Cryer, P. E., and Daughaday, W. H., 1969, Regulation of growth hormone secretion in acromegaly, *J. Clin. Endocrinol. Metab.* 29:386–393.

Cummiskey, J., Guilleminault, C., Del Rio, G., and Silvestri, R., 1983, The effects of flurazepam on sleep studies in patients with chronic obstructive pulmonary disease, *Chest* 84:143–147.

Curran, T., and Morgan, J. I., 1985, Superinduction of c-fox by nerve growth factor in the presence of peripherally active benzodiazepines, *Science* 229:1265–1268.

Czeisler, C. A., Zimmerman, J. C., Ronda, J. M., Moore-Ede, M. C., and Weitzman, E. D., 1980, Timing of REM sleep is coupled to the circadian rhythm of body temperature in man, *Sleep* 2:329–346.

Czeisler, C. A., Richardson, G. S., Coleman, R. M., Zimmerman, J. C., Moore-Ede, M. C., Dement, W. C., and Weitzman, E. D., 1981a, Chronotherapy: Resetting the circadian clocks of patients with delayed sleep phase insomnia, *Sleep* 4:1–21.

Czeisler, C. A., Richardson, G. S., Zimmerman, J. C., Moore-Ede, M. C., and Weitzman, E. D., 1981b, Entrainment of human circadian rhythms by light–dark cycles: A reassessment, *Photochem. Photobiol.* 34:239–247.

Czeisler, C. A., Moore-Ede, M. C., and Coleman, R. M., 1982, Rotating shift work schedules that disrupt sleep are improved by applying circadian principles, *Science* 217:460–463.

Czeisler, C. A., Kronauer, R. E., Ronda, J. M., and Rios, C. D., 1985, Sleep deprivation in constant light phase advance shifts and shortens the free-running period of the human circadian timing system, *Sleep Res.* 14:252.

Czeisler, C. A., Allan, J. S., Strogatz, S. H., Ronda, J. M., Sanchez, R., Rios, D., and Kronauer, R. E., 1986, Bright light resets the human circadian pacemaker, independent of the timing of the sleep–wake cycle, *Science* 233:667–671.

Czernik, A., Petrack, B., Kalinsky, H., Psychos, S., Cash, W., Tsai C., and Reinhart, R., 1982, CGS 8216: Receptor binding characteristics of a potent benzodiazepine antagonist, *Life Sci.* **30**:363–372.

Daan, S., Beersma, D. G. M., and Borbely, A. A., 1984, Timing of human sleep: Recovery process gated by a circadian pacemaker, *Am. J. Physiol.* **246**:R161-R178.

Dahlgren, K., 1981, Adjustment of circadian rhythms and EEG sleep functions to day and night sleep among permanent night workers and rotating shift workers, *Psychophysiology* **18**:381–391.

Dahlstrom, A., and Fuxe, K., 1964, Evidence for the existence of monoamine-containing neurons in the central nervous system, I. Demonstration of monoamine in the cell bodies of the brain stem, *Acta Physiol. Scand.* **62**(232):1–55, 1964

Daly, D. D., and Yoss, R. E., 1956, The treatment of narcolepsy with methyl phenylpiperidylacetate: A preliminary report, *Proc. Staff Meetings Mayo Clinic* **31**:620–625.

Daly, J. W., 1982, Adenosine receptors: Targets for future drugs, *J. Med. Chem.* **25**:197–207.

Dantzer, R. and Perio, A., 1982, Behavioral evidence for partial agonist properties of RO-15-1788, a benzodiazepine receptor antagonist, *Eur. J. Pharmacol.* **81**:655–658.

D'Armiento, M., Bigi, F., Pontecorvi, M., Centanni, M., and Reda, G., 1984, Diazepam-stimulated GH secretion in normal subjects: Relation to oestradiol plasma levels, *Horm. Metab. Res.* **16**:155.

Daughaday, W. H., 1975, Regulation of growth by endocrines, *Ann. Rev. Physiol.* **37**:211–244.

Daughaday, W. H., 1985, The anterior pituitary, in: *Williams Textbook of Endocrinology* (J. D. Wilson and D. W. Foster, eds.), Saunders, Philadelphia, pp. 568–613.

Daughaday, W. H., Othmer, E., and Kipnis, D. M., 1969, Hypersecretion of growth hormone during REM deprivation, Abst.: 126, 1969 51st Mtg. Endocrine Soc., New York.

Davis, K. L., and Yamamura, H. I., 1978, Cholinergic underactivity in human memory disorders, *Life Sci.* **23**:1729–1733.

Davis, V. E., 1973, Neuroamine-derived alkaloids: A possible common denominator in alcoholism and related drug dependencies, *Ann. NY Acad. Sci.* **215**:111–115.

Davis, V. E., and Walsh, M. J., 1970, Alcohol, amines, and alkaloids: A possible biochemical basis for alcohol addiction, *Science* **167**:1005–1007.

Davis, W. C., and Ticku, M., 1981, Ethanol enhances [³H]diazepam binding at the benzodiazepine–gamma-aminobutyric acid receptor–ionophore complex, *Mol. Pharmacol.* **20**:287–294.

Dawson, S., Kaplan, J., Semel, C., Green, R., Woodrow, K., Gillin, J. C., and Wyatt, R. J., 1974, Sleep changes in chronic schizophrenics: Effects of 5-hydroxytryptophan (5-HTP), *Sleep Res.* **3**:37.

Deguchi, T., and Axelrod, J., 1972, Induction and superinduction of serotonin N-acetyltransferase by adrenergic drugs and denervation in rat pineal organ, *Proc. Natl. Acad. Sci. USA* **69**:2208–2211.

de Jonghe, F., Ameling, E. H., Jonkers, F., Folkers, C., and Schwartz, R. V., 1984, Flurazepam and temazepam in the treatment of insomnia in a general hospital population, *Pharmacopsychiatry* **17**:133–135.

De Koninck, J., Quera Salva, M., Besset, A., and Billiard, M., 1986, Are REM cycles in narcoleptic patients governed by an ultradian rhythm? *Sleep* **9**:162–166.

De Lacerda, L., Kowarski, A., Johanson, A., Athanasiou, R., and Miceon, C., 1973, Integrated concentration and circadian variation of plasma testosterone in normal men, *J. Clin. Endocrinol. Metab.* **37**:366–371.

Delitala, G., Frulio, T., Pacifico, A., and Maioli, M., 1982, Participation of cholinergic muscarinic receptors in glucagon and arginine mediated growth hormone secretion in man, *J. Clin. Endocrinol. Metab.* **55**:1231–1233.

Delitala, G., Grossman, A., and Besser, G. M., 1983a, Opiate peptides control growth hormone through a cholinergic mechanism in man, *Clin. Endocrinol. (Oxf)* **18**:401–406.

Delitala, G., Maioli, M., Pacifico, A., Brianda, S., Palermo, M., and Manelli, M., 1983b, Cholinergic receptor control mechanisms for L-dopa, apomorphine, and clonidine-induced growth hormone secretion in man, *J. Clin. Endocrinol. Metab.* **57**:1145–1149.

De Lorenzo, R. J., Burdette, S., and Holderness, J., 1981, Benzodiazepine inhibition of the calcium–calmodulin protein kinase system in brain membrane, *Science* **213**:546–549.

Delorme, F., 1966, Monoamines et sommiels. Etude polygraphique nueropharmacologique et histochimique des etats de sommeil ches le chat. These Universite de Lyon, Imprimerie LMD.

Dement, W. C., 1960, The effect of dream deprivation, *Science* **131**:1705–1707.

Dement, W. C., 1964, Experimental dream studies, *Sci. Psychoanal.* **7**:129–184.

Dement, W., 1965, Recent studies on the biological role of REM sleep, *Am. J. Psychiatry* **122**:404–408.

Dement, W. C., 1969, The biological role of REM sleep, in: *Sleep Physiology and Pathology*, J. B. Lippincott, Philadelphia, pp. 245–265.

Dement, W. C., and Fisher, C., 1963, Experimental interference with the sleep cycle, *Can. Psychiatr. Assoc. J.* **8**:400–405.

Dement, W., and Kleitman, N., 1957, Cyclic variations in EEG sleep and their relation to eye movements, body motility, and dreaming, *Electroencephalogr. Clin. Neurophysiol.* **9**:673–690.

Dement, W. C., and Mitler, M. M., 1974, An introduction to sleep, in: *Basic Sleep Mechanisms* (O. Petre-Quadens and J. D. Schlag, eds.), Academic Press, New York, pp. 271–296.

Dement, W., Greenberg, S., and Klein, R., 1966a, The effect of partial REM sleep deprivation and delayed recovery, *J. Psychiatr. Res.* **4**:141–152.

Dement, W., Rechtschaffen, A., and Gulevich, G., 1966b, The nature of the narcoleptic sleep attack, *Neurology (Minneap.)* **16**:18–33.

Dement, W., Zarcone, V., Ferguson, J., Cohen, H., Pivik, T., and Barchas, J., 1969, Some parallel findings in schizophrenic patients and serotonin-depleted cats, in: *Schizophrenia: Current Concepts and Research* (S. Sankar, ed.), PJD Publications, Hicksville, NY, pp. 775–809.

Dement, W. C., Carskadon, M., and Ley, R., 1973a, The prevalence of narcolepsy, II, *Sleep Res.* **2**:147.

Dement, W., Guilleminault, C., and Mitler, M., 1973b, Cataplectic attack: Polygraphic recording in man and experimental induction in cat, *Neurology (Minneap)* **23**:403–404.

Dement, W., Holman, R., and Guilleminault, C., 1976, Neurochemical and neuropharmacological foundations of sleep disorders, *Psychopharmacol. Commun.* **2**:77–90.

Dement, W. C, Carskadon, M. A., Mitler, M. M., Phillips, R. L., and Zarcone, Jr., V. P., 1978, Prolonged use of flurazepam: A sleep laboratory study, *Behav. Med.* **5**:25–31.

Dement, W. C., Seidel, W., and Carskadon, M. A., 1982, Daytime alertness, insomnia and benzodiazepines, *Sleep* **5**:528–545.

Dement, W. C., Seidel, W., and Carskadon, M., 1984, Issues in the diagnosis and treatment of insomnia, *Psychopharmacology* **2**(suppl.):11–43.

De Paula, A. J. M., 1984, Comparative study of lormetazepam and flurazepam in the treatment of insomnia, *Clin. Ther.* **6**:500–508.

Derbez, R., and Grauer, H., 1967, A sleep study and investigation of a new hypnotic compound in a geriatric population, *Can. Med. Assoc. J.* **97**:1388–1393.

Des Andres, I., Guttierrez-Rivas, E., Vava, E., and Reinoso-Suarez, F., 1976, Indepen-dence of sleep–wakefulness cycle in an implanted head "encephale isolé," Neurosci. Lett. 2:13–18.

Desir, D., Cauter, E. V., Golstein, J., Fang, V. S., Leclerq, R., Refetoff, S., and Copinschi, G., 1980, Circadian ultradian variations of ACTH and cortisol secretion, Horm. Res. 13:302–316.

Detre, T., Himmelhock, J., Swartzburg, M., Anderson, D. M., Byck, R., and Kupfer,D. J., 1972, Hypersomnia and manic-depressive disease, Am. J. Psychiatry 128:1303–1305.

Diaz-Guerrero, R., Gottlieb, J. S., and Knott, J. R., 1946, The sleep of patients with manic-depressive psychosis, depressive type: An electroencephalographic study, Psychosom. Med. 8:300–404.

Diaz-Guerrero, R., Gottleib, J. S., and Knott, J. R., 1966, The sleep of patients with manic depression, Br. J. Psychiatry 112:1263–1267.

Dickens, C., 1837, The Posthumous Papers of the Pickwickian Club, Chapman & Hall, Lon-don.

Dirlich, G., Kammenloher, A., Schultz, H., Lund, R., Doerr, P., and von Zerssen, D., 1981, Temporal coordination of rest–activity cycle, body temperature, urinary-free cor-tisol, and mood in a patient with 48 unipolar depressive cycles in clinical and time-cue free environments, Biol. Psychiatry 16:163–179.

Doig, R. J., Mummery, R. V., Willis, M. R., and Elkes, A., 1966, Plasma cortisol levels in depression, Br. J. Psychiatry 112:1263–1267.

Dollery, C. T., Hamilton, C. A., and Maling, T. J. B., 1977, Changes in sleep pattern, blood pressure, heart rate and plasma noradrenaline after nighttime administration of slow release clonidine, Br. J. Clin. Pharmacol. 4:634.

Dolly, F. R., and Block, A. J., 1982, Effect of flurazepam on sleep-disordered breathing and nocturnal oxygen desaturation in asymptomatic subjects, Am. J. Med. 73:239–243.

Dolly, F. R., and Block, A. J., 1983, Medroxyprogesterone acetate and COPD: Effect on breathing and oxygenation in sleeping and awake patients, Chest 84:394–398.

Domino, E. F., and Corssen, G., 1967, Central and peripheral effects of muscarinic cholinergic blocking agents in man, Anaesthesiology 28:568–574.

Douglas, W. W., 1970, Histamine and antihistamines 5-hydroxytryptamine and antago-nists, in: The Pharmacological Basis of Therapeutics (L. S. Goodman and A. Gilman, eds.), Macmillan, London, pp. 621–662.

Douglas, W. W., 1980, Histamine and 5-hydroxytryptamine (serotonin) and their antago-nists, in: The Pharmacological Basis of Therapeutics (A. G. Gilman, L. S. Goodman, and A. Gilman, eds.), Macmillan, New York, pp. 609–646.

Downes, H., Perry, R. S., Ostlund, R. E., and Karler, R., 1970, A study of the excitatory effects of barbiturates, J. Pharmacol. Exp. Ther. 175:692–699.

Dragstedt, L. L., 1959, Causes of peptic ulcer, JAMA 169:203–209.

Dreifuss, F. E., and Flynn, D. V., 1984, Narcolepsy in a horse [Letter], J. Am. Vet. Med. Assoc. 184:131–132.

Drucker-Colin, R., and Bernal-Pedraza, J., 1983, Kainic acid lesions of gigantocellular at-egmental field (FTG) neurons does not abolish REM sleep, Brain Res. 272:387–391.

Drucker-Colin, R. R., Spanis, C. W., Shkurovich, M., and Ugartechea, J. C., 1975, Central neuroprotein regulation of REM sleep. Presented at the Second International Sleep Research Congress, Edinburgh, June 30–July 4, 1975.

Dudl, R. J., Ensinck, J. W., Palmer, H. E., and Williams, R. H., 1973, Effect of age on growth hormone secretion in man, J. Clin. Endocrinol. Metab. 37:11–16.

Duncan, W. C., Pettigrew, K. A., and Gillin, J. C., 1979, REM architecture changes in bipolar and unipolar patients, Am. J. Psychiatry 136:1412–1427.

Dundee, J. W., 1954, The influence of body-weight, sex and age on the dosage of thiopentone, *Br. J. Anaesth.* **26**:164–173.

Dundee, J. W., Howard, A. J., and Isaac, M., 1971, Alcohol and the benzodiazepines: The interaction between intravenous ethanol and chlordiazepoxide and diazepam, *Q. J. Stud. Alcohol* **32**:960–968.

Dunleavy, D. K. F., Maclean, A. W., and Oswald, I., 1971, Debrisoquine, quanethidine, propranolol and human sleep, *Psychopharmacologia* **21**:101–110.

Dunleavy, D. L., Brezinova, V., Oswald, I., Maclean, A. W., and Tinker, M., 1972, Changes during weeks in effects on tricyclic drugs on the human sleeping brain, *Br. J. Psychiatry* **120**:663–672.

Dunleavy, D. L., Oswald, I., Brown, and P., Strong, J. A., 1974, Hyperthyroidism, sleep and growth hormone, *Electroencephalogr. Clin. Neurophysiol.* **36**:259–263.

Duron, B., 1972, La fonction respiratoire pendant le sommeil physiologique, *Bull. Physiopathol. Respir.* **8**:1277–1288.

Durrigl, V., Buranji, I., and Stojanovic, V., 1973a, Characteristics of paradoxical sleep in schizophrenic patients, in: *Sleep: Physiology, Biochemistry, Psychology, Pharmacology, Clinical Implications*, Karger, Basel.

Durrigl, V., Rogina, V., Stojanovic, V., Hajnsek, F., Gubarev, N., and Jovanovic, U. J., 1973b, Drugs—a study of two substances, in: *The Nature of Sleep* (U. J. Jonvanovic, ed.), Fischer-Verlag, Stuttgart, pp. 203–208.

Dushenko, T. W., and Sterman, M. B., 1984, Hemisphere-specific deficits on cognitive/perceptual tasks following REM sleep deprivation, *Int. J. Neurosci.* **25**:25–45.

Duvoisin, R. C., 1967, Cholinergic–anticholinergic antagonism in parkinsonism, *Arch. Neurol.* **17**:124–136.

Eastman, C. J., and Lazarus, L., 1973, Growth hormone release during sleep in growth retarded children, *Arch. Dis. Child.* **48**:502–507.

Eckernas, S. A., Sahlstrom, L., and Aquilonius, S. M., 1977, *In vivo* turnover rate of acetylcholine in rat brain parts at elevated steady-state concentration of plasma choline, *Acta Physiol. Scand.* **101**:404–410.

Edinger, J. D., Stout, A. L., and Hoelscher, T. J., 1986, MMPI defined subtypes of insomniacs, *Sleep Res.* **15**:118.

Editorial, 1984, Rapid eye movement (REM) sleep: Cholinergic mechanisms? *Psychol. Med.* **14**:501–506.

Ehret, C. F., Potter, U. R., and Dobra, K. W., 1975, Chronotypic action of theophylline and of pentobarbital as circadian Zeitbeibers in the rat, *Science* **188**:1212–1215.

Ehret, C. F., Groh, K. R., and Meinart, J. C., 1980, Considerations of diet in alleviating jet lag, in: *Chronobiology: Principles and Applications to Shifts in Schedules* (L. E. Schwing, and F. Halberg, eds.), Sijthoff and Nordhoff, Rockville, MD, pp. 393–401.

Ekbom, K. A., 1945, Restless legs, *Acta Med. Scand.* **158S**:4–122.

Ekbom, K. A., 1960, Restless legs syndrome, *Neurology* **10**:868–873.

Ekbom, K., 1975, Growing pains and restless legs, *Acta Paediatr. Scand.* **64**:264–266.

Ellingsen, P. A., 1983, Double-blind trial of triazolam 0.5 mg vs. nitrazepam 5 mg in outpatients, *Acta Psychiatr. Scand.* **67**:154–158.

Ellman, S. J., Spielman, A. J., Luck, D., Steiner, S. S., and Halperin, R., 1978, REM deprivation: A review, in: *The Mind in Sleep: Psychology and Psychophysiology* (A. M. Arkin, J. S. Antrobus, and S. J. Ellman, eds.), Laurence Earlbaum Assoc., Hillsdale, NJ, pp. 419–457.

Elomaa, E., and Johansson, G. G., 1980, Rapid eye movement stage of sleep participates in the generation of the nocturnal meal pattern in the rat, *Physiol. Behav.* **24**:331–336.

Elsenga, S., and Van den Hoffdakker, R., 1983, Clinical effects of sleep deprivation and clomipramine in endogenous depression, *J. Psychiatr. Res.* **17**:361–374.

Engle-Friedman, M., Baker, E. A., and Bootzin, R. R., 1985, Reports of wakefulness during EEG identified stages of sleep, *Sleep Res.* **14**:152.

Englen, M., Milon, H., and Wurzner, H. P., 1980, Brain catecholamines and sleep states in offspring of caffeine treated rats, *Experientia* 36:1105–1106.

Enright, J. T., 1980, *The Timing of Sleep and Wakefulness*, Springer, New York.

Erickson, C. K., and Burnam, W. L., 1971, Cholinergic alteration of ethanol-induced sleep and death in mice, *Agents Actions* **2**:8–13.

Erickson, C. K., and Matchett, J. A., 1974, Correlation of brain amine changes with ethanol induced sleeptime in mice, *Adv. Exp. Med. Biol.* **59**:419–430.

Erickson, C. K., Tyler, T. D., Beck, L. K., and Duensing, K. L., 1980, Calcium enhancement of alcohol and drug-induced sleeping time in mice and rats, *Pharmacol. Biochem. Behav.* **12**:651–656.

Erlich, S. S., and Apuzzo, L. J., 1985, The pineal gland: Anatomy, physiology, and clinical significance, *J. Neurosurg.* **63**:321–341.

Erlich, S. S., and Itabushi, H. H., 1986, Narcolepsy: A neuropathologic study, *Sleep* **9**:126–132.

Ersmark, B., and Lidvall, H., 1973, Trial with amantine in narcolepsy, *Psychopharmacologia* **28**:308.

Eskin, A., and Takahashi, J. S., 1983, Adenylate cyclase activation shifts the phase of a circadian pacemaker, *Science* **220**:82–84.

Evans, J. I., and Oswald, I., 1966, Some experiments in the chemistry of narcoleptic sleep, *Br. J. Psychiatry* **112**:401–404.

Evans, J. I., MacLean, A. M., Ismail, A. A. A., and Love, D., 1971a, Circulating levels of plasma testosterone during sleep, *Proc. Royal Soc. Med.* **64**:841–842.

Evans, J. I., MacLean, A. W., Ismail, A. A. A., and Love, D., 1971b, Concentration of plasma testosterone in normal men during sleep, *Nature* **229**:261–262.

Fabre, L. F., and Crismon, L., 1985, Efficacy of fluoxetine in outpatients with major depression, *Curr. Ther. Res.* **37**:115–123.

Fabre, Jr., L. F., Gross, L., Pasigajen, V., and Metzler, C., 1977, Multiclinic double-blind comparison of triazolam and flurazepam for seven nights in patients with insomnia, *J. Clin. Pharmacol.* **17**:402–409.

Fahndrich, E., 1981, Effects of sleep deprivation on depressed patients of different nosological groups, *Psychiatry Res.* **5(3)**:277–285.

Falck, B., Hillarp, N. A., Thieme, G., and Torp, A., 1962, Fluorescence of catecholamine and related compounds condensed with formaldehyde, *J. Histochem. Cytochem.* **10**:348–354.

Faull, K. F., Barchas, J. D., Foutz, A. S., Dement, W. C., and Holman, R. B., 1982, Monoamine metabolite concentrations in the cerebrospinal fluid of normal and narcoleptic dogs, *Brain Res.* **242**:137–143.

Faull, K. F., Zeller-DeAmicis, L. C., Radde, L., Bowersox, S. S., Baker, T. L., Kilduff, T. S., and Dement, W. C., 1986a, Biogenic amine concentrations in the brains of normal and narcoleptic canines: Current status, *Sleep* **9**:107–110.

Faull, K. F., Thiemann, S., King, R. T., and Guilleminault, C., 1986b, Monoamine interactions in narcolepsy and hypersomnia: A preliminary report, *Sleep* **9**:246–249.

Faure, J., 1962, La phase "paradoxale" du sommeil chez le lapin (ses relations neurohormonales), *Rev. Neurol.* **106**:190–197.

Feinberg, I., 1968 The ontogenesis of human sleep and the relationship of sleep variables to intellectual function, *Compr. Psychiatry* **9**:138–147.

Feinberg, I., 1969a, Sleep in organic brain conditions, in: *Sleep: Physiology and Pathology* (A. Kales, ed.), Lippincott Co., Philadelphia, pp. 131–147.

Feinberg, I., 1969b Recent sleep research: Findings in schizophrenia and and some implications for the mechanisms of action of chlorpromazine and for the neurophysiology delirium, in: *Schizophrenia: Current Concepts and Research* (D. V. Siva-Sanker, ed.), PJD, Hicksville, NY, pp. 739–750.

Feinberg, I., 1974, Changes in sleep cycle patterns with age, *J. Psychiatry Res.* **10:**283–306.

Feinberg, I., 1976, Functional implications of changes in sleep-physiology with age, in: *Aging*, Vol. 3, *The Neurobiology of Aging* (S. Gershon and R. Terry, eds.), Raven Press, New York, pp. 23–41.

Feinberg, I., and Carlson, V. R., 1968, Sleep variables as a function of age in man, *Arch. Gen. Psychiatry* **18:**239–250.

Feinberg, I., Koresko, R. L., and Heller, N., 1967, EEG sleep patterns as a function of normal and pathological aging in man, *J. Psychiatr. Res.* **5:**107–144.

Feinberg, I., Wender, P. H., Koresko, R. L., Gottleib, F., and Piehuta, J. A., 1969, Differential effects of chlorpromazine and phenobarbital on EEG sleep patterns, *J. Psychiatr. Res.* **7:**101–109.

Feinberg, I., Hibi, S., Cavness, C., and March, J., 1974a, Absence of REM rebound after barbiturate withdrawals, *Science* **185:**534–535.

Feinberg, I., Hibi, S., Braun, M., Cavness, C., Westerman, G., and Small, A., 1974b, Sleep amphetamine effects in MBDS and normal subjects, *Arch. Gen. Psychiatry* **31:**723–731.

Feinberg, I., Fein, G., and Floyd, T. C., 1980, EEG patterns during and following extended sleep in young adults, *Electroencephalogr. Clin. Neurophysiol.* **50:**467–476.

Feinberg, M., Carroll, B. J., King, D., and Greden, J. F., 1984, The effect of dexamethasone on sleep: Preliminary results in eleven patients, *Biol. Psychiatry* **19:**771–775.

Feinberg, M. E., Gillin, J. C., Carroll, B. J., Greden, J. F., and Zis, A. P., 1982, EEG studies of a sleep in the diagnosis of depression, *Biol. Psychiatry* **17:**305–316.

Feldberg, W., and Sherwood, S. L., 1954, Injections of drugs into the lateral ventricle of the cat, *J. Physiol.* (London) **123:**148–167.

Feldstein, A., 1973, Ethanol-induced sleep in relation to serotonin turnover and conversion to 5-hydroxyindoleacetaldehyde, 5-hydroxytrytophol, and 5-hydroxyindoleacetic acid, *Ann. NY Acad. Sci.* **215:**71–76.

Feldstein, A., Chang, F. H., and Kucharski, J. M., 1970, Tryptophol, 5-hydroxytryptophol and 5-methoxytryptophol induced to sleep in mice, *Life Sci.* **9:**323–329.

Felger, H. L., 1971, Chlorprothixene-enforced sleep for newly admitted patients with acute mental decomposition, *Dis. Nerv. Syst.* **32:**46–51.

Fevre, M., Segel, T., Marks, J. F., and Boyar, R. M., 1978, LH and melatonin secretion patterns in pubertal boys, *J. Clin. Endocrinol. Metab.* **47:**1383–1387.

Figurelli, F. A., 1958, Delirium tremens: Reduction of mortality and morbidity with promacine, *JAMA* **166:**747–750.

File, S., Lister, R. F., and Nutt, D., 1982, The anxiogenic action of benzodiazepine antagonists, *Neuropharmacology* **21:**1033–1037.

Fillingim, J. M., 1982, Double-blind evaluation of temazepam, flurazepam, and placebo in geriatric insomniacs, *Clin. Ther.* **4:**369–379.

Finkelstein, J. W., Boyar, R. M., Roffwarg, H. P., Kream, J., and Hellman, L., 1972, Age-related change in the twenty-four-hour spontaneous secretion of growth hormone, *J. Clin. Endocrinol. Metab.* **35:**665–670.

Fischer-Perroudon, C., Mouret, J., and Jouvet, M., 1974, Sur un cas d'agrypnie (4 mois sans sommeil) au cours d'une maladie de Morvan. Effet favorable du 5-hydroxytryptophane, *Electroencephalogr. Clin. Neurophysio.* **36**:1–18.

Fisher, E., and von Mering, S., 1903, Uber eine neue Klasse von Schlafmitteln, *Ther. Ggw.* **44**:97.

Fisher, R. J. H., and Dean, B. C., 1985, A multi-centre, double-blind trial in general practice, *Pharmatherapeutica* **4**:231–236.

Fiss, H., Lavie, P., and Hesselbrock, V., 1983, Psychopathological correlates of sleep apnea, hypopnea, narcolepsy, and nocturnal myoclonus: A comparative study, *Sleep Res.* **12**:305.

Fletcher, E. C., and Levin, D. C., 1984, Cardiopulmonary hemodynamics during sleep in subjects with chronic obstructive pulmonary disease: The effect of short- and long-term oxygen, *Chest* **85**:6–14.

Fletcher, E. C., and Martin, R. J., 1982, Sexual dysfunction and erectile impotence in chronic obstructive pulmonary disease, *Chest* **81**:413–421.

Fletcher, E., Lavoi, M., Zenner, G., Malitz, W., and Nickeson, D., 1984, Protriptyline in the treatment of sleep apnea, *Am. Rev. Respir. Dis.* **129**:A59.

Fletcher, E. C., Miller, J., Schaaf, J. W., and Fletcher, J., 1987, Urinary catecholamines before and after tracheostomy in patients with obstructive sleep apnea and hypertension, *Sleep* **10**:35–44.

Flick, M. R., and Block, A. J., 1977, Continuous *in-vivo* monitoring of arterial oxygenation in chronic obstructive lung disease, *Ann. Intern. Med.* **86**:725–730.

Florio, V., Scotti, A., Carolis, A., and Longo, V. G., 1968, Observations on the effect of D, 1-parachlorophenylalanine on the electroencephalogram, *Physiol. Behav.* **3**:861–863.

Fontaine, R., Chouinard, G., and Annable, L., 1984, Rebound anxiety in anxious patients after abrupt withdrawal of benzodiazepine treatment, *Am. J. Psychiatry* **141**:848–852.

Foreman, P. J., Stahl, J., Hobbins, T. E., Paskewitz, D. A., and Gross, H. S., 1986, Sleep apnea in five patients evaluated for nocturnal penile tumescence, *Md. Med. J.* **35**:46–48.

Foret, J., and Benoit, O., 1978, Study of sleep of shift workers with alternating schedules: Adaptation and recovery in case of rapid shift rotation of 3–4 days (author's trans.), in: *The Pharmacological Basis of Therapeutics* (A. G. Gilman, L. S. Goodman, and A. Gilman, eds.), Macmillan, New York, pp. 71–82.

Foret, J., and Lantin, G., 1972, The sleep of train drivers: An example of the effects of irregular work schedules on sleep, in: *Aspects of Human Efficiency* (W. P. Colquhoun, ed.), The English University Press, London, pp. 273–282.

Fornal, C., and Radulovacki, M., 1981, Sleep suppressant action of quipazine: Relation to central serotonergic stimulation, *Pharmacol. Biochem. Behav.* **15**:937–944.

Fornal, C., and Radulovacki, M., 1982a, Sleep suppressant action of fenfluramine in rats: Evidence against the involvement of presynaptic serotonergic mechanism, *J. Pharmacol. Exp. Ther.* **225**:675–681.

Fornal, C., and Radulovacki, M., 1982b, Methysergide blocks the sleep suppressant action of quipazine in rats, *Psychopharmacology* **76**:255–259.

Fornal, C., and Radulovacki, M., 1983, Sleep suppressant action of fenfluramine in rats. II. Evidence against the involvement of presynaptic serotonergic mechanism, *J. Pharmacol. Exp. Ther.* **225**:675–681.

Fornal, C., Wojcik, W. J., and Radulovacki, M., 1982b, Alpha-flupenthixol increases slow-wave sleep in rats: Effect of dopamine receptor blockade, *Neuropharmacology* **21**:323–325.

Fornal, C., Markus, R., and Radulovacki, M., 1984, Muramyl dipeptide does not induce slow-wave sleep or fever in rats, *Peptides* **5**:91–95.

Foster, F. G., Kupfer, D. J., Coble, P., and McPartland, R. J., 1976, Rapid eye movement sleep density: An objective indicator in severe medical-depressive syndromes, *Arch. Gen. Psychiatry* **133**:1119–1123.

Foulkes, D., Pivik, T., Aherns, J. G., and Swanson, E. M., 1968, Effects of dream deprivation on dream content: An attempted cross night replication, *Psychophysiology* **4**:386–387.

Fowler, L. K., 1977, Temazepam (Euhypnos) as a hypnotic: A twelve-week trial in general practice, *J. Int. Med. Res.* **5**:295–296.

Fram, D. H., Murphy, D. L., Goodwin, F. K., Brodie, H. K., Bunney, W. E., and Snyder, F., 1970, L-DOPA and sleep in depressed patients, *Psychophysiology* **7**:316–317.

Fram, D., Gillin, J. C., Wyatt, R. J., and Snyder, F., 1972, The waking action of histidine: Evidence to the contrary, *Psychophysiology* **9**:85.

Frankel, B. L., Patten, B. M., and Gillin, J. C., 1974, Restless legs syndrome: Sleep-electroencephalographic and neurological findings, *JAMA* **230**:1302–1303.

Fraschini, F., Collu, R., and Martini, L., 1971, Mechanisms of inhibitory action of pineal principles on gonodotropin secretion, in: *Ciba Foundation Symposium on the Pineal Gland* (G. E. Wolstenholme and J. Knight, eds.), Churchill-Livingstone, London, pp. 259–273.

Freedman, R., Hauri, P., Coursey, R., and Frankel, B., 1978, Behavioral treatment of insomnia: A collaborative study, *Sleep Res.* **7**:179.

Freud, S., 1954, Project for a scientific psychology (1895), in: The *Origins of Psychoanalysis: Letters to Wilhelm Fliess, Drafts and Notes, 1887–1902* (M. Bonaparte, A. Freud, and E. Kres, eds.), Basic Books, New York, p. 400.

Friedman, M. B., Erickson, C. K., and Leslie, S. W., 1980, Effects of acute and chronic ethanol administration on whole mouse brain synaptosomal calcium influx, *Biochem. Pharmacol.* **29**:1903–1908.

Fry, J. M., Pressman, M. R., DiPhillipo, M. A., and Forst-Paulus, M., 1986, Treatment of narcolepsy with codeine, *Sleep* **9**:269–274.

Fujita, A. S., Conway, W., and Zorick, F., 1981, Surgical corrections of anatomic abnormalities in obstructive sleep apnea syndrome: Uvulopapatopharyngoplasty, *Otolaryngol. Head Neck Surg.* **89**:923–934.

Fullerton, D. T., Wenzel, F. J., Lohrenz, F. N., and Fahs, H., 1968a, Circadian rhythm of adrenal cortical activity in depression. I, *Arch. Gen. Psychiatry* **19**:674–682.

Fullerton, D. T., Wenzel, F. J., Lohrenz, F. N., and Fahs, H., 1968b, Circadian rhythm of adrenal cortical activity in depression. II, *Arch. Gen. Psychiatry* **19**:682–688.

Gagnon, P., and De Koninck, J., 1984, Reappearance of EEG slow waves in extended sleep, *Electroencephr. Clin. Neurophysiol.* **58**:155–160.

Gaillard, J. M., and St. Hilaire-Kafi, S., 1985, Sleep, depression and the effects of antidepressant drugs, *Acta Psychiatr. Belg.* **85**:561–567.

Gallagher, B. B., 1971, Regulation of cortisol secretion in Parkinson's syndrome and narcolepsy, *J. Clin. Endocrinol. Metab.* **32**:796–801.

Gallagher, T. F., Yoshida, K., Fukushima, D. K., Weitzman, E. D., and Hellman, L., 1973, ACTH and cortisol secretory patterns in man, *J. Clin. Endocrinol. Metab.* **36**:1058–1068.

Garattini, S., Mennini, T., Bendotti, C., Invernizzi, R., and Samanin, R., 1986, Neurochemical mechanism of action of drugs which modify feeding via the serotoninergic system, *Appetite* **7(S)**:15–38.

Garay, S. M., Turino, G. M., and Goldring, R. M., 1981, Sustained reversal of chronic hypercapnia in patients with aveolar hypoventilation syndromes: Long-term maintenance with noninvasive nocturnal mechanical ventilation, *Am. J. Med.* **70**:269–278.

Garay, S. M., Rapoport, D. M., Epstein, H., Sorkin, B., and Goldring, R. M., 1983, Hypercapnia, in post-tracheostomy obstructive sleep apnea, *Am. Rev. Respir. Dis.* **127**:235.

Gastaut, H., Tassinari, C. A., and Duron, B., 1966, Polygraphic study of the episodic diurnal and nocturnal (hypnotic and repiratory) manifestations of the Pickwick Syndrome, *Brain Res.* **2**:167–186.

Gastaut, H., Duron, B., Tassinari, C., Lyagoubi, S., and Saier, J., 1969, Mechanisms of the respiratory pauses accompanying slumber in the Pickwickian syndrome, *Acta Nerv. Super.* **11**:209–215.

Geddes, D. M., Rudolf, M., and Saunders, K. B., 1976, Effect of nitrazepam and flurazepam on the ventilatory response to carbon dioxide, *Thorax* **31**:548–551.

Gelineau, J., 1880, De la Narcolepsie, *Gas. D. Hop.* (Paris) **53**:626–628.

George, C. F., West, P., and Kryger, M. H., 1986, Trial of nomifensine in obstructive sleep apnea, *Sleep Res.* **15**:123.

George, F. R., Elmer, G. I., and Collins, A. C., 1982, Indomethacin significantly reduces mortality due to acute ethanol overexposure, *Substance Alcohol Actions/Misuse* **3**:267–274.

Gereau, S., Sher, A. E., Glovinsky, P. B., Burack, B., Thorpy, M. J., and Ledereich, P. S., 1986, Results of UPPP in patients selected by Muller maneuver, *Sleep Res.* **15**:124.

Gerner, R. H., Post, R. M., Gillin, J. C., and Bunney, W. E., 1979, Biological and behavioral effects of one night's sleep deprivation in depressed patients and normals, *J. Psychiatr. Res.* **15**:21–40.

Gessa, G. L., Biggio, G., Fadda, F., Corsini, G. U., and Tagliamonte, A. J., 1974, Effect of the oral administration of tryptophan-free amino acid mixtures on serum tryptophan, brain tryptophan and serotonin metabolism *J. Neurochem.* **22**:869–870.

Gessner, P. K., and Gessner, T., 1973, The interaction of barbital and testosterone, relative to their hypnotic effects, *Arch. Int. Pharmacodyn.* **201**:52–58.

Ghabrial, H., Desmond, P. V., Watson, K. J. R., Gijsbers, A. J., Harman, P. J., Breen, K. J., and Mashford, M. L., 1986, The effects of age and chronic liver disease on the elimination of temazepam, *Eur. J. Clin. Pharmacol.* **30**:93–97.

Giles, D. G., Roffwarg, H. P., Schlesser, M. A., and Rush, A. J., 1986, Which endogenous depressive symptoms relate to REM latency reduction? *Biol. Psychiatry* **21**:473–482.

Gill, B., 1977, *Lindbergh Alone*, Harcourt Brace Jovanovich, New York.

Gillin, J. C., 1983, The sleep therapies of depression, *Prog. Neuropsychopharmacol. Biol. Psychiatry* **7**:351–364.

Gillin, J. C., and Wyatt, R. J., 1975, Schizophrenia. Perchance a dream? *Int. Rev. Neurobiol.* **17**:297–342.

Gillin, J. C., Jacobs, L. S., Fram, D. H., and Snyder, F., 1972a, Acute effect of a glucocortoid on normal human sleep, *Nature* **237**:398–399.

Gillin, J., Post, R., Wyatt, Snyder, F., Goodwin, F., and Bunney, W. E., 1972b, Infusion of threodihydroxyphenylserine (DOPS) and 5-hydroxytryptophan (5HTP) during human sleep, *Sleep Res.* **1**:45.

Gillin, J. C., Post, R. M., Wyatt, R. J., Goodwin, F. K., Snyder, F., and Bunney, W. E., 1973, REM inhibitory effect of L-DOPA infusion during human sleep, *Electroencephalogr. Clin. Neurophysiol.* **35**:181–186.

Gillin, J. C., Jacobs, L. S., Snyder, F., and Henkin, R. I., 1974a, Effects of decreased adrenal corticosteriods: Changes in sleep in normal subjects and patients with adrenal cortical insufficiency, *Electroencephalogr. Clin. Neurophysiol.* **36**:283–289.

Gillin, J. C., Jacobs, L. S., Snyder, F., and Henkin, R. I., 1974b, Effects of ACTH on the sleep of normal subjects and patients with Addison's disease, *Neuroendocrinology* **15**:21–31.

Gillin, J. C., Fram, D. H., Wyatt, R. J., Henkin, R. I., and Snyder, F., 1975a, L-Histidine: Failure to affect the sleep–waking cycle in man, *Psychopharmacologia* **40**:305–311.

Gillin, J. C., van Kammen, D. P., Graves, J., and Murphy, D., 1975b, Differential effects of D- and L-amphetamine on the sleep of depressed patients, *Life Sci.* **17**:1233–1240.

Gillin, J. C., Mazure, C., Post, R. M., Jimerson, D., and Bunney, W. E., Jr., 1977, An EEG sleep study of a bipolar (manic-depressive) patient with a nocturnal switch process, *Biol. Psychiatry* **12**:711–718.

Gillin, J. C., Mendelson, W. B., Sitaram, N., and Wyatt, R. J., 1978a, The neuropharmacology of sleep and wakefulness, *Ann. Rev. Pharmacol. Toxicol.* **18**:563–579.

Gillin, J. C., Sitaram, N., Mendelson, W. B., and Wyatt, R. J., 1978b,Physostigmine alters onset but not duration of REM sleep in man, *Psychopharmacology* **58**:111–114.

Gillin, J. C., Sitaram, N., and Duncan, W. C., 1979a, Muscarinic supersensitivity: A possible model for the sleep disturbance of primary depression? *Psychiatry Res.* **1**:17–22.

Gillin, J. C., Duncan, W., Pettigrew, K. D., Frankel, B. L., and Snyder, F., 1979b, Successful separation of depressed, normal, and insomniac subjects by EEG sleep data, *Arch. Gen. Psychiatry* **36**:85–90.

Gillin, J. C., Duncan, W., Murphy, D. L., Post, R. M., Goodwin, F. K., Wyatt, R. J., and Bunney, W. E. J., 1981, Age related changes in sleep in depressed and normal subjects, *Psychiatry Res.* **4**:73–78.

Gillin, J. C., Sitaram, N., and Mendelson, W. B., 1982, Acetycholine, sleep, and depression, *Hum. Neurobiol.* **1**:211–219.

Gillin, J. C., Sitaram, N., Wehr, T., Duncan, W., Post, R., Murphy, D. L., and Mendelson, W. B., 1984, Sleep and affective illness, in: *Neurobiology of Mood Disorders* (R. M. Post and J. C. Ballenger, eds.), pp. 157–189.

Gillin, J. C., Kelsoe, J., Risch C., Darko, D., Kalir, H., and Janowsky, D., 1985, Cholinergic supersensitivity in depression? (Abstr. 518.2) Fourth World Congress of Biological Psychiatry, p. 387.

Gillin, J. C., Kripke, D. F., Butters, N., Grant, I., Irwin, M., Naimie, M. D., and Schuckit, M., 1986, A longitudinal study of sleep in primary alcoholism, *Sleep Res.* **15**:92.

Gilman, L., 1958, *Insomnia and Its Relation to Dreams*, J. B. Lippincott, Philadelphia, p. 237.

Gitlow, S. E., Bentkover, S. H., Dziedzic, S. W., and Khazan, N., 1973, Persistence of abnormal REM sleep response to ethanol as a result of previous ethanol ingestion, *Psychopharmacologia* **33**:135–140.

Gitlow, S. E., Dziedzic, S. W., and Dziedzic, L. B., 1977, Persistent abnormalities in central nervous system function (long-term tolerance) after brief ethanol administration, *Drug Alcohol Depend.* **2**:453–468.

Glenn, W. W. L., Phelps, M., and Gersten, L. M., 1978, Diaphragm pacing in the management of central alveolar hypoventilation, in: *Sleep Apnea Syndromes* (C. Guilleminault and W. C. Dement, eds.), Alan R. Liss, Inc., New York, pp. 333–345.

Glenn, W. W. L., Hogan, J. F., Loke, J. S. O., Ciesielski, T. E., Phelps, M. L., and Rowedder R., 1984, Ventilatory support by pacing of the conditioned diaphragm in quadriplegia, *New Engl. J. Med.* **310**:1150–1155.

Glick, S. M., Roth, J., Yalow, R. S., and Berson, S. A., 1965, The regulation of growth secretion, *Recent Prog. Horm. Res.* **21**:241–283.

Godbout, R., and Montplasir, J., 1986, All day performance variations in normal and narcoleptic subjects, *Sleep* **9**:200–204.

Goetze, U., and Tolle, R., 1981, Antidepressant effect of partial sleep deprivation during the first half of the night, *Psychiatry Clin. (Basel)* **14**:129–149.

Goldberg, M. R., Hollister, A. S., and Robertson, D., 1983, Influence of yohimbine on blood pressure, autonomic reflexes and plasma catecholamines in humans, *Hypertension* **5**:772–778.

Goldstein, D. B., and Chin J. H., 1981, Interaction of ethanol with biological membranes, *Fed. Proc.* **40**:2073–2076.

Goldstein, R., and Pavel, S., 1981, REM sleep suppression in cats by melatonin, *Brain Res. Bull.* **7**:723–724.

Golstein, J., Van Cauter, E., Linkowski, P., Vanhaelst, L., and Mendlewicz, J., 1980, Thyrotropin nyctochemeral pattern in primary depression: Differences between unipolar and bipolar women, *Life Sci.* **27**:1695–1703.

Golstein, J., Cauter, E. V., Desir, D., Neol, P., Spire, J. P., Refetoff, S., and Copinschi, G., 1983, Effects of "jet lag" on hormonal patterns. IV. Time shifts increase growth hormone release, *J. Clin. Endocrinol. Metab.* **56**:433–440.

Goodman, W. K., Charney, D. S., Price, L. H., Woods, S. W., and Heninger, G. R., 1986, Ineffectiveness of clonidine in the treatment of the benzodiazepine withdrawal syndrome: Report of three cases, *Am. J. Psychiatry* **143**:900–903.

Goodwin, D. W., and Hill, S. Y., 1975, The chronic effects of alcohol and other psychoactive drugs on intellect, learning and memory, in: *Alcohol, Drugs and Brain Damage* (J. Rankin, ed.), Alcohol Drug Research Foundation, Ontario, Canada, pp. 55–70.

Gordon, C. R., and Lavie, P., 1984, Effect of adrenergic blockers on the dog's sleep–wake pattern, *Physiol. Behav.* **32**:345–350.

Graber, A. L., Givens, J. R., Nicholson, W. E., Island, D. P., and Liddle, G. W., 1965, Persistence of diurnal rhythmicity in plasma ACTH concentrations in cortisol-deficient patients, *J. Clin. Endocrinol. Metab.* **25**:804–807.

Green, A. R., and Curzon, G., 1968, Decrease of 5-hydroxytryptamine in the brain provoked by hydrocortisone and its prevention of allopurinal, *Nature* **220**:1095–1097.

Green, A. R., Youdin, M. B. H., and Grahame-Smith, D. G., 1976, Quipazine: Its effects on rat brain 5-hydroxytryptamine metabolism, monoamine oxidase activity and behavior, *Neuropharmacology* **15**:173–179.

Green, W. J., and Stajduhar, P. P., 1966, The effect of ECT on the sleep–dream cycle in a psychotic depression, *J. Nerv. Ment. Dis.* **143**:123–134.

Greenberg, D. A., Cooper, E. C., and Carpenter, C. L., 1984, Calcium entry activators: Distinct sites of dihydropyridine and aminopyridine action, *Neurosc. Lett.* **50**:279–282.

Greenberg, R., and Pearlman, C., 1967, Delirium tremens and dreaming, *Am. J. Psychiatry* **124**:133–142.

Greenberg, R., and Pearlman, C. A., 1970, L-dopa, parkinsonism, and sleep, *Psychophysiology* **7**:314.

Greenblatt, D. J., 1979, Reduced serum albumin concentration in the elderly: A report from the Boston collaborative drug surveillance program, *J. Am. Geriatr. Soc.* **27**:20–22.

Greenblatt, D. J., 1983, Benzodiazepine oxidation versus conjugation. The effects of old age and metabolic inhibitors, in: *Treatment of Sleep Disorders*, Sandoz, Boston, pp. 16–23.

Greenblatt, D. J., and Greenblatt, M., 1972, Which drug for alcohol withdrawal? *J. Clin. Pharmacol.* **12**:429–431.

Greenblatt, D. J., and Shader, R. I., 1977, Nonprescription psychotropic drugs, in: *Pharmacology in the Practice of Medicine* (M. E. Jarvik, ed.), Appleton-Century-Crofts, New York, pp. 345–357.

Greenblatt, D. J., and Shader, R. I., 1978, Dependence, tolerance, and addiction to benzodiazepines: clinical and pharmacokinetic considerations, *Drug Metab. Rev.* **8**:13–28.

Greenblatt, D. J., Divoll, M., Harmatz, J. S., MacLaughlin, D. S., and Shader, R. I., 1981, Kinetics and clinical effects of flurazepam in young and elderly non-insomniacs, *Clin. Pharmacol. Res.* **30**:475–486.

Greenwood, M., Friedel, J., Bond, A. J., Curzon, G., and Lader, M. H., 1974, The acute effects of intravenous infusion of L-tryptophan in normal subjects, *Clin. Pharmacol. Ther.* **16**:455–464.

Grelak, R. P., Clark, R., Stump, J. M., and Vernier, V. G., 1970, In vivo conversion of [^{3}H]-L-tryptophan into [^{3}H]serotonin in brain areas of adrenalectomized rats, *Science* **169**:201–204.

Gresham, S. C., Webb, W. B., and Williams, R. L., 1963, Alcohol and caffeine: Effect on inferred visual dreaming, *Science* **140**:1226–1227.

Gresham, S. C., Agnew, W. F., Jr., and Williams, R. L., 1965, The sleep of depressed patients, *Arch. Gen. Psychiatry* **13**:503–507.

Griesinger, W., 1868, Berliner medicinisch-psychologische Gesellschaft, *Arch. Psychiatr. Nervenkr.* **1**:200–204.

Griffiths, W. J., Lester, B. K., Coulter, J. D., and Williams, H. L., 1972, Tryptophan and sleep in young adults, *Psychophysiology* **9**:345–356.

Grob, P., and Harvey, J. C., 1958, Effects in man of the anticholinesterase compound sarin (isopropyl methyl phosphoro-flouridate), *J. Clin. Invest.* **37**:350–368.

Gross, M. M., Goodenough, D., Tobin, M., Halpert, E., Lepore, D., Perlstein, A., and Sirota, M., 1966, Sleep disturbances and hallucinations in the acute alcoholic psychosis, *J. Nerv. Ment. Dis.* **142**:493–514.

Gross, M. M., Goodenough, D. R., Hastey, J., and Lewis, E., 1973, Experimental study of sleep in chronic alcoholics before and after four days of heavy drinking, with a non-drinking companion, *Ann. NY Acad. Sci.* **215**:254–275.

Gruen, P. H., Sachar, E. J., Altman, N., and Sassin, J., 1975, Growth hormone responses to hypoglycemia in postmenopausal women, *Arch. Gen. Psychiatry* **32**:31–33.

Guilhaume, A., Benoit, O., and Richardet, J. M., 1981, Deficit en sommeil lent profond et nanisme de frustration, *Arch. Fr. Pediatr.* **38**:25–27.

Guilhaume, A., Benoit, O., Gourmelen, M., and Richardet, J. M., 1982, Relationship between sleep stage IV deficit and reversible HGH deficiency in psychosocial dwarfism, *Pediatr. Res.* **16**:299–303.

Guilleminault, C., 1982, Sleep and breathing, in: *Sleep and Waking* (C. Guilleminault, ed.), Addison-Wesley, Menlo Park, CA, pp. 155–182.

Guilleminault, C., 1986, Narcolepsy (Editorial), *Sleep* **9**:99.

Guilleminault, C., and Flagg, W., 1984, Effect of baclofen on sleep-related periodic leg movements, *Ann. Neurol.* **15**:234–239.

Guilleminault, C., Dement, W. C., Wilson, R., and Zarcone, V., 1972, Respiration problems and sleep disorders, *Sleep Res.* **1**:151.

Guilleminault, C., Cathala, J. P., and Castaigne, P., 1973a, Effects of 5-hydroxytryptophan on the sleep of a patient with a brain stem lesion, *Electroencephalogr. Clin. Neurophysiol.* **34**:177–184.

Guilleminault, C., Raynal, D., Wilson, R., and Dement, W., 1973b, Continuous polygraphic recording in narcoleptic patients, *Sleep Res.* **2**:152.

Guilleminault, C., Smythe H., and Dement, W., 1973c, Cataplexy, H-reflex and therapeutic trial, *Sleep Res.* **2**:153.

Guilleminault, C., Carskadon, M., and Dement, W. C., 1974, On the treatment of rapid eye movement narcolepsy, *Arch. Neurol.* **30**:90–93.

Guilleminault, C., Raynal, D., Weitzman, E. D., and Dement, W. C., 1975a, Sleep-related periodic myoclonus in patients complaining of insomnia, *Trans. Am. Neurol. Assoc.* **100**:19–22.

Guilleminault, C., Montplasir, J., Zarcone, V., and Dement, W. C., 1975b, Excessive daytime sleepiness (EDS) patients in a sleep disorder clinic, *Sleep Res.* **4**:217.

Guilleminault, C., Phillips, R., and Dement, W. C., 1975c, A syndrome of hypersomnia with automatic behavior, *Electroencephalogr. Clin. Neurophysiol.* **38**:403–413.

Guilleminault, C., Spiegel, R., and Dement, W. C., 1977, A propos des insomnies, *Confin. Psychiatr.* **15**:151–172.

Guilleminault, C., Van den Hoed, J., and Mitler, M. M., 1978, Clinical overview of the sleep apnea syndromes, in: *Sleep Apnea Syndromes* (C. Guilleminault and W. C. Dement, eds.), Alan R. Liss, New York, pp. 1–12.

Guilleminault, C., Simmons, F. B., Motta, J., Cummiskey, J., Roseking, M., Schroeder, J. S., and Dement, W. C., 1981, Obstructive sleep apnea syndrome and tracheostomy: Long-term follow-up experience, *Arch. Intern. Med.* **141**:985–988.

Guilleminault, C., McQuitty, J., Ariaguo, R. L., Challamel, M. J., Kerobkin, R., and McClead, R. E., 1982, Congenital central alveolar hypoventilation syndrome in six infants, *Pediactrics* **70**:684–694.

Guilleminault, C., Silvestri, R., Mondini, S., and Coburn, S., 1984, Aging and sleep apnea: Action of benzodiazepine, acetozolamide, alcohol and sleep deprivation in a healthy elderly group, *J. Gerontol.* **39**:655–661.

Guilleminault, C., Quera Salva, M. A., Mancuso, J., and Hayes, B., 1986a, Narcolepsy, cataplexy, heart rate, and blood pressure, *Sleep* **9**:222–226.

Guilleminault, C., Mancuso, J., Quera Salva, M. A., Hayes, B., Mitler, M., Poirier, G., and Montplasir, J., 1986b, Viloxazine hydrochloride in narcolepsy: A preliminary report, *Sleep* **9**:275–279.

Guldner, F. H., 1985, Structure and neural connections of the suprachiasmatic nucleus, in: *Circadian Rhythms in the Central Nervous System* (P. H. Redfern, I. C. Campbell, J. A. Davies, and K. F. Martin, eds.), VCH, Deerfield, FL, pp. 30–44.

Gulevich, G., Dement, W., and Johnson, L. 1966, Psychiatric and EEG observations on a case of prolonged (264 hours) wakefulness, *Arch. Gen. Psychiatry* **15**:29–35.

Gunderson, C. H., Dunne, P. B., and Feyer, T. L., 1973, Sleep deprivation seizures, *Neurology (Minneap.)* **23**:678–686.

Gunne, L. M., Lidvall, H. F., and Widen, L., 1971, Preliminary clinical trial with L-dopa in narcolepsy, *Psychopharmacologia* **19**:204–206.

Gursey, D., and Olson, R. E., 1961, Depression of serotonin and norepinephrine levels in brain stem of rabbit by ethanol on noradrenaline, dopamine, or 5-hydroxytryptamine levels in brain, *Acta Pharmacol. Toxicol.* **18**:278–280.

Haefely, W., Kulsar, R., Mohler, H., Pieri, L., Polc, P., and Schaffner, R., 1975, Possible involvement of GABA in the central actions of benzodiazepines, *Adv. Biochem. Psychopharmacol.* **14**:131–151.

Haider, I., 1968, Patterns of insomnia in depressive illness: A subjective evaluation, *Br. J. Psychiatry* **114**:1127–1132.

Halasz, B., 1969, The endocrine effects of isolation of the hypothalamus from the rest of the brain, in: *Frontiers in Neuroendocrinology* (W. F. Ganong and L. Martini, eds.), Oxford University Press, New York, pp. 307–342.

Haley, J., 1963, *1963 Strategies of Psychotherapy*, Grune & Stratton, New York, pp. 1–240.

Hallman, H., and Jonsson, G., 1984, Pharmacological modification of the neurotoxic action of the noradrenaline neurons, *Eur. J. Pharmacol.* **103**:269–278.

Halushka, P. V., and Hoffman, P. C., 1970, Alcohol addiction and tethydropapaveroline, *Science* **169**:1104–1105.

Hambrecht, F. T., 1980, Applications of neural controls in humans, *Ann. Biomed. Eng.* **8**:333–338.

Harman, E. M., Wynne, J. W., and Block, A. J., 1981, Effect of weight loss on sleep disordered breathing (SDB) and desaturation in morbidly obese males, *Am. Rev. Respir. Dis.* **123**:69.

Harper, J., 1981, Gelineau's narcolepsy, *Lancet* **1**:92.

Harris, P. F., Overstreet, D. H., and Orbach, J., 1982, Disruption of passive avoidance memory by REM sleep deprivation: Methodological and pharmacological considerations, *Pharmacol. Biochem. Behav.* **17**:1119–1122.

Harris, R. A., and Hood, W. F., 1980, Inhibition of synaptosomal calcium uptake by ethanol, *J. Pharmacol. Exp. Ther.* **213**:562–568.

Hartman, P., and Scrima, L., 1986, Arousals associated with muscle activity in the legs (mal) in patients with narcolepsy, OSA, nocturnal myoclonus versus normal individuals, *Sleep Res.* **15**:126.

Hartmann, E. L., 1966, Reserpine: Its effect on the sleep–dream cycle in man, *Psychopharmacologia* **9**:242–247.

Hartmann, E., 1968a, Longitudinal studies of sleep and dream patterns in manic-depressive patients, *Arch. Gen. Psychiatry* **19**:312–329.

Hartmann, E., 1968b, The effects of four drugs on sleep in man, *Psychopharmacologia* **12**:346–353.

Hartmann, E., 1969, The biochemistry and pharmacology of the D-state (dreaming sleep), *Exp. Med. Surg.* **27**:105–120.

Hartmann, E., 1970, L-Tryptophan and 5H-tryptophan: Effects on human sleep, *Psychophysiology* **7**:320–321.

Hartmann, E., 1973, *The Functions of Sleep*, Yale University Press, New Haven, CT.

Hartmann, E. L., and Bridwell, T. J., 1970, Effects of AMPT, L-DOPA, and L-tryptophan on sleep in the rat, *Psychophysiology* **7**:313.

Hartmann, E., and Cravens, J., 1973a, The effects of long term administration of psychotropic drugs on human sleep: II. The effects of reserpine, *Psychopharmacologia* **33**:169–184.

Hartmann, E., and Cravens, J., 1973b, The effects of long term administration of psychotropic drugs on human sleep: III. The effects of amitriptyline, *Psychopharmacologia* **33**:185–202.

Hartmann, E., and Cravens, J., 1973c, The effects of long term administration of psychtropic drugs on human sleep: IV. The effects of chlorpromazine, *Psychopharmacologia* **33**:203–218.

Hartmann, E., and Spinweber, C. L., 1979, Sleep induced by L-tryptophan, *J. Nerv. Ment. Dis.* **167**:497–499.

Hartmann, E., Verdone, P., and Snyder, F., 1966, Longitutinal studies of sleep and dreaming patterns in psychiatric patients, *J. Nerv. Ment. Dis.* **142**:117–126.

Hartmann, E., Chung, R., and Chien, C. P., 1971, L-Tryptophan and sleep, *Psychopharmacologia* **19**:114–127.

Hartmann, E., Baekeland, F., and Zwilling, G. R., 1972, Psychological differences between long and short sleepers, *Arch. Gen. Psychiatry* **26**:463–468.

Hartmann, E., Cravens, J., and List, S., 1974a, Hypnotic effects of L-tryptophan, *Arch. Gen. Psychiatry* **31**:394–397.

Hartmann, E., Orzack, M. H., and Branconnier, R., 1974b, Deficits produced by sleep deprivation: Reversal by *d*- and *l*-amphetamine, *Sleep Res.* **3**:151.

Hartmann, E., and Spinweber, C. L., 1979, Sleep induced by L-tryptophan, *J. Nerv. Ment. Dis.* **167**:497–499.

Hartmann, E., Lindsley, J. G., and Spinweber, C., 1983, Chronic insomnia: Effects of tryptophan, flurazepam, secobarbital and placebo, *Psychopharmacology* **80:**138–142.

Hartse, K. M., Roth, T., and Zorick, F. J., 1982, Daytime sleepiness and daytime wakefulness: The effect of instruction, *Sleep* **5:**s107–s118.

Harza, J., 1970, Effect of hemicholinum-3 on slow wave and paradoxical sleep of the cat, *Eur. J. Pharmacol.* **11:**395–397.

Haskell, D., 1975 Letter: Withdrawal from diazepam, *JAMA* **233:**135.

Hauri, P., Treating psychophysiologic insomnia with biofeedback, *Arch. Gen. Psychiatry* **38:**752–758.

Hauri, P., 1986, Presentation to the American Psychiatric Association Annual Meeting, May 10–16, 1986, Washington, D.C.,

Hauri, P., and Cohen, S., 1977, Treatment of insomnia with biofeedback: Final report of study I, *Sleep Res.* **6:**136.

Hauri, P., and Hawkins, D., 1971, Phasic REM, depression, and the relationship between sleeping and waking, *Arch. Gen. Psychiatry* **25:**56–63.

Hauri, P., Chernik, D., Hawkins, D., and Mendels, J., 1974, Sleep of depressed patients in remission, *Arch. Gen. Psychiatry* **31:**386–391.

Hauri, P. J., Percy, L., Hellekson, C., Hartmann, E., and Russ, D., 1982, The treatment of psychophysiologic insomnia with biofeedback: A replication study, *Biofeedback Self-Regul.* **7:**223–235.

Hauri, P., Chernik, D., Hawkins, D., and Mendels, J., 1985, Sleep of depressed patients in remission, *Arch. Gen. Psychiatry* **42:**368–391.

Haus, E., and Halberg, F., 1959, 24-Hour rhythm in susceptibility of C mice to a toxic dose of ethanol, *J. Appl. Physiol.* **14:**878–880.

Havrankova, J., Roth, J., and Brownstein, M. J., 1979, Concentrations of insulin and of insulin receptors in the brain are independent of peripheral insulin levels, *J. Clin. Invest.* **64:**636–642.

Hawkins, D. R., and Mendels, J., 1966, Sleep disturbances in depressive syndromes, *Am. J. Psychiatry* **123:**682–690.

Hawkins, D. R., Mendels, J., Scott, J., Benschm, G., and Teachy, W., 1967, The psychophysiology of sleep in psychotic depression: A longitudinal study, *Psychosom. Med.* **29:**339–344.

Hawkins, D. R., Taub, J. M., Van de Castle, R. L., 1985, Extended sleep (hypersomnia) in young depressed patients, *Am. J. Psychiatry* **142:**905–910.

Hawkins, M., Pravica, M., and Radulovacki, M., 1986, Effects of chronic administration of diazepam and R015-1788 on adenosine A1 and A2 receptors in the rat brain (abstract), Society for Neuroscience Meeting 1986.

Haynes, S. N., Price, M. G., and Simons, J. B., 1975, Stimulus control treatment of insomnia, *J. Behav. Ther. Exp. Psychiatry* **6:**279–282.

Hazra, J., 1970, Effect of hemicholinium-3 on slow-wave and paradoxical sleep of cat, *Eur. J. Pharmacol.* **11:**395–397.

Heath, C., 1889, Minutes from the Clinical Society of London, *Br. Med. J. 358.*

Hedemark, L. L., and Kronenberg, R. S., 1983, Flurazepam attenuates the arousal response to CO_2 during sleep in normal subjects, *Am. Rev. Respir. Dis.* **128:**980–985.

Heiman, E. M., and Christie, M., 1986, Lithium aggravated nocturnal myoclonus and restless legs syndrome, *Am. J. Psychiatry* **143:**1191–1192.

Heise, G. A., 1987, Facilitation of memory and cognition by drugs, *Trends Pharmacol. Sci.* **8:**65–68.

Hellman, L., Nakada, R., Curti, J., Weitzman, E. D., Kream, J., Roffwarg, H., and Ellman, S., 1970a, Cortisol is secreted episodically by normal man, *J. Clin. Endocrinol. Metab.* **30:**411–422.

Hellman, L., Weitzman, E. D., Roffwarg, H., Fukushima, D. K., Yoshida, K., and Gallagher, T. F., 1970b, Cortisol is secreted episodically in Cushing's syndrome, *J. Clin. Endocrinol. Metab.* **30**:686–689.

Henkin, R. I., Gill, J. R., Warmotts, J. R., Carr, A. A., and Bartter, F. C., 1963, Steroid dependent increase in nerve conduction velocity in adrenal insufficiency, *J. Clin. Invest.* **42**:941.

Henkin, R. I., and Bartter, F. C., 1966, Studies on olfactory thresholds in normal man and in patients with adrenal cortial insufficiency: The role of adrenal cortical steroids and of serum sodium concentration, *J. Clin. Invest.* **45**:1631–1639.

Henkin, R. L., and Daly, R. L., 1968, Auditory detection and perception in normal man and in patients with adrenal cortical insufficiency: Effect of adrenal cortical steroids, *J. Clin. Invest.* **47**:1269–1280.

Hernandez-Peon, R., Chavez-Ibana, G., Morgane, P. J., and Timo-Iaria, C., 1963, Limbic cholinergic pathways involved in sleep and emotional behavior, *Exp. Neurol.* **8**: 93–111.

Hernandez-Peon, R., O'Flaherty, J. J., Mazzuchelli-O'Flaherty, A. L., and O'Flaherty, A. C., 1967, Sleep and other behavioral effects induced by acetylcholinergic stimulation of basal temporal cortex and striate structures, *Brain Res.* **4**:243–267.

Hernandez-Peon, R., Drucker, R. R., Del Angel, A. R., Chavez, B., and Sarrano, P., 1969, Brain catecholamines and serotonin in rapid sleep deprivation, *Physiol. Behav.* **4**:659–661.

Hershman, J. M., and Pittman, J. A., 1971, Utility of the radioimmunoassay of serum thyrotrophin in man, *Ann. Intern. Med.* **74**:481–490.

Hess, W. R., 1929, Hirnreizversuche uber den mechanismus des Schlafes, *Arch. Psychiatr. Nervenkr.* **86**:287–292.

Hess, W. R., 1944, Das Schlafsyndrom alsfolge diencephaler Reizung, *Helv. Physiol. Pharmacol. Acta* **2**:305–344.

Heston, W. D., Erwin, V. G., Anderson, S. M., and Robbins, H., 1974, A comparison of the effects of alcohol on mice selectively bred for differences in ethanol sleep-time, *Life Sci.* **14**:365–370.

Hiatt, J. F., Floyd, T. C., Katz, P. H., and Feinberg, I., 1985, Further evidence of abnormal non-rapid-eye-movement in schizophrenia, *Arch. Gen. Psychiatry* **42**:797–802.

Higuchi, T., Takahashi, Y., Takashi, K., Nimi, Y., and Miyasita, A., 1979, Twenty-four hour secretory patterns of growth hormone, prolactin, and cortisol in narcolepsy, *J. Clin. Endocrinol. Metab.* **49**:197–204.

Hilakivi, I., 1983, The role of beta- and alpha-adrenoceptors in the regulation of the stages of the sleep–waking cycle in the cat, *Brain Res.* **277**:109–118.

Hilakivi, I., and Leppavuori, A., 1984, Effects of methoxamine, an alpha-1 adrenoceptor agonist and prazosin, an alpha-1 antagonist on the stages of the sleep–waking cycle in the cat, *Acta Physiol. Scand.* **120**:363–372.

Hill, M. W., Guilleminault, C., and Simmons, F. B., 1978, Fiber-optic and EMG studies in hypersomnia–sleep apnea syndrome, in: *Sleep Apnea Syndrome* (C. Guilleminault and W. C. Dement, eds.), Alan R. Liss, New York, pp. 249–258.

Hindmarch, I., 1984 Subjective aspect of the effects of benzodiazepines on sleep and early morning behavior, *Ir. J. Med. Sci.* **153**:272–278.

Hindmarch, I., and Ott H., 1984 Sleep, benzodiazepines and performance: Issues and comments, *Psychopharmacology (Suppl.)* **1**:194–202.

Hiner, B. C., Roth, H. L., and Peroutka, S. J., 1986, Antimigraine drug interactions with 5-hydroxytryptamine la receptors, *Ann. Neurol.* **19**:511–513.

Hinton, J. M., 1963, A comparison of the effects of six barbiturates and a placebo on insomnia and motility in psychiatric patients, *Br. J. Pharmacol.* **20**:319–325.

Hirsch, J. D., and Kochman, R. L., 1982, Coupling at putative calcium channels with brain benzodiazepine receptors, *Soc. Neurosci. Abst.* **8:**574.

Hishikawa, Y., and Kaneko, Z., 1965, Electroencephalographic study on narcolepsy, *Electroencephalogr. Clin. Neurophysiol.* **18:**249–259.

Hishikawa, Y., Nahai, K., Ida, H., Nakai, K., Ioa, H., and Kaneko, Z., 1965, The effect 12,05,12of imipramine, desmethylimipramine and chloropromazine on the sleep–wakefulness 15,05,12cycle of the cat, *Electroencephal. Clin. Neurophysiol.* **19:**518–521.

Ho, A., 1972, Sex hormones and sleep of women, *Sleep Res.* **1:**184.

Ho, K. Y., Evans, W. S., and Thorner, W. O., 1985, Disorders of prolactin and growth hormone secretion, *Clin. Endocrinol. Metab.* **14:**1–32.

Hobson, J. A., 1983, Sleep mechanisms and pathophysiology: Some clinical implications of the reciprocal interaction hypothesis of sleep cycle control, *Psychosom. Med.* **45:**123–140.

Hobson, J. A., McCarley, R. W., and Wyzinski, P. W., 1975, Sleep cycle oscillations: Reciprocal discharge by two brainstem neuronal groups, *Science* **18:**55–58.

Hobson, J. A., McCarley, R. W., and McKenna, T. M., 1976, Cellular evidence bearing on the pontine brain stem hypothesis of desynchronized sleep control, *Progr. Neurobiol.* **6:**279–376.

Hobson, J. A., Lydic, R., and Baghdoyan, N., 1986, Evolving concepts of sleep cycle generation: From brain centers to neuronal populations, *Behav. Brain Sci.* **9:**371–391.

Hoffman, J. S., and Domino, E. F., 1969, Comparative effects of reserpine on the sleep cycles of man and cat, *J. Pharmacol. Exp. Ther.* **170:**190–198.

Hoffman, P. L., and Tabakoff, B., 1985, Ethanol's action on brain biochemistry, in: *Alcohol and the Brain: Chronic Effects* (D. H. van Thiel and R. E. Tarter, eds.), Plenum Press, New York, pp. 19–68.

Hokfelt, T., Fehfeld, J. F., Skirboll, L., Ivemark, B., Goldstein, M., and Markey, K., 1980, Evidence for coexistence of dopamine and CCK in mesolimbic neurons, *Nature* **285:**476–478.

Holman, B., and Snape, B. M., 1985, Effects of ethanol on 5-hydroxytryptamine release from rat corpus striatum *in vivo, Alcohol* **2:**249–253.

Holmes, J. H., and Gaon, M. D., 1956, Observations on acute and multiple exposure to anticholinesterase agents, *Trans. Am. Clin. Climatol. Assoc.* **68:**86–101.

Holmes, S. W., and Sugden, D., 1982, Effects of melatonin on sleep and neurochemistry in the rat, *Br. J. Pharmacol.* **76:**95–101.

Honda, Y., Takahashi, K., Takahashi, S., Azumi, K., Irie, M., Tsushima, T., and Shizume, K., 1969, Growth hormone secretion during nocturnal sleep in normal subjects, *J. Clin. Endocrinol. Metab.* **29:**20–29.

Honda, Y., Juji, T., Matusuki, K., Naohara, T., Satake, M., Inoko, H., and Someya, T., 1986a, HLA-DR2 and Dw2 in narcolepsy and in other disorders of excessive somnolence without cataplexy, *Sleep* **9:**133–142.

Honda, Y., Doi, Y., Ninomiya, R., and Ninomiya, C., 1986b, Increased frequency of non-insulin-dependent diabetes mellitus among narcoleptic patients, *Sleep* **9:**254–259.

Honma, K., Kenji, W., and Hiroshiga, T., 1979, Effects of parachlorophenylalanine and 5, 6-dihydroxytryptamine on the free-running rhythms of locomotor activity and plasma corticosterone in the rat exposed to continuous light, *Brain Res.* **169:**531–544.

Horne, J. A., and Ostberg, O., 1977, Individual differences in human circadian rhythms, *Biol. Psychol.* **5:**179–190.

Horseman, N. D., Meinert, J. C., and Ehret, C. F., 1979, Corticosteroid injections phase-shift the circadian thermoregulatory rhythm of rats, *Am. Zool.* **19:**896.

Howerton, T. C., Marks, M. J., and Collins, A. C., 1982, Norepinephrine gamma-aminobutyric acid, and choline reuptake kinetics and the effects of ethanol in long-sleep and short-sleep, *Substance Alcohol Actions/Misuse* **3:**89–99.

Howse, P. M., Rayner, P. H. W., Williams, J. W., and Rudd, B. T., 1974, Growth hormone secretion during sleep in short children, *Arch. Dis. Child.* **49**:246.

Huang, L. M., and Barker, J. L., 1980, Pentobarbital: Stereospecific actions of (+) and (−) isomers revealed on cultured mammaliam neurons, *Science* **207**:195–197.

Hudgel, D. W., and Robertson, D. W., 1984, Nasal resistance during wakefulness and sleep in normal man, *Acta Otolaryngol. (Stockh.)* **98**:130–135.

Hufford, D. 1982, *The Terror That Comes in the Night*, University of Pennsylvania Press, Philadelphia, p. 23.

Hume, K. I., and Mills, J. N., 1975, A split sleep investigation of the relative effects of time of day and duration of prior wakefulness on the sleep process, *Sleep Res.* 4:226.

Hunt, W. A., 1985, *Alcohol and Biological Membranes*, The Guilford Press, New York.

Hunt, W. A., and Dalton, T. K., 1976, Regional brain acetylcholine levels in rats acutely treated with ethanol or rendered ethanol dependent, *Brain Res.* **109**:628–631.

Hunt, W. A., and Majchrowicz, E., 1974, Alterations in the turnover of brain norepinephrine and dopamine in the alcohol-dependent rat, *J. Neurochem.* **23**:549–552.

Hunter, W. M., Friend, J. A., and Strong, J. A., 1966, The diurnal pattern of growth hormone concentration in adults, *J. Endocrinol. Metab.* **34**:139–146.

Hurwitz, N., 1969, Predisposing factors in adverse reactions to drugs, *Br. Med. J.* **1**:536.

Hyland, R. H., Hutcheon, M. A., Perl, A., Bowes, G., Anthonisen, N. R., and Zamel, N., 1981, Upper airway occlusion induced by diaphragm pacing for primary aveolar hypoventilation: Implications for the pathogenesis of obstructive sleep apnea, *Am. Rev. Respir. Dis.* **124**:180–185.

Ichikawa, Y., Nishikai, M., Kawagoe, M., Yoshida, K., and Homma, M., 1972, Plasma corticotropin, cortisol and growth hormone responses to hypoglycemia in the morning and evening, *J. Clin. Endocrinol. Metab.* **34**:895–898.

Idzikowski, C., and Mills, F. J., 1986a, Ritanserin causes sustained increase in slow wave sleep, presentation at Collegium Int. Neuro-Psychopharmacology 15th CINP, 1986 Dec. 14–17, 1986, San Juan, PR.

Idzikowski, C., and Mills, F. J., 1986b, Ritanserin antagonizes the effects of nitrazepam on sleep, presentation at Collegium Int. Neuro-Psychopharmacology 15th CINP Congress, Dec. 14–17, 1986, San Juan, PR.

Iijima, S., Sugita, Y., Teshima, Y., and Hishikawa, Y., 1986, Therapeutic effects of mazindol on narcolepsy, *Sleep* **9**:265–268.

Ikematsu, T., 1964, Study of snoring, 4th report: Therapy, *J. Jap. Otorhine–laryngol.* **64**:434–435.

Illig, R., Stahl, M., Hendricks, I., and Hecker, A., 1971, Growth hormone release during slow wave sleep, *Helv. Paediatr. Acta* **26**:655–663.

Imura, H., and Kato, Y., 1974, Role of monoamines in the control of growth hormone and prolactin secretion in man and rats, in: *Psychoneuroendocrinology* (N. Hatotani, ed.), Karger, Basel, p. 657.

Ingbar, S. H., 1985, The thyroid gland, in: *Williams Textbook of Endocrinology* (J. D. Wilson and D. W. Foster, eds.), Saunders, Philadelphia, pp. 682–815.

Innes, I. R., and Nickerson, M., 1970, Drugs inhibiting the action of ACTH on structures innervated by prostaganglionic parasympathetic nerves (antimuscarinic or atropinic drugs), in: *The Pharmacologic Basis of Therapeutics* (L. S. Goodman and A. Gilman, eds.), Macmillan, New York, pp. 524–548.

Inoue, S., Honda, K., Komoda, Y., Uchizono, K., Ueno, R., and Hayaishi, O., 1984, Differential sleep-promoting effects of five sleep substances nocturnally infused in unrestrained rats, *Proc. Natl. Acad. Sci. USA* **81**:6240–6244.

Institute of Medicine, 1979a, Supplement to *Sleeping Pills, Insomnia and Medical Practice*, National Academy of Sciences, Washington, D.C., pp. 1–46.

Institute of Medicine, 1979b, *Sleeping Pills, Insomnia and Medical Practice*, National Academy of Sciences, Washington, D.C., pp. 47–62.

Irie, M., Sakuma, M., Tsushima, T., Shizume, K., and Nakao, K., 1967, Effect of nicotinic acid administration on plasma growth hormone concentration, *Proc. Soc. Biol. Med.* **126**:708–711.

Irwin, M., Fuentenebro, F., Marder, S. R., and Yuwiler, A., 1986, L-5-Hydroxytryptophan-induced delirium, *Biol. Psychiatry* **21**:673–676.

Iskander, T. W., and Kaebling, R., 1970, Catecholamines, a dream sleep model and depression, *Am. J. Psychiatry* **127**:43–50.

Issa, F. G., and Sullivan, C. E., 1984, Upper airway closing pressures in obstructive sleep apnea, *J. Appl. Physiol.* **57**:520–527.

Issa, F. G., and Sullivan, C. E., 1986, Reversal of central sleep apnea using nasal CPAP, *Chest* **90**:165–171.

Iverson, L. L., 1985, Super-potent serotonin blockers, *Nature* **316**:107–108.

Jacobs, B. L., 1985, Overview of the activity of brain monoaminergic neurons across the sleep–wake cycle, in: *Sleep: Neurotransmitters and Neuromodulators* (A. Wauquier, J. M. Gaillard, J. M. Monti, and M. Radulovacki, eds.), Raven Press, New York, pp. 1–14.

Jacobs, L. S., Green, R., Gillin, J. C., Wyatt, R. J., and Snyder, F. A., 1976, A toxic psychosis and sleep changes in a patient receiving phenelzine, *J. Hawaiian Med. Soc.* **35**:109–111.

Jacobs, L. S., Mendelson, W. B., Rubin, R. T., and Bauman, J. E., 1978, Failure of nocturnal prolactin suppression by methysergide to entrain changes in testosterone in normal men, *J. Clin. Endocrinol. Metab.* **46**:560–561.

Jacobson, E., 1938, *Progressive Relaxation*, University of Chicago Press, Chicago.

Jacobson, E., 1964, *Anxiety and Tension Control*, Lippincott, Philadelphia.

James, S. P., and Mendelson, W. B., 1987, The effect of low dose melatonin on normal sleep, *Sleep Res.* **16**:95.

Janowsky, D., El-Yousef, M. K., and Davis, J. M., 1972, A cholinergic–adrenergic hypothesis of mania and depression, *Lancet* **2**:632–635.

Jasper, H. H., and Tessier, J., 1971, Acetylcholine liberation from cerebral cortex during paradoxical sleep, *Science* **172**:601–602.

Jernajczyk, W., 1986, Latency of eye movement and other REM sleep parameters in bipolar depression, *Biol. Psychiatry* **21**:465–472.

Jick, H., Stone, D., Shapiro, S., and Lewis, G. P., 1969, Clinical effects of hypnotics, *JAMA* **209**:2013–2015.

Joaquim, P. A., Goetz, R., Hanion, C., Davies, M., Thompson, J., Chambers, W. J., and Tabrizi, M. A., 1982, Sleep architecture and REM sleep measures in prepubertal children with major depression, *Arch. Gen. Psychiatry* **39**:932–939.

Johns, M. W., Egan, P., Gay, T. J. A., and Masterson, S. P., 1970, Sleep habits and symptoms in male medical and surgical patients, *Br. Med. J.* **2**:509–512.

Johns, M. W., Masterson, J. P., Paddle-Ledinek, J. E., Winidoff, M., and Makinek, M., 1975, Delta-wave sleep and thyroid function in healthy young men, Presented at the Second Int. Sleep Research Cong., Edinburgh, Scotland, June 30–July 4, 1975.

Johnson, J. H., and Sawyer, C. H., 1971, Adrenal steroids and the maintenance of a circadian distribution of paradoxical sleep in rats, *Endocrinology* **89**:507–512.

Johnson, L. C., 1969, Psychological and physiological changes following total sleep deprivation, in: *Sleep: Physiology and Pathology* (A. Kales, ed.), Lippincott, Philadelphia, pp. 206–220.

Johnson, L. C., and Chernik, D. A., 1982, Sedative hypnotics and human performance, *Psychopharmacology* **76**:101–113.

Johnson, L. C., Slye, E. S., and Dement, W., 1965, Electroencephalographic and automatic activity during and after prolonged sleep deprivation, *Electroencephalogr. Clin. Neurophysiol.* **27**:415–423.

Johnson, L. C., Burdick, A., and Smith, J., 1970, Sleep during alcohol intake and withdrawal in the chronic alcoholic, *Arch. Gen. Psychiatry* **22**:406–418.

Jones, B. E., 1969, Catecholamine-containing neurons in the brain stem of the cat and their role in waking, Imprimerie des Beauzarts J. Tixier & Fils, Lyon.

Jones, B. E., Bolillier, P., Pin, C., and Jouvet, M., 1973, The effect of lesions of catecholamine-containing neurons upon monoamine content of the brain and EEG and behavioral waking in the cat, *Brain Res.* **58**:157–177.

Jones, B. E., Harper, S. T., and Halaris, A. E., 1977, Effects of locus ceruleus lesions upon cerebral monoamine content, sleep–wakefulness states and the response to amphetamine in the cat, *Brain Res.* **124**:473–496.

Jones, D., Kelwala, S., Bell, J., Duke, S., Jackson, E., and Sitaram, N., 1985, Cholinergic REM sleep induction response correlation with endogenous major depressive subtype, *Psychiatry Res.* **14**:99–110.

Jones, H. S., and Oswald, I., 1968, Two cases of healthy insomnia, *Electroencephalogr. Clin. Neurophysiol.* **24**:378–380.

Jouvet, M., 1962, Recherches sur les structures nerveuses et les mecanismes responsables des differentes phases du sommeil physiologique, *Arch. Ital. Biol.* **100**:125–206.

Jouvet, M., 1965, Paradoxical sleep—a study of its nature and mechanisms, *Prog. Brain Res.* **18**:20–62.

Jouvet, M., 1967, Mechanisms of the states of sleep: A neuropharmacological approach, in: *Sleep and Altered States of Consciousness* (F. O. Euarts and H. L. Williams, eds.), Williams & Williams, Baltimore, pp. 86–126.

Jouvet, M., 1969, Biogenic amines and the states of sleep, *Science* **163**:32–41.

Jouvet, M., 1972, The role of monoamines and acetylcholine-containing neurons in the regulation of the sleep–waking cycle, *Ergeb. Physiol.* **64**:166–307.

Jouvet, M., and Delorme, F., 1965, Locus ceruleus et sommeil paradoxal, *Compt. Rend. Soc. Biol. (Paris)* **159**:895–899.

Jouvet, M., and Michel, F., 1959, Correlations electromyographiques du sommeil chez le chat decortique et mesencephalique chronique, *Comp. Rend. Soc. Biol. (Paris)* **153**: 422–425.

Jouvet, M., and Renault, J., 1966, Insomnie persistente après lesions des noyaux raphe chez le chat, *Compt. Rend. Soc. Biol. (Paris)* **160**:1461–1465.

Jouvet, M., Bobillier, P., Pujol, J. F., and Renault, J., 1966, Effets des lesions du systeme du raphe sur le sommeil et la sertonine cerebrale, *Compt. Rend. Soc. Biol. (Paris)* **160**:2343–2350.

Jouvet, M., Mouret, J., Chorvet, G., and Siffre, M., 1974, Toward a 48–hour day, in: *Experimental Biocircadian Rhythm in Man in the Neurosciences: Third Study Program* (F. Schmitt and F. Worden, eds.), MIT Press, Cambridge, MA, pp. 491–497.

Jovanovic, U. J., 1977, The sleep profile in manic-depressive patients in the depressive phase: Studies to compare these patients with healthy human subjects, *Waking Sleeping* **1**:199–210.

Judd, H. L., Parker, D. C., Siler, T. M., and Yen, S. S. C., 1974, The nocturnal use of plasma testosterone in pubertal boys, *J. Clin. Endocrinol. Metab.* **38**:710–713.

Juji, T., Satake, M., Honda, Y., and Doi, Y., 1984, HLA antigens in Japanese patients with narcolepsy, *Tissue Antigens* **24**:316–319.

Jus, K., Bouchard, M., Jus, A. K., Villeneuve, A., and Lachance, R., 1973, Sleep EEG studies in untreated, long term schizophrenic patients, *Arch. Gen. Psychiatry* **29**:386–390.

Kabuto, M., Namura, I., and Saitoh, Y., 1986, Nocturnal enhancement of plasma melatonin could be suppressed by benzodiazepines in humans, *Endocrinol. Jpn.* **33**:405–414.

Kaim, S. C., 1974, Prevention of delirium tremens: Use of phenothiazines versus drugs cross-dependent with alcohol, in: *The Phenothiazines and Structurally Related Drugs* (C. J. Cons and E. Usdin, eds.), Raven Press, New York, pp. 685–690.

Kaim, S. C., and Klett, C. J., 1972, Treatment of delirium tremens: A comparative evaluation of four drugs, *Q. J. Stud. Alcohol* **33**:1065–1072.

Kaim, S. C., Klett, C. J., and Rothfeld, B., 1969, Treatment of the acute alcohol withdrawal state: A comparison of four drugs, *Am. J. Psychiatry* **125**:1640–1646.

Kaitin, K. I., Kilduff, T. S., and Dement, W. C., 1986. Sleep fragmentation in canine narcolepsy, *Sleep* **9**:116–119.

Kales, A., Hoedemaker, F. S., Jacobson, A., and Lichenstein, E. L., 1964, Dream deprivation: An experimental reappraisal, *Nature* **204**:1337–1338.

Kales, A., Heuser, G., Jacobson, A., Kales, J. D., Hanley, J., Zweizig, J. R., and Paulson, M. J., 1967, All night sleep studies in hypothyroid patients, before and after treatment, *J. Clin. Endocrinol. Metab.* **27**:1593–1599.

Kales, A., Beall, G. N., Bajor, G. F., Jackson, A., and Kales, J. R., 1968, Sleep studies in asthmatic adults—relationship to sleep stage and time of night, *J. Allergy Clin. Immunol.* **41**:164–173.

Kales, A., Heuser, G., Kales, J. D., Rickles, W. H., Jr., Rubin, R. T., Scharf, M. B., and Ungerleider, J. T., 1969a, Drug dependency. Investigation of stimulants and depressants, *Ann. Intern. Med.* **70**:591–614.

Kales, A., Malmstrom, E. J., Scharf, M. B., and Rubin, R. T., 1969b, Psychophysiological and biochemical changes following use and withdrawal of hypnotics, in: *Sleep: Physiology and Pathology* (A. Kales, ed.), Lippincott, Philadelphia, pp. 331–343.

Kales, A. T. L., Killer, E. J., Naitoh, P., Preston, T. A., and Malstrom, E. J., 1970, Sleep patterns following 205 hours of sleep deprivation, *Psychosom. Med.* **32**:189–200.

Kales, A., Bixler, E. O., Tan, T., Scharf, M. B., and Kales, J. D., 1974a, Chronic hypnotic drug use: Ineffectiveness, drug-withdrawal insomnia, and dependence, *JAMA* **227**:513–517.

Kales, A., Bixler, E. O., and Kales, J. D., 1974b, Role of the sleep research and treatment facility: Diagnosis, treatment and education, in: *Advances in Sleep Research* (E. Weitzman, ed.), Spectrum, Flushing, NY, pp. 391–417.

Kales, A., Kales, J. D., and Humphrey, F. J., 1975a, Sleep and dreams, in: *Comprehensive Textbook of Psychiatry II* (A. M. Freedman, H. I. Kaplan, and B. J. Sadock, eds.), Williams & Wilkins, Baltimore, pp. 114–128.

Kales, A., Kales, J. D., Bixler, E. O., and Scharf, M. B., 1975b, Effectiveness of hypnotic drugs with prolonged use of flurazepam and pentobarbital, *Clin. Pharmacol. Ther.* **18**:356–363.

Kales, A., Kales, J. D., Soldatos, C. R., Kotas, K., and Santen, R., 1975c, Effects of thioridazine (Mellaril) on anterior pituitary secretion: Changes in testosterone and prolactin, presented at the Second International Sleep Research Congress, Edinburgh, June 30–July 4, 1975.

12,05,12Kales, A., Hauri, P., Bixler, E. D., and Silberfarb, P., 1976a, Effectiveness of intermediate- 15,05,12term use of secobarbital, *Clin. Pharmacol. Ther.* **20**:541–545.

Kales, A., Caldwell, A. B., Bixler, E. O., Healy, S., Kales, J. D., and Preston, T. A., 1976b, MMPI scales in insomnia: A comparison of Hershey and Los Angeles studies, *Sleep Res.* **5**:144.

Kales, A., Kales, J., Bixler, E. O., Scharf, M. B., and Russek, E., 1976c, Hypnotic efficacy of triazolam: Sleep laboratory evaluation of intermediate term effectiveness, *J. Clin. Pharmacol.* **16**:399–406.

Kales, A., Bixler, E. O., Scharf, M., and Kales, J. D., 1976d, Sleep laboratory studies of flurazepam: A model for evaluating hypnotic drugs, *Clin. Pharmacol. Ther.* **19**: 576–583.

Kales, A., Scharf, M. B., and Kales, J. D., 1978a, Rebound insomnia: A new clinical syndrome, *Science* **201**:1039–1041.

Kales, A., Bixler, E. O., Caldwell, A. B., Healy, S., Preston, T. A., and Kales, J. D., 1978b, Further evaluation of MMPI findings in insomnia: Comparison of insomniac patients and normal controls, *Sleep Res.* **7**:189.

Kales, A., Soldatos, C. R., Cadieux, R., Bixler, E. O., Tan, T., and Scharf, M. B., 1979, Propranolol in the treatment of narcolepsy, *Ann. Intern. Med.* **91**:741–743.

Kales, A., Soldatos, C. R., Bixler, E. O., Caldwell, A., Cadieux, R. J., Verrechio, J. M., and Kales, J. D., 1982a, Narcolepsy–cataplexy II. Psychosocial consequences and associated psychopathology, *Arch. Neurol* **39**:169–171.

Kales, A., Bixler, E. O., Soldatos, C. R., Vela-Bueno, A., Caldwell, A. B., and Cadieux, R. J., 1982b, Biopsychobehavioral correlates of insomnia, part 1: Role of sleep apnea and nocturnal myoclonus, *Psychosomatics* **23**:589–600.

Kales, A., Soldatos, C. R., Bixler, E. O., Vela-Bueno, A., Jacoby, J., and Kales, J. D., 1982c, Quazepam and flurazepam: Long-term use and extended withdrawal, *Clin. Pharmacol. Ther.* **32**:781–788.

Kales, A., Soldatos, C. R., Bixler, E. O., and Kales, J. D., 1983, Early morning insomnia with rapidly eliminated benzodiazepines, *Science* **220**:95–97.

Kales, J., Kales, A., Bixler, E. O., and Slye, E. S., 1971, Effects of placebo and flurazepam on sleep patterns in insomniac subjects, *Clin. Pharmacol. Ther.* **12**:691–697.

Kalucy, R. S., Crisp, A. H., Chard, T., and Chen, C., 1975, Nocturnal hormonal profiles in obese anorexia nervosa and normal subjects, presented at Second International Sleep Research Congress, Edinburgh, June 30–July, 4, 1975.

Kamberi, I. A., Mical, R. S., and Porter, J. C., 1971, Effects of melatonin and serotonin on the release of FSH and prolactin, *Endocrinology* **88**:1288–1293.

Kaneko, Y., Takahashi, Y., Kaneko, M., and Kumashio, H., 1978, Therapeutic usefulness of ergotamine for narcolepsy, *Am. J. Psychiatry* **35**:873–874.

Kannengiesser, M. H., Hunt, P. F., and Raynaud, J. P., 1976, Comparative action of fenfluramine on the uptake and release of serotonin and dopamine, *Eur. J. Pharmacol.* **35**:35–43.

Kanno, O., and Clarenbach, P., 1985, Effect of clonidine and yohimbine on sleep in man: Polygraphic study and EEG analysis by normalized slope descriptors, *Electroencephalog. Clin. Neurophysiol.* **60**:478–484.

Kapen, S., Boyar, R., Hellman, L., Tucker, K., and Weitzman, E. D., 1972, Changes in the sleep stage pattern during the menstrual cycle of normal females, *Sleep Res.* **1**:186.

Kapen, S., Boyar, R., Perlow, M., Hellman, L., and Weitzman, E. D., 1973, Luteinizing hormone: Changes in secretory pattern during sleep in adult women, *Life Sci.* **13**:693–701.

Kapen, S., Boyar, R. M., Finkelstein, J. W., Hellman, L., and Weitzman, E. D., 1974, Effect of sleep–wake cycle reversal on LH secretory pattern in puberty, *J. Clin. Endocrinol. Metab.* **39**:283–289.

Kapen, S., Boyar, R., Hellman, L., and Weitzman, E. D., 1975, Inhibition of LH secretion during the nighttime hours: A subgroup of the anmenorrhea–galactorrhea syndrome, presented at the Second International Sleep Research Congress Edinburgh, June 30–July 4, 1975.

Kaplan, J., Dawson, S., Vaughan, T., Green, R., and Wyatt, R. J., 1974, Effect of prolonged chlorpromazine administration on the sleep of chronic schizophrenics, *Arch. Gen. Psychiatry* **31**:62–66.

Karacan, I., 1986, Erectile dysfunction in narcoleptic patients, *Sleep* **9**:227–231.

Karacan, I., Rosenbloom, A. L., Williams, R. L., Finley, W. W., and Hursch, C. J., 1971, Slow wave sleep deprivation in relation to plasma growth hormone concentration, *Behav. Neuropsychiatry* 2:11–14.

Karacan, I., Rosenbloom, A. L., Lononon, J. H., Williams, R. L., and Salis, P. J., 1975, Growth hormone levels during morning and afternoon naps, *Behav. Neuropsychiatry* 6:67–69.

Karczmar, A. G., 1975, Cholinergic influences on behavior, in: *Cholinergic Mechanisms* (P. G. Waser, ed.), Raven Press, New York, pp. 501–529.

Kastin, A. J., Ehrensing, R. H., Schalch, D. S., and Anderson, M. S., 1972, Improvement in mental depression with decreased thyrotropin response after administration of thyrotropin releasing hormone, *Lancet* 2:740–742.

Kato, R., Chiesara, E., and Frontino, G., 1962, Influence of sex difference on the pharmacological action and metabolism of some drugs, *Biochem. Pharmacol.* 11:221–227.

Katsantonis, G. P., Walsh, J. K., Schweitzer, P. K., and Friedman, W. H., 1985, Further evaluation of uvulopalatopharyngoplasty in the treatment of obstructive sleep apnea syndrome, *Otolaryngol. Head Neck Surg.* 93:244–250.

Kaufman, L. S., 1983, Parachlorophenylalanine does not affect pontine–geniculate–occipital waves in rats despite significant effects on other sleep–waking parameters, *Exp. Neurol.* 80:410–417.

Kawamura, H., and Sawyer, C. H., 1965, Elevation in brain temperature during paradoxical sleep, *Science* 150:912–913.

Kay, D. C., Blackburn, A. B., Buckingham, J. A., and Karacan, I., 1965, Human pharmacology of sleep, in: *Pharmacology of Sleep* (R. L. Williams and I. Karacan, eds.), John Wiley and Sons, New York, pp. 83–210.

Kaya, N. 1984, Sectioning the hyoid bone as a therapeutic approach for obstruction sleep apnea, *Sleep* 7:77–78.

Kearley, M. D., Wynne, J. W., Block, A. J., Boysen, P. G., Lindsey, S., and Martin, C., 1980, The effect of low flow oxygen on sleep-disordered breathing and oxygen desaturation, *Chest* 78:682–685.

Kendel, K., Beck, U., Wita, C., Hohneck, E., and Zimmerman, H., 1972, Der Einfluss von L-dopa auf den Nachtschlaf bei Patienten mit Parkinson-syndrom, *Arch. Psychiatr. Nervenkr.* 216:82–100.

Kepner, C. A., Lippa, A. S., Benson, D. I., Sano, M. C., and Beer, B., 1979, Resolution of two biochemically and pharmacologically distant benzodiazepine receptors, *Pharmacol. Biochem. Behav.* 11:457–462.

Kerkhofs, M., Hoffmann, G., De Martelaere, V., Linkowski, P., and Mendlewicz, J., 1985, Sleep EEG recordings in depressive disorders, *J. Affective Dis.* 9:47–53.

Keshavan, M. S., and Crammer, J. C., 1985, Clonidine in benzodiazepine withdrawal, *Lancet* 1:1325–1326.

Kessler, S., Guilleminault, C., and Dement, W., 1974, A family study of narcoleptics, *Acta Neurol. Scand.* 50:503–512.

Khaleque, A., and Rahman, A., 1982, Sleep disturbances and health complaints of shift workers, *J. Human Ergon.* 11:155–164.

Kiianmaa, K., and Tabakoff, B., 1983, Neurochemical correlates of tolerance and strain differences in the neurochemical effects of ethanol, *Pharmacol. Biochem. Behav.* 18S1:383–388.

Kijne, B., Aggernaes, H., Fog-Meller, F., Andersen, H. H., Nissen, J., Kirkegaard, C., and Bjorum, N., 1982, Circadian variation of serum thyrotropin in endogenous depression, *Psychiatry Res.* 6:277–282.

Kilduff, S., 1986, Bowersox, S. S., Kaitin, K., Baker, T. L., Ciaranello, R. D., and Dement,

W. C., 1986, Muscarinic cholinergic receptors and the canine model of narcolepsy, *Sleep* **9**:102–106.

Kim, J. H., Manuelidis, E. E., Glenn, W. W. L., Fukuda, Y., Cole, D. S., and Hogan, J. F., 1983, Light and electron microscopic studies of phrenic nerves after long-term electrical stimulation, *J. Neurosurg.* **58**:84–91.

Kim, J. S., Sherman, L., Kolodny, H. D., Benjamin, F., and Singh, A., 1971, Attenuation by haloperidol of human serum growth hormone (HGH) response to insulin, *Clin. Res.* **19**:718.

King, D., and Jewett, R. S., 1971, The effects of alpha methyl tyrosine on sleep and brain norepinephrine in cats, *J. Pharmacol. Exp. Ther.* **177**:188–194.

Kirmil-Gray, K., Coates, T. J., Thoresen, C. E., Rosekind, M. R., and Price, V. A., 1978, Treating insomnia in adolescents, *Sleep Res.* **7**:237.

Kjellman, B. F., Beck-Frilis, J. B., Ljunggren, J. G., and Wetterberg, L., 1984, Twenty-four-hour serum levels of TSH in affective disorders, *Acta Psychiatr. Scand.* **69**:491–502.

Klaff, L. J., Barron, J. L., Levitt, N. S., Ling, N., and Millar, R. P., 1982, Somatostatin-28 inhibits thyroid-stimulating hormone release in man, *S. Afr. Med. J.* **62**:929–930.

Klasi, J., 1922, Uber die therapeutische Anwendung der Dauernarhose mittles Somnifens bei Schizophrenen Zentralblatt fur die Gesante, *Neurol. Psychiatrie* **74**:557–592.

Klein, H. E., and Seibold, B., 1985, DST In healthy volunteers and after sleep deprivation, *Acta Psychiatr. Scand.* **72**:16–19.

Klein, K. E., Herrmann, R., Kuklinski, P., and Wegmann, H., 1977, Circadian performance rhythms: Experimental studies in air operation, in: *Vigilance: Theory, Operational Performance, and Physiological Correlates,* (R. R. Mackie, ed.), Plenum Press, New York, pp. 111–132.

Kleinberg, D. L., Noel, G. L., and Frantz, A. G., 1971, Chlorpromazine stimulation and 12,05,12L-dopa suppression of plasma prolactin in man, *J. Clin. Endocrinol. Metab.* **33**:873–876.

Kleitman, N., 1963, *Sleep and Wakefulness,* University of Chicago Press, Chicago.

Klotz, U., Avant, G. R., Hoyumpa, A., Schenker, S., and Wilkinson, G. R., 1975, The effects of age and liver disease on the disposition and elimination of diazepam in adult man, *J. Clin. Invest.* **55**:347–359.

Knopf, R. F., Conn, J. W., Fajans, S. S., Floyd, J. C., Guntsche, E. M., and Rull, J. A., 1965, Plasma growth hormone response to intravenous administration of amino acids, *J. Clin. Endocrinol. Metab.* **25**:1140–1144.

Knott, P. J., and Curzon, G., 1972, Free tryptophan in plasma and brain tryptophan metabolism, *Nature* **239**:452–253.

Knowles, J. B., and MacLean, A. W., 1985, A critical evaluation of models of depression, Presentation at Fourth World Congress of Biological Psychiatry, Philadelphia, Sept. 8–13, 1985.

Knowles, J., Waldron, J., and Cairns, J., 1979, Sleep preceding the onset of a manic episode, *Biol. Psychiatry* **14**:671–675.

Knowles, J. B., Laverty, S. G., and Kuechler, H. A., 1968, The effects of alcohol on REM sleep, *Q. J. Stud. Alcohol* **29**:342–349.

Knowles, J. B., Southmayd, S. E., Delva, N., MacLean, A. W., Cairns, J., and Letemendia, F. J., 1979, Five variations of sleep deprivation in a depressed woman, *Br. J. Psychiatry* **135**:403–410.

Knowles, J. B., Southmayd, S. E., Delva, N., Prowse, A., Maclean, A. W., Cairns, J., and Letemendia, F. J., 1981, Sleep deprivation: Outcome of controlled single case studies of depressed patients, *Can. J. Psychiatry* **26**:330–333.

Koella, W. P., 1969, Neurohumoral aspects of sleep control, *Biol. Psychiatry* **1**:161–177.

Koella, W. P., Feldstein, A., and Czieman, J. S., 1968, The effect of para-chlorophenylalanine on the sleep of cats, *Electroencephalogr. Clin. Neurophysiol.* **25**:481–490.

Koelle, G. B., 1986, Otto Loewi 1873–1961, *Trends Pharmacol. Sci.* **7**:290–291.

Koerger, R. K., Torkelson, R., Haven, G., Donaldson, J., Cohen, S. M., and Case, M., 1984, Increased cerebrospinal fluid 5-hydroxytrptamine and 5-hydroxyindoleacetic acid in Klein–Levin syndrome, *Neurology* **34**:1597–1600.

Kogi, K., 1982, Sleep problems in night and shift work, *J. Hum. Ergon.* **11**:217–231.

Kolko, D. J., 1984, Behavioral treatment of excessive daytime sleepiness in an elderly woman with multiple medical problems, *J. Behav. Ther. Psychiatry* **15**:341–345.

Koranyi, E. K., and Lehman, H. E., 1960, Experimental sleep deprivation in schizophrenic patients, *Arch. Gen. Psychiatry* **2**:534–544.

Kostowski, W., Giacalone, E., Garattini, S., and Valzelli, L., 1968, Studies on behavioural and biochemical changes in rats after lesions of midbrain raphe, *Eur. J.Pharmacol.* **4**:371–376.

Kotagal, S., Rathnow, S. R., Chu, J. Y., O'Connor, D. M., Cross, J., and Sterneck, R. L., 1985, Letter to the editor: Nocturnal myoclonus, a sleep disturbance with leukemia, *Dev. Med. Child Neurol.* **27**:124–127.

Koulu, M., Lammintausta, R., Kangas, L., and Dahlstrom, S., 1979, The effect of methysergide, pimozide, and sodium valporate on the diazepam-stimulated growth hormone secretion in man, *J. Clin. Endocrinol. Metab.* **48**:119–122.

Koulu, M., Lammintausta, R., and Dahlstrom, S., 1980, Effects of some gamma-aminobutyric acid (GABA)-ergic drugs on the dopaminergic control of human growth hormone secretion, *J. Clin. Endocrinol. Metab.* **51**:124–129.

Koulu, R., Huupponen, R., Pihlajamaki, K., and Makinen, P., 1985, Suppressive effect of naloxone on diazepam stimulated human growth hormone (GH) secretion, *Acta Endocrinol. (Suppl. 270)* **109**:140.

Kovacevic-Ristanovic, Spire, J., Jadot, C., and Noel, P., 1978, Time shift (jet lag) and sleep, *Sleep Res.* **7**:306.

Koyama, T, Lowy, M. T., and Meltzer, H. Y., 1987, 5-Hydroxytryptophan-induced cortisol response and CSF 5-HIAA in depressed patients, *Am. J. Psychiatry* **144**:334–337.

Kramer, M., Roth, T., and Trindar, J., 1971, Noise Disturbance and Sleep Department Transportation Report No. FAA-NO-70-16.

Krieger, D. T., and Gewitz, G. P., 1974, Recovery of hypothalamic–pituitary–adrenal function growth hormone responsiveness and sleep EEG pattern in a patient following removal of an adrenal cortical adenoma, *J. Clin. Endocrinol. Metab.* **38**:1075–1082.

Krieger, D. T., and Glick, S. M., 1974, Sleep EEG stages and plasma growth hormone concentration in states of endogenous and exogenous hypercortisolemia or ACTH elevation, *J. Clin. Endocrinol. Metab.* **39**:986–1000.

Krieger, D. T., and Rizzo, F., 1971, Circadian periodicity of plasma II-hydroxycorticosteroid levels in subjects with partial and absent light perception, *Neuroendocrinology* **8**:165–179.

Krieger, D. T., Kreuzer, J., and Rizzo, F. A., 1969, Constant light: Effect on circadian pattern and phase reversal of steroid and electrolyte levels in man, *J. Clin. Endocrinol. Metab.* **29**:1634–1638.

Krieger, D. T., Albin, J., Paget, S., and Glick, S. M., 1972, Failure of suppression of nocturnal growth hormone rise by acute corticosteroid administration, *Horm. Metab. Res.* **4**:463–466.

Krieger, I., and Mellinger, R.C., 1971, Pituitary function in the deprivation syndrome, *J. Pediatr.* **79**:216–225.

Krieger, J., Mangin, P., and Kurtz D., 1980, Les Modifications respiratories au cours sommeil du age normal, *Rev. EEG Neurophysiol.* **10**:177–185.

Kripke, D. F., and Garfinkel, L., 1984, Excess nocturnal deaths related to sleeping pill and tranquilizer use, *Lancet* **8368**:99.

Kripke, D. F., and Wyborney, V. G., 1980, Lithium slows rat circadian activity rhythms, *Life Sci.* **26**:1319–1321.

Kripke, D. F., Mullaney, D. J., Atkinson, M., and Wolf, S., 1978, Circadian rhythm disorders in manic-depressives, *Biol. Psychiatry* **13**:335–344.

Kripke, D. F., Simons, R. N., Garfinkel, L., and Hammond, E. C., 1979, Short and long sleep and sleeping pills, *Arch. Gen. Psychiatry* **36**:103–116.

Kripke, D. F., Ancoli-Isreal, S., and Okudaira, N., 1982, Sleep apnea and nocturnal myoclonus in the elderly, *Neurobiol. Aging* **3**:329–336.

Krishnan, R. R., Volow, M. R., Miller, P. P., and Carwile, S. T., 1984, Narcolepsy: Preliminary retrospective study of psychiatric and psychosocial aspects, *Am. J. Psychiatry* **141**:428–432.

Kronauer, R. E., Czeisler, C. A., Pilato, S. F., Moore-Ede, M. C., and Weitzman, E. D., 1982, Mathematical model of the human circadian system with two interacting oscillators, *Am. J. Physiol.* **242**:r3–r17.

Krueger, J., 1986, Immunology and sleep: 1986 Presentation at Assoc. of Professional Sleep Societies, First Annual Meeting, Columbus, Ohio, June 15–20, 1986.

Krueger, J. M., Bacsik, J., and Garcia-Arraras, J., 1980, Sleep-promoting material from human urine and its relation to factor S from brain, *Am. J. Physiol.* **238**:111–123.

Krueger, J. M., Pappenheimer, J. R., and Karnovsky, M. L., 1982, The composition of sleep promoting factor isolated from human urine, *J. Biol. Chem.* **257**:1664–1669, 1982.

Kuhn, D. M., Wolf, W. A., and Youdim, M. B. H., 1986, Serotonin neurochemistry revisited: A new look at some old axioms, *Neurochem. Int.* **8**:141–154.

Kumashiro, H., Sato, M., Hirata, J., Baba, O., and Otsaki, S., 1971, Sleep apnea and sleep regulating mechanism: A case effectively treated with monochlorimipramine, *Folia Psychiatr. Neurol. Jpn.* **25**:41–49.

Kunugi, H., 1970, All night sleep EEG in chronic schizophrenia (Engl. abstr.), *Seihin Shinkeigaku Zasshi* **71**:226–227.

Kupfer, D. J., 1976, REM latency: A psychobiological marker for primary depressive disease, *Biol. Psychiatry* **11**:159–174.

Kupfer, D. J., and Bowers, M. B., 1972, REM sleep and central monoamine oxidase inhibition, *Psychopharmacologia* **27**:183–190.

Kupfer, D. J., and Foster, F. G., 1972, Interval between onset of sleep and rapid eye movement sleep as an indicator of depression, *Lancet* **2**:684–686.

Kupfer, D. J., and Foster, F. G., 1973, Sleep and activity in a psychotic depression, *J. Nerv. Ment. Dis.* **156**:341–348.

Kupfer, D. J., and Foster, F. G., 1975, The sleep of psychotic patients: Does it all look alike? in: *The Biology of the Major Psychosis: A Comparative Analysis* (D. X. Freedom, ed.), Raven Press, New York, pp. 143–164.

Kupfer, D. J., and Heninger, E. R., 1972, REM activity as a correlate of mood changes throughout the night (EEG patterns in a patient with a 48 hr cyclic mood disturbance), *Arch. Gen. Psychiatry* **27**:368–373.

Kupfer, D. J., and Reynolds, C. F., 1983, A critical review of sleep and its disorders from a developmental perspective, *Psychiat. Devel.* **4**:367–386.

Kupfer, D. J., Wyatt, R. J., and Snyder, F., 1970, Comparison between electroencephalographic and systematic nursing observations of sleep in psychiatric patients, *J. Nerv. Mental Dis.* **151**:361–368.

Kupfer, D. J., Himmelhoch, J., Schwartzburg, M., Anderson, C., Byck, R., and Detre, P., 1972, Hypersomnia in manic-depressive disease, *Dis. Nerv. Syst.* **33**:720–724.

Kupfer, D. J., Foster, F. G., and Detre, T. P., 1973, Sleep continuity changes in depression, *Dis. Nerv. Syst.* **34**:192–195.

Kupfer, D. J., Reynolds, C. F., Weiss, B. L., and Foster, F. C., 1974, Lithium carbonate and sleep in affective disorders: Further considerations, *Arch. Gen. Psychiatry* **30**:79–84.

Kupfer, D. J., Spiker, D. C., Coble, P. A., and Shaw, D. H., 1978, Electroencephalographic sleep recordings and depression in the elderly, *J. Am. Geriatr. Soc.* **26**:53–57.

Kupfer, D. J., Edwards, D. J., Spiker, D. G., Holzer, B. C., and Coble, P., 1979, MAO activity and EEG sleep in primary depression, *Psychiatry Res.* **1**:241–247.

Kupfer, D. J., Gillin, J. C., Coble, P. A., Spiker, D. G., Shaw, D., and Holtzer, B., 1980a, REM sleep, naps, and depression, *J. Psychiatr. Res.* **5**:17–25.

Kupfer, D. J., Hanin, I., and Spiker, D. G., 1980b, EEG sleep and tricyclic plasma levels in primary depression, *Psychopharmacol. Bull.* **16**:35–36.

Kupfer, D. J., Jarrett, D. B., and Frank, E., 1984a, Relationship among selected neuroendocrine and sleep measures in patients with recurrent depression, *Biol. Psychiatry* **19**:1525–1535.

Kupfer, D. J., Ulrich, R. F., Coble, P. A., Jarrett, D. B., Grochocinski, U., Doman, J., and Matthews, G., 1984b, Application of automated REM and slow-wave sleep analysis: II. Testing the assumptions of the two-process model of sleep regulation in normal and depressed subjects, *Psychiatry Res.* **13**:335–343.

Kupfer, D. J., Reynolds, C. F., Grochocinski, V. J., Ulrich, R. F., and McEachran, A., 1986, Aspects of short REM latency in affective states: A revisit, *Psychiatry Res.* **17**:49–59.

Kushida, C. A., Baker, T., and Dement, W. C., 1985, Electroencephalographic correlates of cataplectic attacks in narcoleptic canines, *Electroencephalog. Clin. Neurophysiol.* **61**:61–70.

Kvist, J., and Kirkegaard, C., 1980, Effect of repeated sleep deprivation on clinical symptoms and the TRH test in endogenous depression, *Acta Psychiat. Scand.* **62**:494–502.

Laguzzi, R. F., Adrien, J., Bourgoin, S., and Hamon, M., 1979, Effects of intraventricular injection of 6-hydroxydopamine in the developing kitten, *Brain Res.* **160**:445–459.

Lahmeyer, H. W., Poznanski, E. O., and Bellur, S. N., 1983, EEG sleep in depressed adolescents, *Am. J. Psychiatry* **140**:1150–1153.

Lake, C. R., Coleman, M. D., Ziegler, M. G., and Murphy, D. L., 1979, Fenfluramine and its effects on the sympathetic nervous system in man, *Curr. Med. Res. Opin.* **6**:63–72.

Lal, S., De la Vega, C. E., Sourkes, T. L., and Friesen, H. G., 1973, Effect of apomorphine on growth hormone, prolactin, luteinizing hormone and follicle-stimulating hormone levels in human serum, *J. Clin. Endocrinol. Metab.* **37**:719–724.

Lal, S., Mendis, T., Cervantes, P., Guyda, H., and DeRivera, J. L., 1979, Effect of benztropine on haloperidol-induced prolactin secretion, *Neuropsychobiology* **5**:327–331.

Lamacq, L., 1987, A Propos de quelque cas de narcolepsie, *Rev. Med.* **17**:699–714.

Lancranjan, I., Ohnhaus, E., Marbach, P., Wirz-Justice, A., Del Pozo, E., and Audibert, A., 1979, Neurotransmitters—control of growth hormone (GH) and prolactin (PRL) secretion: The adrenergic and serotonergic modulation of GH and PRL in man, *Int. J. Neurol.* **13**:37–52.

Langdon, N., Lock, C., Welsh, K., Vergani, D., Dorow, R., Wachtel, H., and Palenschat, D., 1986a Immune factors in narcolepsy, *Sleep* **9**:143–148.

Langdon, N., Shindler, J., Parkes, J. D., and Bandak, S., 1986b, Fluoxetine in the treatment of cataplexy, *Sleep* **9**:371–373.

Lanoir, J., Ternaux, J. P., Pons, C., and Lagarde, J. M., 1981, Long-term effects of a tryptophan-free diet of serotonin metabolism and sleep–waking balance in rats, *Exp. Brain Res.* **41:**346–357.

Laposata, E. A., and Lange, L. G., 1986, Presence of nonoxidative ethanol metabolism in human organs commonly damaged by ethanol abuse, *Science* **231:**497–499.

Laron, Z., Doron, M., and Amikam, B., 1970, Plasma growth hormone in men and women over 70 years of age, in: *Medicine and Sport* (E. Jokl and M. Habbelinck, eds.), University Park Press, Baltimore, pp. 126–131.

Lasegue, C., 1881, Le Delire alcoholique n'est pas un delire, mais un réve, *Arch. Gen. Med.* **88:**513–536.

Lavie, P., 1983, Incidence of sleep apnea in a presumably healthy working population: A significant relationship with excessive daytime sleepiness, *Sleep* **6:**312–318.

Lavie, P., 1984, Nothing new under the moon: Historical accounts of sleep apnea syndrome, *Arch. Intern. Med.* **144:**2025–2028.

Lavie, P., Gertner, R., Zomer, J., and Podoshin, L., 1981, Breathing disorders in sleep associated with "microarousals" in patients with allergic rhinitis, *Acta Otolaryngol.* **92:**529–533.

Lawton, M. P., and Cahn, B., 1963, The effects of diazepam (Valium) and alcohol on psychomotor performance, *J. Nerv. Ment. Dis.* **133:**550–554.

Le Gassicke, J., Ashcroft, G. W., Eccleston, D., Evans, J. I., Oswald, I., and Ritson, E. B., 1965, The clinical state, sleep, and amine metabolism of a tranylcypromine ("Parnate") addict, *Br. J. Psychiatry* **111:**357–364.

Leaf, A., and Liddle, G. W., 1974, Summarization of the effects of hormones on water and electrolyte metabolism, in: *Textbook of Endocrinology* (R. H. Williams ed.), W. B. Saunders Co., Philadelphia, pp. 938–947.

Leckman, J. F., and Gershon, E. S., 1975, A genetic model of narcolepsy, *Br. J. Psychiatry* **127:**276–279.

Leckman, J. F., Anderson, G. M., Cohen, D. J., Ort, S., Harcherik, D. F., Hoder, E. L., and Shaywitz, B. A., 1984, Whole blood serotonin and tryptophan levels in Tourette's disorder: Effects of acute and chronic clonidine treatment, *Life Sci.* **35:**2497–2503.

Leebaw, W. F., Lee, L. A., and Woolf, P. D., 1978, Dopamine affects basal and augmented pituitary hormone secretion, *J. Clin. Endocrinol. Metab.* **47:**480–487.

Leeb-Lundberg, F., Snowman, A., and Olsen, R., 1980, Barbiturate receptor sites are coupled to benzodiazepine receptors, *Proc. Natl. Acad. Sci. USA* **77:**7468–7472.

Lefur, G., Mizoule, J., Burgevin, M. C., Gerris, O., Heaulame, M., Gantlier, A., and Guerteney, C., 1981, Multiple benzodiazepine receptors: Evidence of dissociation between anticonflict and anticonvulsant properties by PK 8165 and PK 9083 (two quinoline derivatives), *Life Sci.* **28:**1439–1448.

Legendre, R., and Pieron, H., 1910, Des resultats histophysiologiques de l'injection intra-occipito-atlantoidedienne des liquides insomniques, *Compt. Rend. Soc. Biol. (Paris)* **68:**1108–1109.

Lehmann, W., and Liljenberg, B., 1981, Effect of temazepam and temazepam-ethanol on sleep, *Eur. J. Pharmacol.* **20:**201–205.

Leibowitz, M., and Sunshine, A., 1978, A long-term hypnotic efficacy and safety of triazolam and flurazepam, *J. Clin. Pharmacol.* **18:**302–309.

Lenard, H. G., and Schulte, F. J., 1972, Polygraphic sleep study in craniopagus twins (where is the sleep transmitter?), *J. Neurol. Neurosurg. Psychiatry* **35:**756–762.

Leslie, S. W., Friedman, M. B., Wilcox, R. E., and Elrod, S. V., 1980, Acute and chronic effects of barbiturates on depolarization-induced calcium influx into rat synaptosomes, *Brain Res.* **185:**409–417.

Lester, B. K., and Guerrero-Figueroa, R., 1966, Effects of some drugs on electroencephalographic fast activity and dream time, *Psychophysiology* **2**:224–236.

Lester, B. K., Coulter, J. D., Cosden, L. C., and Williams, H. L., 1971, Chlorpromazine and human sleep, *Psychopharmacologia* **20**:280–287.

Lester, B. K., Rundell, O. H., Cowden, L. C., and Williams, H. L., 1973, Chronic alcoholism, alcohol and sleep, *Adv. Exp. Med. Biol.* **35**:261–279.

Levander, S., and Sachs, C., 1985, Vigilance performance and automatic function in narcolepsy: Effects of central stimulants, *Psychophysiology* **22**:24–32.

Levin, D., Bertelson, A. D., and Lacks, P., 1984, MMPI differences among mild and severe insomniacs and good sleepers, *J. Pers. Assess.* **48**:126–129.

Levin, E. R., Sharp, B., and Carlson, H. E., 1984, Failure to confirm consistent stimulation of growth and hormone by diazepam, *Horm. Res.* **19**:86–90.

Levin, M., 1959, Aggression, guilt and cataplexy, *Am. J. Psychiatry* **116**:133–136.

Levy, A. B., Bucher, P., and Votolato, N., 1985, Myoclonus, hyperreflexia and diaphoresis in patients on phenelzine–tryptophan combination treatment, *Can. J. Psychiatry* **30**:434–436.

Lewis, M. J., Groom, G. V., Barber, R., and Henderson, A. H., 1981, The effects of propanolol and acebutolol on the overnight plasma levels of anterior pituitary and related hormones, *Br. J. Clin. Pharmacol.* **12**:737–742.

Lewis, S. A., and Evans, J. I., 1969, Some effects of chlorpromazine on human sleep, *Psychopharmacologia* **14**:342–348.

Lewis, S. A., Oswald, I., and Dunleavy, D. L. F., 1971, Chronic fenfluramine, administration: Some cerebral effects, *Br. Med. J.* **3**:67–70.

Leysen, J. E., Van Gompel, P., Gommeren, W., Woestenborghs, R., and Janssen, P. A., 1986, *Psychopharmacology* **88**:434–444.

Liddle, G. W., 1974, The adrenal cortex, in: *Textbook of Endocrinology* (R. H. Williams, ed.), Saunders, Philadelphia, pp. 233–283.

Liljequist, S., and Engel, J. A., 1984, The effects of GABA and benzodiazepine receptor antagonists in the anti-conflict actions of diazepam or ethanol, *Pharmacol. Biochem. Behav.* **21**:521–525.

Lin, T. U., and Tucci, J. R., 1974, Provocative tests of growth-hormone release, *Ann. Intern. Med.* **80**:464–469.

Lincoln, G., 1983, Melatonin as a seasonal time-cue: A commercial story, *Nature* **302**:755.

Linkowski,P., Mendlewicz, J., Leclercq, R., Brasseur, M., Hubain, P., Goldstein, J., and Van Cauter, E., 1985, The 24-hour profile of adrenocorticotropin and cortisol in major depressive illness, *J. Clin. Endocrinol. Metab.* **61**:429–438.

Linnoila, M., 1978, Psychomotor effects of drugs and alcohol on healthy volunteers and psychiatric patients, *Adv. Pharmacol. Ther.* **8**:235–249.

Linnoila, M., and Mattila, M. J., 1973, Drug interaction on psychomotor skills related to driving: Diazepam and alcohol, *Eur. J. Clin. Pharmacol.* **5**:186–194.

Linnoila, M., Seppala, T., and Mattila, M. J., 1974, Acute effect of antipyretic analgesics, alone or in combination with alcohol, on human psychomotor skills related to driving, *Br. J. Pharmacol.* **1**:477–484.

Linnoila, M., Ewin, W., and Logue, P. E., 1980, Efficacy and side effects of flurazepam and a combination of amobarbital and secobarbital in insomniac patients, *J. Clin. Psychol.* Feb.:117–123.

Lipman, R. L., Taylor, A. L., Schenk, A., and Mintz, D. H., 1972, Inhibition of sleep-related growth hormone release by elevated fatty acids, *J. Clin. Endocrinol. Metab.* **35**:592–594.

Lippa, A. S., Coupet, J., Greenblatt, N., Klepner, A., and Beer, B., 1979a, A synthetic non-benzodiazepine ligand for benzodiazepine receptors, *Pharmacol. Biochem. Behav.* **11**:99–106.

Lippa, A. S., Critchett, D. J., Sano, C., Klepner, C. A., Greenblatt, E. N., Coupet, J., and Beer, B., 1979b, Benzodiazepine receptors: Cellular and behavioral characteristics, *Pharmacol. Biochem. Behav.* **10**:831–843.

Lippa, A. S., Meyerson, L. R., and Beer, B., 1982, Molecular sustrates of anxiety: Clues from the heterogeneity of benzodiazepine receptors, *Life Sci.* **31**:1409–1417.

Llinas, R., and Jahnsen, H., 1982, Electrophysiology of mammalian thalamic neurons *in vitro*, *Nature* **197**:406–408.

Lloyd, K. G., Morselli, P. L., Depoortere, H., Fournier, O., Zivkovic, B., Scatton, B., and Broekkamp, C., 1983, The potential use of GABA agonists in psychiatric disorders: Evidence from studies with progabide in animal models and clinical trials, *Pharmacol. Biochem. Behav.* **18**:957–966.

Lo, M. M. S., Trifiletti, R. R., and Snyder, S. H., 1983, Physical separation and characterization of two central benzodiazepine receptors, in: *Pharmacology of Benzodiazepines* (E. Usdin, P. Skolnick, J. F., Tallman, D. Greenblatt, and S. M. Paul, eds.), Macmillan, London, pp. 165–173.

Long, J. B., and Holaday, J. W., 1985, Blood-brain barrier: Endogenous modulation by adrenal-cortical function, *Science* **227**:1580–1585.

Loomis, A. L., Harvey, E. N., and Hobart, G. A., 1937, Cerebral states during sleep, as studied by human brain potentials, *J. Exp. Psychol.* **21**:127–144.

Loosen, P., Achenhell, M., Athen, D., Bechmann, H., Benkert, O., Dittmer, T., and Hippius, H., 1974, The therapy of endogenous depression by sleep deprivation. 2. Comparisons of psychopathologic and biochemical parameters, *Arzneim. Forsch.* **24**:1075–1077.

Lowy, F. H., Cleghorn, J. M., and McClure, D. S., 1971, Sleep patterns in depression, *J. Nerv. Ment. Dis.* **153**:10–26.

Luby, E. D., and Caldwell, D. F., 1967, Sleep deprivation and EEG slow wave activity in chronic schizophrenia, *Arch. Gen. Psychiatry* **17**:361–384.

Luby, E. D., and Gottlieb, J. S., 1966, Sleep deprivation, in: *American Handbook of Psychiatry* (S. Arieti, ed.), Basic Books, New York, p. 406.

Lucke, G., and Glick, S. M., 1971a, Experimental modification of the sleep-induced peak growth hormone secretion, *J. Clin. Endocrinol. Metab.* **32**:729–736.

Lucke, C., and Glick, S. M., 1971b, Effect of medroxyprogesterone acetate on the sleep-induced peak of growth hormone, *J. Clin. Endocrinol. Metab.* **33**:851–853.

Lucke, C., Hoeffken, B., and Morgner, K., 1974, L-DOPA induced growth hormone secretion. Comparison with insulin tolerance test, arginine infusion and sleep induced GH secretion, *Acta Endocrinol.* **77**:241–249.

Lucke, C., Hoeffken, B., and Muhlen, A., 1976, Studies on the postponed growth hormone secretion following the infusion of somatostatin, *Acta Endocrinol. (Copenhagen)* **82**:460–466.

Lugaresi, E., Coccagna, G., and Ceroni, G. B., 1968a, Syndrome de Pickwick et syndrome d'hypoventimation alveolaire primaire, *Ann. Med. Psychol.* **1**:777.

Lugaresi, E., Goccagna, G., Ceroni, G., and Arnbroselti, C., 1968b, Restless legs syndrome and nocturnal myoclonus, in: *The Abnormalties of Sleep in Man*, Aulo Gaggi, Bologna, pp. 285-294.

Lugaresi, E., Cirignotta, F., Coccagna, G., and Baruzzi, A., 1982, Snoring and the obstructive apnea syndrome, *Electroencephalogr. Clin. Neurophysiol. (Suppl.)* **35**:421–430.

Lund, R., 1974, Personality factors and the desynchronization of circadian rhythms, *Psychosom. Med.* **36**:224–228.

Lund, R., and Berger, M., 1981, REM latency and duration in subgroups of depressive disorders, presented at Annual Meeting, Association for the Psychophysiological Study of Sleep, June, 1981, Hyannis Port, MA.

Lundquist, G., 1961, Delirium tremens: A comparative study of pathogenesis, course and prognosis with delirium tremens, *Acta Psychiatr. Scand.* **36**:443–466.

Luttinger, D., Nereroff, C. B., Mason, G. A., Frye, G. D., and Breese, G. R., 1981, Enhancement of ethanol-induced sedation and hypothermia by centrally administered neurotensin, beta-endorphin and bombesin, *Neuropharmacology* **20**:305–309.

Luttinger, D., Frye, G. D., and Bissette, G., 1982, Effects of neurotensin on the actions of barbituarites and ethanol, *Ann. NY Acad. Sci.* **400**:259–267.

Lynch, H. J., Wurtman, R. J., Moskowitz, M. A., Archer, M. C., and Ho, M. H., 1975, Daily rhythm in human urinary melanin, *Science* **187**:169–171.

Maas, J. W., and Mednieks, M., 1971, Hydrocortisone-mediated increase of norepinephrine uptake by brain slices, *Science* **171**:178–179.

MacIndoe, J. H., and Turkington, R. W., 1973, Stimulation of human prolactin secretion by intravenous infusion of L-tryptophan, *J. Clin. Invest.* **52**:1972–1978.

MacLean, A. W., and Cairns, J., 1982, Dose–response effects of ethanol on the sleep of young men, *J. Stud. Alcohol* **43**:434–444.

MacWilliam, J. A., 1923, Some applications of physiology to medicine, III. Blood pressure and heart action in sleep and dreams, *Br. Med. J.* **II**: 1196–1200.

Mace, J. W., Gotlin, R. W., and Beck, P., 1972, Sleep related human growth hormone (GH) release: A test of physiologic growth hormone secretion in children, *J. Clin. Endocrinol. Metab.* **34**:339–341.

Maclusky, N. J., Chaptal, C., Lieberburg, I., and McEwen, B. S., 1976, Properties and subcellular interrelationships of presumptive estrogen receptor macromolecules in the brains of neonatal and prepubertal female rats, *Brain Res.* **114**:158–165.

Madsen, B. W., and Rossi, L., 1980, Sleep and Michealis–Menten elimination of ethanol, *Clin. Pharmacol. Ther.* **27**:114–119.

Maggini, C., Murri, M., and Sacchatti, G., 1969, Evaluation of the effectiveness of temazepam on the insomnia of patients with neurosis and endogenous depression, *Arzneimittelforsch* **19**:1647–1652.

Mailman, R. B., Frey, G. D., Mueller, R. A., and Breese, G. R., 1980, The effects of thyrotropin-releasing hormone (TRH) and other drugs on the actions of alcohol, *Adv. Exp. Med. Biol.* **126**:509–522.

Maitre, M., Chesielski, S., Lehmann, A., Kemp, E., and Mandel, P., 1974, Protective effect of adenosine and nicotinamide against audiogenic seizures, *Biochem. Pharmacol.* **23**:2807–2816.

Majewska, M. D., Harrison, N. L., Schwartz, R. D., Barker, J. L., and Paul, S. M., 1986, Steroid hormone metabolites are barbiturate-like modulators of the GABA receptor, *Science* **232**:1004–1007.

Makipour, H., Iber, F. L., and Hartmann, E., 1972, Effects of L-tryptophan on sleep in hospitalized insomniac patients, paper presented at Annual Meeting of the Association for Psychophysiological Study of Sleep, Lake Minnewaska, New Mexico, 1972.

Malarkey, W. B., and Mendall, J. R., 1976, Failure of serotonin inhibitor to effect nocturnal GH and prolactin secretion in patients with Duchenne muscular dystrophy, *J. Clin. Endocrinol. Metab.* **43**:889–892.

Malmo, R. B., and Bilanger, D., 1967, Related physiological and behavioral changes: What are their determinants? in: *Sleep and Altered States of Consciousness* (S. S. Kety, E. V. Evarts, and H. C. Williams, eds.), Williams & Wilkins, Baltimore, pp. 288–313.

Mamelak, M., and Webster, P., 1981, Treatment of narcolepsy and sleep apnea with gammahydroxybutrate: A clinical and polysomnographic case study, *Sleep* **4**:105–111.

Mamelak, M., Escriu, J. M., and Stokan, O., 1977, The effects of gamma-hydroxybutyrate on sleep, *Biol. Psychiatry* **12**:273–287.

Mamelak, M., Csima, A., and Price, B., 1984, A comparative 25-night sleep laboratory study on the effects of quazepam and triazolam on chronic insomniacs, *J. Clin. Pharmacol.* **24**:65–75.

Mamelak, M., Scharf, M. B., and Woods, M., 1986, Treatment of narcolepsy with hydroxybutyrate. A review of clinical and sleep laboratory findings, *Sleep* **9**:285–289.

Mancia, G., and Zanchetti, A., 1980, Cardiovascular regulation during sleep, in: *Physiology and Sleep* (J. Orem and C. D. Barnes, eds.), Academic Press, New York, pp. 1–56.

Mancillas, J. R., Siggins, G. R., and Bloom, F. E., 1986, Systematic ethanol: Selective enhancement of responses to acetylcholine and somatostatin in hippocampus, *Science* **231**:161–163.

Mandell, A. J., and Mandell, M. P., 1969, Peripheral hormonal and metabolic correlates of rapid eye movement sleep, *Exp. Med. Surg.* **27**:224–236.

Mandell, M. P., Mandell, A. J., and Jacobson, A., 1964 Biochemical and neurophysiological studies of paradoxical sleep, in: *Recent Advances in Biological Psychiatry* (J. Wortis, ed.), pp. 115–122.

Mandell, A. J., Chaffey, B., Brill, P., Mandell, M. P., Rodnick, J., Rubin, R. T., and Sheff, R., 1966, Dreaming sleep in man: Changes in urine volume and osmolality, *Science* **151**:1158–1560.

Marangos, P. J., Patel, J., Skolnick, P., and Paul, S. M., 1983, Endogenous "benzodiazepine-like" agents, in: *Pharmacology of Benzodiazepines* (E. Usdin, P. Skolnick, J. Tallman, D. Greenblatt, S. M. Paul, eds.), Macmillan, London, pp. 519–527.

Marantz, R., and Rechtschaffen, A., 1967, Effect of alpha-methylparatyrosine on sleep in the rat, *Percept. Mot. Skills* **25**:805–808.

Marantz, R., Rechtshaffen, A., Lovell, R. A., and Whitehead, P. K., 1968, Effect of alpha-methyltyrosine on the recovery from paradoxical deprivation in the rat, *Commun. Behav. Biol.* **A2**:161–164.

Marchant, M., 1729, Observation botanique, *Histoire de l'Academie Royale des Sciences (Paris)* 35–36.

Marchini, E. J., Coates, T. J., Magistad, J. G., and Waldum, S. J., 1983, What do insomniacs do, think, and feel during the day? A preliminary study, *Sleep* **6**:147–155.

Marczynski, T. J., Yamaguchi, N., Ling, G. M., and Grodzinska, L., 1964, Sleep induced by the administration of melatonin (5-methoxy-N-acetyltryptamine) to the hypothalamus in unrestrained cats, *Experientia* **20**:435–437.

Mark, J. D., and Brooks, J. G., 1984, Sleep-associated airway problems in children, *Pediat. Clin. North Am.* **31**:907–918.

Marshall, J. F., Levitan, D., and Stricker, E. M., 1976, Activation-induced restoration of sensorimotor functions in rats with dopamine-depleting brain lesions, *J. Comp. Physiol. Psychol.* **90**:536–546.

Martilla, J. K., Hammel, R. J., Alexander, B., and Lustiak, R., 1977, Potential untoward effects of long-term use of flurazepam in geriatric patients, *J. Am. Pharaceut. Assoc.* **17**:692–695.

Martin, J. B., 1974, The role of hypothalamic and extrahypothalamic structures in the control of growth hormone secretion, in: *Advances in Human Growth Hormone Research*, DHEW Pub. No. NIH74612 (S. Raite, ed.), USDHEW, Washington, D.C., pp. 223–255.

Martin, P., Majchrowicz, E., Tamborska, E., Marietta, C., Mukherjee, A. B., and Eckardt, M. J., 1985, Response to ethanol reduced by past thiamine deficiency, *Science* **227**:1365–1369.

Martin, R. J., Pennock, B. F., Orr, W. C., Sanders, M. H., and Rogers, R. M., 1980, Respiratory mechanics and timing during sleep in occlusive sleep apnea, *J. Appl. Physiol.* **48**:432–437.

Martin, R. J., Sanders, M. H., Gray, B. A., and Pennock, B. E., 1982, Acute and long-term ventilatory effects of hyperoxia in the adult sleep apnea syndrome, *Am. Rev. Respir. Dis.* **125:**175–180.

Matsumoto, K., Sasagawa, N., and Kawamori, M., 1978, Studies of fatigue of hospital nurses due to shift work—with special reference to night shifts and short off-duty [author's trans.], *Sangyo-Igaku* **20:**81–93.

Matte, A. C., 1981, Growth hormone and isolation-induced aggression in wild male mice, *Psychopharm. Aggression Social Behav.* **14:**85–87.

Matthews, M. J., Parker, D. C., Rebar, R. W., Jones, K. L., Rossman, L., Carey, D. E., and Yen, S. S. C., 1982, Sleep-associated gonadotrophin and oestradiol patterns in girls with precocious sexual development, *Clin. Endocrinol.* **17:**601–607.

Matussek, N., Romisch, P., and Achenheil, M., 1977, MHPG excretion during sleep deprivation in endogenous depression, *Neuropsychobiology* **31:**23–29.

Maurice, M., 1975, *Shift Work: Economic Advantages*, Int'l. Labor Organization, Geneva.

Mayer, W., and Scherer, I., 1975, Phase shifting effect of caffeine in the circadian rhythm of *Phaseolus coccineus* L. Z., *Naturforsch. Teil* **C30:**855–856.

Mayer-Gross, W., Slater, E., and Roth, M., 1960, *Clin. Psychiatry* **211:**381–395.

McCallum, R. W., Sowers, J. R., Hershman, J. M., and Sturdevant, R. A., 1976, Metoclopramide stimulates prolactin secretion in man, *J. Clin. Endocrinol. Metab.* **42:**1148–1152.

McCarley, R. W., and Hobson, J. A., 1975, Neuronal excitability modulation over the sleep cycle: A structural and mathematical model, *Science* **189:**58–60.

McCarley, R. W., and Massaquoi, S. G., 1985, The REM sleep limit cycle model and depression, presentation to the Fourth World Congress of Biological Psychiatry Philadelphia, Sept. 8–13, 1985.

McCarley, R. W., and Masssaquoi, S. G., 1986, Further discussion of a model of the REM sleep oscillator, *Am. J. Physiol.* **251:**R1030–1036.

McClure, D. J., 1966, The diurnal variation of plasma cortisol levels in depression, *J. Psychosom. Res.* **10:**189–195.

McDonald, R. K., Sollberger, A. R., Mueller, P. S., and Sheard, M. H., 1969, The effect of small doses of human ACTH on serum corticosteroid levels in man, *Proc. Soc. Exp. Biol. Med.* **131:**1091–1094.

McEvoy, R. D., and Thornton, A. T., 1984, Treatment of obstructive sleep apnea syndrome with nasal continuous positive airway pressure, *Sleep* **7:**313–325.

McEwen, B. S., 1985, Steroids and brain function, *TIPS* **6:**22–26.

McGeer, E., and McGeer, P. L., 1976, Neurotransmitter metabolism in the aging brain, in: *Neurobiology of Aging* (R. D. Terry and S. Gershon, eds.), Raven Press, New York, pp. 389–403.

McGhie, A., 1966, The subjective assessment of sleep patterns in psychiatric illness, *Br. J. Med. Psychol.* **39:**221–230.

McGinty, D. J., 1985, Physiological equilibrium and the control of sleep states, in: *Brain Mechanisms of Sleep* (D. J. McGintym, A. Morrison, R. Drucker-Colin, and Parmeggian, eds.), Raven Press, New York, pp. 361–384.

McGinty, D. J., and Harper, R. M., 1976, The dorsal raphe neurons: Depression of firing during sleep in cats, *Brain Res.* **101:**569–575.

McPartland, R. J., Kupfer, R. J., Coble, P., Shaw, D. H., and Spiker, D. G., 1979, An automated analysis of REM sleep in primary depression, *Biol. Psychiatry* **14:**767–776.

Meddis, R., Pearson, A., and Langford, G., 1973, An extreme case of healthy insomnia, *Electroencephalogr. Clin. Neurophysiol.* **35:**213–214.

Medical Letter, 1981, The choice of benzodiazepines, *Med. Lett.* **23:**41–43.

Mefford, I. N., Baker, T. L., 1983, Boehme, R., Foutz, A. S., Ciaranello, R. D., Barchas, J.

D., and Dement, W. C., 1983, Narcolepsy: Biogenic amine deficits in an animal model, *Science* **220**:629–632.

Meier-Ewert, K., Matsubayashi, K., and Benter, L., 1985, Propranolol: Long-term treatment in narcolepsy–cataplexy, *Sleep* **8**:95–104.

Meites, J., and Clemens, J. A., 1972, Hypothalamic control of prolactin secretion, *Vitam. Horm.* **30**:165–221.

Melichor, C. L., 1982, TIQs block the development of environment dependent tolerance to ethanol, in: *Beta-carbolines and Tetrahydrolsoquinolines* (A. Liss, ed.), Alan Liss, New York, pp. 377–385.

Mellinger, G. D., and Balter, M. B., 1983, Prevalence of insomnia and drug treatment, abstract at NIMH Consensus Development Conference, "Drugs and Insomnia," Nov. 15–17, 1983, Bethesda, MD.

Mello, N. K., and Mendelson, J. H., 1970, Behavioral studies of sleep patterns in alcoholics during intoxication and withdrawal, *J. Pharmacol. Exp. Ther.* **175**:94–112.

Meltzer, H. Y., Lowy, M., Robertson, A., Goodnick, P., and Perline, R., 1984, Effect of 5-hydroxytryptophan on serum cortisol levels in major affective disorders. III. Effect of antidepressants and lithium carbonate, *Arch. Gen. Psychiatry* **41**:391–397.

Mendels, J., and Chernik, D. A., 1972, The effect of L-tryptophan on sleep in man, *Sleep Res.* **1**:66.

Mendels, J., and Chernik, D. A., 1975, Sleep and changes and affective illness, in: *The Nature and Treatment of Depression* (F. F. Flach and S. C. Draghi, eds.), Wiley, New York, pp. 309–333.

Mendels, J., and Hawkins, D. R., 1967a, Sleep and depression: A controlled EEG study, *Arch. Gen. Psychiatry* **15**:744–754.

Mendels, J., and Hawkins, D. R., 1967b, Sleep and depression: A follow-up study, *Arch. Gen. Psychiatry* **16**:536–542.

Mendels, J., and Hawkins, D. R., 1968, Sleep and depression: Further consideration, *Arch. Gen. Psychiatry* **19**:445–452.

Mendels, J., and Hawkins, D. R., 1971, Sleep and depression. IV longitudinal studies, *J. Nerv. Ment. Dis.* **153**:251–272.

Mendelson, W. B., 1980, *The Use and Misuse of Sleeping Pills. A Clinical Guide*, Plenum Press, New York, pp. 1–215.

Mendelson, W. B., 1982, Studies of human growth hormone secretion in sleep and waking, *Int. Rev. Neurobiol.* **23**:367–389.

Mendelson, W. B., 1984, The BZ receptor and sleep, *Psychiatr. Dev.* **3**:161–177.

Mendelson, W. B., 1985, Pharmacological treatment of insomnia, in: *American Psychiatric Association Annual Review* (Vol. IV), (R. E. Hales and A. J. Frances, eds.), APA Press, Washington, pp. 379–394.

Mendelson, W. B., 1986, The reciprocal interaction model of sleep: A look at a vigorous ten year old, *Behav. Brain Sci.* **9**:371–373.

Mendelson, W. B., and Hill, S. Y., 1976, A dose–response study of the acute effects of ethanol on the sleep of rats, *Sleep Res.* **5**:1976.

Mendelson, W. B., and Hill, S. Y., 1978, Effects of the acute administration of ethanol on the sleep of the rat: A dose response study, *Pharmacol. Biochem. Behav.* **8**:723–726.

Mendelson, W. B., Reichman, J., and Othmer E., 1975a, Serotonin inhibition and sleep, *Biol. Psychiatry* **10**:459–464.

Mendelson, W. B., Jacobs, L. S., Reichman, J. D., Othmer, E., Cryer, P. E., Trivedi, B., and Daughaday, W. H., 1975b, Methysergide: Suppression of sleep-related prolactin secretion and enhancement of sleep-related growth hormone secretion, *J. Clin. Invest.* **56**:690–697.

Mendelson, W. B., Gillin, J. C., and Wyatt, R. J., 1977, *Human Sleep and Its Disorders*, Plenum Press, New York, pp. 147–210.

Mendelson, W. B., Buchsbaum, M. S., Murphy, D. L., Wyatt, R. J., and Gillin, J. C., 1978a, Platelet monoamine oxidase activity and human sleep, *Commun. Psychopharmacol.* **2**:539–544.

Mendelson, W. B., Majchrowicz, E., Mirmirani, N., Dawson, S., Gillin, J. C., and Wyatt, R. J., 1978b, Sleep during chronic ethanol administration withdrawal in rats, *J. Stud. Alcohol.* **39**:1213–1223.

Mendelson, W. B., Jacobs, L. S., Sitaram, N., Wyatt, R. J., and Gillin, J. C., 1978c, Methscopolamine inhibition of sleep-related growth hormone secretion, *J. Clin. Invest.* **61**:1683–1690.

Mendelson, W. B., Gillin, J. C., Dawson, S. D., Lewy, A. J., and Wyatt, R. J., 1980a, Effects of melatonin and propranolol on sleep of the rat, *Rain Res.* **201**:240–244.

Mendelson, W. B., Gillin, J. C., Pisner, G., and Wyatt, R. J., 1980b, Arginine vasotocin and sleep in the rat, *Brain Res.* **182**:246–249.

Mendelson, W. B., Garnett, D., and Gillin, J. C., 1981a, Flurazepam-induced sleep apnea syndrome in a patient with insomnia and mild sleep-related respiratory changes, *J. Nerv. Ment. Dis.* **169**:261–264.

Mendelson, W. B., Slater, S., Gold, P., and Gillin, J. C., 1981b, The effect of growth hormone administration on human sleep: A dose–response study, *Biol. Psychiatry* **15**:613–618.

Mendelson, W. B., Lantigua, R. A., Wyatt, R. J., Gillin, J. C., and Jacobs, L. S., 1981c, Piperidine enhances sleep-related and insulin-induced growth hormone secretion: Further evidence for a cholinergic secretory mechanism, *Clin. Endocrinol. Metab.* **52**:409–415.

Mendelson, W. B., Gillin, J. C., and Wyatt, R. J., 1982a, The search for circulating sleep-promoting factors, in: *Advances in Pharmacology and Therapeutics II* (H. Yoshida, Y. Hagihava, and S. Ebash, eds.), Pergamon Press, New York, pp. 227–240.

Mendelson, W. B., Cohen, R. M., Campbell, I. C., Murphy, D. L., Gillin, J. C., and Wyatt, R. J., 1982b, Lifetime monoamine oxidase inhibition and sleep, *Pharmacol. Biochem. Behav.* **16**:429–431.

Mendelson, W. B., Weingartner, H., Greenblatt, D. J., Garnett, D., and Gillin, J. C., 1982c, A clinical study of flurazepam, *Sleep* **5**:350–360.

Mendelson, W. B., Paul, S. M., and Skolnick, P., 1982d, Does the benzodiazepine receptor play a role in sleep? Studies of stereospecificity, *Sleep Res.* **11**:65.

Mendelson, W. B., Cain, M., Cook, J. M., Paul, S. M., and Skolnick, P., 1983a, A benzodiazepine receptor antagonist decreases sleep and reverses the hypnotic actions of flurazepam, *Science* **219**:414–416.

Mendelson, W. B., Davis, T., Paul, S. M., and Skolnick, P., 1983b, Do benzodiazepine receptors mediate the anticonflict action of pentobarbital? *Life Sci.* **32**:2241–2247.

Mendelson, W. B., Jacobs, L. S., and Gillin, J. C., 1983c, Negative feedback suppression of sleep-related growth hormone secretion, *J. Clin. Endocrinol. Metab.* **56**:486–487.

Mendelson, W. B., Kuruvilla, A., Watlington, T., Goehl, K., Paul, S. M., and Skolnick, P., 1983d, Sedative and electroencephalographic actions of Erythro-9-(2-hydroxy-3-nonly)-adenine (EHNA): Relationship to inhibition, *Psychopharmacology* **79**:126–129.

Mendelson, W. B., Martin, J. V., Paul, S. M., Skolnick, P., and Cook, J., 1983e, Effects of a relatively stable beta-carboline on sleep in the rat, *Sleep Res.* **12**:111.

Mendelson, W. B., Wyatt, R. J., and Gillin, J. C., 1983f, Whither the sleep factors, in: *Sleep Disorders—Basic and Clinical Research* (M. Chase, ed.), Spectrum Press, New York, pp. 281–305).

Mendelson, W. B., Skolnick, P., Martin, J. V., Luu, M. D., Wagner, R., and Paul, S. M., 1984a, Diazepam-stimulated increases in the synaptosomal uptake of 45Ca $^{2+}$ Reversal by dihydropyridine calcium channel antagonists, *Eur. J. Pharmacol.* **104:**181–183.

Mendelson, W. B., Owen, C., Skolnick, P., Paul, S. M., Martin, J. V., Ko, G., and Wagner, R., 1984b, Nifedipine blocks sleep induction by flurazepam in the rat, *Sleep* **7:**64–68.

Mendelson, W. B., Garnett, D., Gillin, J. C., and Weingartner, H., 1984c, The experience of insomnia and daytime and nighttime functioning, *Psychiatry Res.* **12:**235–250.

Mendelson, W. B., Garnett, D., and Linnoila, M., 1984d, Do insomniacs have impaired daytime functioning? *Biol. Psychiatry* **19:**1261–1263.

Mendelson, W. B., Martin, J. V., Wagner, R., Roseberry, C., Skolnick, P., Weissman, B. A., and Squires, R., 1985a, Are the toxicities of pentobarbital and ethanol mediated by the GABA-benzodiazepine receptor ionophore complex? *Eur. J. Pharmacol.* **108:**63.

Mendelson, W. B., Martin, J. V., Wagner, R., and Skolnick, P., 1985b, Are the subtypes of benzodiazepine receptors associated with different functions? *Sleep Res.* **14:**43.

Mendelson, W. B., Martin, J. V., Wagner, R., and Skolnick, P., 1985c, Awakening effect of the benzodiazepine B10 is blocked by CGS 8216, *Sleep Res.* **14:**44.

Mendelson, W. B., Martin, J. V., and Wagner, R., 1986a, A calcium agonist potentiates hypnotic effects of flurazepam, *Sleep Res.* **15:**38.

Mendelson, W. B., Martin, J. V., Perlis, M., and Wagner, R., 1986b, Do alterations in chloride flux mediate sleep induction by hypnotics? *Sleep Res.* **15:**36.

Mendelson, W. B., Martin, J. V., Wagner, R., Perlis, M., Majewska, M. D., and Paul, S. M., 1986c, Sleep induction by an adrenal steroid, abstract, 15th Congress, Collegium Internationale Neuro-Psychopharmacologicum, Dec. 14–17, 1986, San Juan, PR.

Mendelson, W. B., James, S. P., Garnett, D., Sack, D. A., and Rosenthal, N. E., 1986d, A psychophysiological study of insomnia, *Psychiatry Res.* **19:**267–284.

Mendelson, W. B., Martin, J. V., Perlis, M., and Wagner, R., 1986e, Lack of effect of nifedipine on sleep induction by pentobarbital, *Sleep Res.* **15:**37.

Mendelson, W. B., Martin, J. V., Wagner, R., Milton, J. G., James, S. P., Garnett, D., and Wehr, T. A., 1986f, Do depressed patients have decreased delta power in the sleep EEG? *Sleep Res.* **15:**146.

Mendelson, W. B., Martin, J. V., Perlis, M., and Wagner, R., 1987a, Arousing effects of triazolam injected into the dorsal raphe nuclei, *Sleep Res.* **16:** 106.

Mendelson, W. B., Sack, D. A., James, S. P., Martin, J. V., Wagner, R., Garnett, D., Milton, J., and Wehr, T. A., 1987b, Frequency analysis of the sleep EEG in depression, *Psychiatry Res.* **21:**89–94.

Mendelson, W. B., Rosenthal, N. E., and James, S. P., 1987c, Melatonin administration and nocturnal sleep in insomniacs, *Sleep Res.* **16:**109.

Mendelson, W. B., Martin, J. V., Perlis, M., Giesen, H., Wagner, R., and Rapoport, S. I., 1987d, Sleep-related apneas in adult rats, *Sleep Res.* **16:** 390.

Mendelson, W. B., 1987e, Medications in the treatment of sleep disorders, in: *Psychopharmacology: A Decade of Progress* (H. Meltzer, ed.), Raven Press, New York, in press.

Mendelson, W. B., Martin, J. V., Perlis, M., and Wagner, R., 1987f, Sleep and benzodiazepine receptor sub-types, *J. Neural Transmission*, in press.

Mendelson, W. B., Stephens, H., Giesen, H., and James, S. P., 1987g, Hypnotic effects on arousal threshold to different stimuli and on perception of being asleep, *Sleep Res.* **16:**in press.

Mendlewicz, J., Kerkhofs, M., Hoffman, G., and Linkowski, P., 1984a, Dexamethasone suppression test and REM sleep in patients with major depressive disorder, *Brit. J. Psychiatry* **145:**383–388.

Mendlewicz, J., Hoffmann, G., Kerkhofs, M., and Linkowski, P., 1984b, Electroencephalogram and neuroendocrine parameters in pubertal and adolescent depressed children, *J. Affective Dis.* **6**:265–272.

Mendlewicz, J., Linkowski, P., Kerkhofs, M., Desmedt, D., Golstein, J., Copinschi, G., and Cauter, E. V., 1985, Diurnal hypersecretion of growth hormone in depression, *J. Clin. Endocrinol. Metab.* **60**:505–512.

Merritt, J. H., and Geller, I., 1973, Soporific action of ethanol in mice: Possible role of biogenic amines, *Pharmacol. Biochem. Behav.* **1**:271–276.

Mestre, M., Carriot, T., Belin, C., Uzan, A., Renault, C., Dubroeucq, M. C., and Le Fur, G., 1985, Electrophysiological and pharmacological evidence that peripheral type benzodiazepine receptors are coupled to calcium channels in the heart, *Life Sci.* **36**:391–400.

Meyer, J. S., Sakai, F., Karacan, I., Derman, S., and Yamamoto, M., 1980, Sleep apnea, narcolepsy, and dreaming: Regional cerebral hemodynamics, *Ann. Neurol.* **7**:479–485.

Michaelis, E. K., and Myers, S. L., 1979, Calcium binding to brain synaptosomes, *Biochem. Pharmacol.* **28**:2081–2087.

Middlemiss, D. N., and Spedding, M., 1985, A functional correlate for the dihydropyridine binding site in rat brain, *Nature* **314**:94–96.

Milcu, S. M., Pavel, S., and Neascu, C., 1963, Biological and chromatographic characteristics of a polypeptide with pressor and oxytocic activities isolated from bovine pineal gland, *Endocrinology* **72**:563–566.

Miles, L. M., Raynal, D. M., and Wilson, M. A., 1977, Blind man living in normal society has circadian rhythms of 24.9 hours, *Science* **198**:421–423.

Miller, A. I., D'Agostino, A., and Minsky, R., 1963, Effects of combined chlordiazepoxide and alcohol in man, *Q. J. Stud. Alcohol* **24**:9–13.

Miller, R. J., and Freedman, S. B., 1984, Are dihydropyridine binding sites voltage sensitive calcium channels? *Life Sci.* **34**:1205–1221.

Millman, R. P., 1986, Did the fat boy snore? (editorial), *Chest* **89**:621–622.

Mills, J. N., Minors, D. S., and Waterhouse, J. M., 1978, Adaptation to abrupt time shifts of the oscillator(s) controlling human circadian rhythms, *J. Physiol.* **285**:455–470.

Minuto, F., Underwood, L. E., Grimaldi, P., Furlanetto, R. W., Van Wyk, J. J., and Giordano, G., 1981, Decreased serum somatomedin C concentrations during sleep: Temporal relationship to the nocturnal surges of growth hormone and prolactin, *J. Clin. Endocrinol. Metab.* **52**:399–404.

Mirsky, I. A., Piken, P., Rosenbaum, M., and Lederer, H., 1941, Adaptation of central nervous system, *Q. J. Stud. Alcohol* **2**:35–45.

Mishara, B. L., and Kastenbaum, R., 1974, Wine in the treatment of long-term geriatric patients in mental institutions, *J. Am. Geriatr. Soc.* **22**:88–94.

Mitchell, R., and Martin, I. L., 1978, The effects of benzodiazepines on K^{2+}-stimulated release of GABA, *Neuropharmacology* **17**:317–320.

Mitchell, S. W., 1890, Some disorders of sleep, *Am. J. Med. Sci.* **100**:110–127.

Mitler, M. M., and Dement, W. C., 1977, Sleep studies on canine narcolepsy: Pattern and cycle comparisons between affected and normal dogs, *Electroencephalog. Clin. Neurophysiol.* **43**:691–699.

Mitler, M., Phillips, R. L., and Billiard, M., 1975, Long-term effectiveness of temazepam 30 mg HS on chronic insomniacs, *Sleep Res.* **4**:109.

Mitler, M., Van den Hoed, J., Carskadon, M. A., Richardson, G., Park, R., Guilleminault, C., and Dement, W. C., 1979a, REM sleep episodes during the multiple sleep-latency test in narcoleptic patients, *Electroencephalogr. Clin. Neurophysiol.* **46**:479–481.

Mitler, M. M., Carskadon, M. A., Phillips, R. L., Sterling, W. R., Zarcone, V. P., Speigel, R., and Dement, W. C., 1979b, Hypnotic efficacy of temazepam: A long-term sleep laboratory evaluation, *Br. J. Clin. Pharmacol.* **8:**63s–68s.

Mitler, M. M., Gujavarty, K., and Browman, C.P., 1982, Maintenance of wakefulness test: A polysomnographic technique for evaluation treatment efficacy in patients with excessive somnolence, *Electroencephalogr. Clin. Neurophysiol.* **53:**658–661.

Mitler, M. M., Seidel, W. F., Van den Hoed, J., Greenblatt, D., and Dement, W. C., 1984, Comparative hypnotic effects of flurazepam, triazolam, and placebo: A long-term simultaneous nighttime and daytime study, *J. Clin. Psychopharmacol.* **4:**2–13.

Mitler, M. M., Shafor, R., Hajdukovich, R., Timms, R. M., and Browman, C. P., 1986a, Treatment of narcolepsy: Objective studies on methylphenidate, pemoline, and protriptyline, *Sleep* **9:**260–264.

Mitler, M. M., Browman, C. P., Menn, S. J., Gujavarty, K., and Timms, R. M., 1986b, Nocturnal myoclonus: Treatment efficacy of clonazepam and temazepam, *Sleep* **9:**385–392.

Model, D. G., 1973, Nitrazepam-induced respiratory depression in chronic obstructive lung disease, *Br. J. Dis. Chest* **67:**128–130.

Model, D. G., and Berry, D. J., 1974, Effect of chlordiazepoxide in respiratory failure due to chronic bronchitis, *Lancet* **2:**869–870.

Modestin, J. J., Hunger, R. B., and Schwartz, R. B., 1973, Uber die depressogeue wirkung von Physostigmine, *Arch. Psychiatr, Nervenkr.* **218:**67–77.

Mogilnicka, E., 1981, REM sleep deprivation changes behavioral response to catecholaminergic and serotonergic receptor activation in rats, *Pharmacol. Biochem. Behav.* **15:**149–151.

Mohler, H., and Okada, T., 1977, Benzodiazepine receptor: Demonstration in the central nervous system, *Science* **198:**849–851.

Mohler, H., Patel, A. J., and Balazs, R., 1976, Gamma-hydroxybutyrate degradation in the brain *in vivo*: Negligible direct conversion to GABA, *J. Neurochem.* **27:**253–258.

Moja, E. A., Mendelson, W. B., Stoff, D. M., Gillin, J. C., and Wyatt, R. J., 1979, Reduction of REM sleep by a tryptophan-free amino acid diet, *Life Sci.* **24:**1467–1470.

Moja, E. A., Antinoro, E., Cesa-Bianchi, M., and Gessa, G. L., 1984, Increase in stage 4 sleep after ingestion of a tryptophan-free diet in humans, *Pharmacol. Res. Commun.* **16:**909–914.

Molander, L., and Duvhok, C., 1976, Acute effects of oxazepam diazepam and methaqualone, alone and in combination with alcohol on sedation, coordination and mood, *Acta Pharmacol. Toxicol.* **38:**145–160.

Moldofsky, H., 1986, Immunology and sleep, June 15–20, 1986, presented at Association of Professional Sleep Societies, First Annual Meeting, Columbus, OH.

Moldofsky, H., and Lue, F. A., 1980, The relationship of alpha and delta EEG frequencies to pain and mood in fibrositis patients treated with chlorpromazine and L-tryptophan, *Electroencephalog. Clin. Neurophysiol.* **50:**71–80.

Moldofsky, H., Tullis, C., Lue, F. A., Quance, G., and Davidson, J., 1984, Sleep-related myoclonus in rheumatic pain modulation disorder (fibrositis syndrome) and in excessive daytime somnolence, *Psychosom. Med.* **46:**145–151.

Monnier, M., and Hosli, L., 1964, Dialysis of sleep and waking factors in blood of the rabbit, *Science* **146:**794–798.

Monnier, M., Shoenenberger, G. A., Glatt, A., Dudler, L., Mehlose, W., Gachter, R., and Knappova, L., 1975, Distribution of the physiological sleep factor delta in blood and cerebrospinal fluid, Presented at the Second International Sleep Research Congress, Edinburgh, June 30–July 4, 1975.

Monroe, L. J., 1967, Psychological and physiological differences between good and poor sleepers, *J. Abnorm. Psychol.* **72**:255–264.

Montagna, P., Cirignotta, F., and Lugaresi, E., 1983, Letter: Disappearance of palatal myoclonus during sleep, *Sleep* **6**:386–387.

Montagna, P., Sassoli de Bianchi, L, Zucconi, M., Crignotta, F., and Lugaresi, E., 1984, Clonazepam and vibration in restless legs syndrome, *Acta Neurol. Scand.* **69**:428–430.

Monti, J. M., Altier, H., and D'Angelo, L., 1979, Diazepam, GABA agonists and antagonists and the sleep–wakefulness cycle, in: *Pharmacology of the States of Alertness* (P. Passouant and I. Oswald, eds.), Pergamon Press, New York, pp. 65–73.

Montplasir, J., and Godbout, R., 1986a, Nocturnal sleep of narcoleptic patients, *Sleep* **9**:159–161.

Montplasir, J., and Godbout, R., 1986b, Serotoninergic reuptake mechanisms in the control of cataplexy, *Sleep* **9**:280–284.

Montplasir, J., Champlain, J., Young, S. N., Missala, K., Sourkes, T. L., Walsh, J., and Remillard, G., 1982, Narcolepsy and idiopathic hypersomnia: Biogenic amines and related compounds in CSF, *Neurology* **37**:1299–1302.

Moore-Ede, M. C., and Sulzman, F. M., 1981, Internal temporal order, in: *Handbook of Behavioral Neurobiology* (J. Aschoff, ed.), Plenum Press, New York, pp. 215–242.

Moore-Ede, M. C., Sulzman, F. M., and Fuller, C. A., 1982, The clocks that time us, in: *Physiology of the Circadian Timing System*, Harvard University Press, Cambridge, MA.

Morden, B., Conner, R., Mitchell, G., Dement, W., and Levine, S., 1968, Effects of rapid eye movement (REM) sleep deprivation on shock-induced fighting, *Physiol. Behav.* **3**:425–432.

Morgan, H. E., 1973, Introduction to endocrine control systems, in: *Best and Taylor's Physiological Basis of Medical Practice* (J. R. Brobeck, ed.), Williams & Wilkins, Baltimore, p. 72.

Morgan, K., and Oswald, I., 1982, Anxiety caused by a short-life hypnotic, *Br. Med. J.* **284**:942.

Morgan, L. K., 1967, Restless limbs: A commonly overlooked symptom controlled by "Valium," *Med. J. Australia* **2**:589–594.

Morgane, P. J., 1982, Amine pathways and sleep regulation, *Brain Res. Bull.* **9**:743–749.

Morgane, P. J., and Stern, W. C., 1972, Relationship of sleep to neuroanatomical circuits, biochemistry and behavior, *Ann. NY Acad. Sci. USA* **193**:95–111.

Morgane, P. J., and Stern, W. C., 1974, Chemical anatomy of brain circuits in relation to sleep and wakefulness, in: *Advances in Sleep Research* (E. D. Weitzman, ed.), Spectrum Publications, New York, pp. 1–131.

Morland, J., Setekleiv, J., Haffner, J. F., Stromsaether, C. E., Danielson, A., and Holst Wethe, G., 1974, Combined effects of diazepam and ethanol on mental and psychomotor functions, *Acta Pharmacol. Toxicol.* **34**:5–15.

Morley, B. J., Kemp, G. E., and Salvaterra, P., 1979, Alpha-bungarotoxin binding sites in the CNS, *Life Sci.* **24**:859–872.

Morris, G., and Singer, M. T., 1961, Sleep deprivation: Transactional and subjective observations, *Arch. Gen. Psychiatry* **5**:453–465.

Morrison, A., 1889, Somnolence with cyanosis cured by massage, *Practitioner* **42**:277–281.

Moruzzi, G., 1972, The sleep–waking cycle, *Ergeb. Physiol.* **64**:1–165.

Moruzzi, G., and Magoun, H. W., 1949, Brain stem reticular formation and activation of the EEG, *Electroencephalogr. Clin. Neurophysiol.* **1**:455–473.

Mosko, S. S., Holowach, J. B., and Sassin, J. F., 1983, The 24-hour rhythm of core temperature in narcolepsy, *Sleep* **6**:137–146.

Mosko, S. S., Shampain, D. S., and Sassin, J. F., 1984, Nocturnal REM latency and sleep disturbance in narcolepsy, *Sleep* **7**:115–125.

Mossberg, D., Liljeberg, P., and Borg, S., 1985, Clinical conditions in alcoholics during long-term abstinence: A descriptive, longitudinal treatment study, *Alcohol* **2**:551–553.

Motta, J., and Guilleminault, C., 1978, Effects of oxygen administration in sleep-induced apneas, in: *Sleep Apnea Syndrome* (C. Guilleminault and W. C. Dement, eds.), Alan R. Liss, Inc., New York, pp. 137–144.

Mouret, J., Bobillier, P., and Jouvet, M., 1968, Insomnia following parachlorophenylalanine in the rat, *Eur. J. Pharmacol.* **5**:17–22.

Mueller, E. E., 1973, Nervous control of growth hormone secretion, *Neuroendocrinology* **11**:338–369.

Mueller, E., and Pecile, A., 1966, Influence of exogenous growth hormone on endogenous growth hormone release, *Proc. Soc. Exp. Biol. Med.* **122**:1289–1291.

Mueller, E. E., Pecile, A., Felici, M., and Cocchi, D., 1970, Norepinephrine and dopamine injection into lateral brain ventricle of the rat and growth hormone-releasing activity in the hypothalmus and plasma, *Endocrinology* **86**:1376–1382.

Mueller, E. E., Nistico, G., and Scapagnini, U., 1977, Sites of action of monoamines in affecting anterior pituitary function, in: *Neurotransmitters and Anterior Pituitary Function*, Academic Press, New York, pp. 312–323.

Mueller, P. S., Heninger, G. R., and McDonald, R. K., 1969, Insulin tolerance test in depression, *Arch. Gen. Psychiatry* **21**:587–595.

Mullaney, D. J., Johnson, L. C., Naitoh, P., Friedman, J. K., and Globus, G. C., 1977, Sleep during and after gradual sleep reduction, *Psychophysiology* **14**:237–244.

Muratorio, A., and Maggini, C., 1967, Caratteristiche struttuveli del sonno dei depressi, *Riv. Neurol.* **39**:101–107.

Murphy, D. L., 1986, Serotonin neurochemistry: A commentary on some of its quandaries, *Neurochem. Int.* **8**:161–163.

Murphy, D. L., Baker, M., Goodwin, F. K., Miller, H., Kotin, J., and Bunney, W. E., 1974, L-Tryptophan in affective disorders: Indoleamine changes and differential clinical effects, *Psychopharmacologia* **34**:11–20.

Murphy, D. L., Wright, C., Buchsbaum, M. S., Nichols, A., Costa, J. L., and Wyatt, R. J., 1976, *Biomed. Med.* **16**:254–265.

Murphy, D. L., Sunderland, T., and Cohen, R.M., 1984, Monoamine oxidase-inhibiting antidepressants, *Psychiatr. Clin. NA* **7**:549–563.

Murphy, D. L., Mueller, E. A., Garrick, N. A., and Aulakh, C. S., 1986, Use of serotonergic agents in the clinical asessment of central serotonin function, *J. Clin. Psychiatry* **47**:9–15 (supp).

Murphy, J. E., and Ankier, S. I., 1984, A comparison of hypnotic activity of loprazolam, flurazepam and placebo, *Br. J. Clin. Practice* **38**:141–149.

Murphy, K. M., and Snyder, S. H., 1982, Calcium antagonist receptor binding sites labeled with [^{3}H] nitrendipine, *Eur. J. Pharmacol.* **77**::201–202.

Murri, L., Feriozzi, F., Cerone, G., and Piacentino, P., 1971, Triptovano e sonno in schizofrenici cronici, *Rev. Neurobiol.* **17**:184–189.

Murri, L., Cerone, G., Piacentino, P., and Pirro, R., 1972, 5-idrossitriptofane e sonno in schizofrenici cronici, *Rev. Neurobiol.* **17**:427–432.

Murri, L., Cerone, G., Feriozzi, F., Mencini, G. M., and Nurzja, A., 1973, Effetto del triptofano sull 'armone somatotropo durante il sonno in schizofrenici, *Boll. Soc. Ital. Biol. Sper.* **49**:1490–1495.

Muzet, A., Johnson, L. C., and Spinweber, C. I., 1982, Benzodiazepine hypnotics increase heart rate during sleep, *Sleep* **5**:256–261.

Muzio, J. N., Roffwarg, H. P., and Kaufman, E., 1966, Alterations in the nocturnal sleep cycle resulting from LSD, *Electroencephalogr. Clin. Neurophysiol.* **21**:313–324.

Myslobodsky, M. S., and Mansour, R., 1979, Hypersynchronisation and sedation produced by GABA-transaminase inhibitors and picrotoxin: Does GABA participate in sleep control? *Waking Sleeping* **3**:245–254.

Naber, D., Wirz-Justice, A., Kafka, M. S., and Wehr, T. A., 1981, Circadian rhythm in rat brain opiate receptor, *Neurosci. Lett.* **21**:45–50.

Naftolin, F., Yes, S. S. C., Perlman, D., Tsai, C. C., Parker, D. C., and Vargo, T., 1973, Nocturnal patterns of serum gonadotropins during the menstrual cycle, *J. Clin. Endocrinol. Metab.* **37**:6–10.

Nagayama, H., Takagi, A., Sakurai, Y., Yoshimoto, S., Nishiwaki, K., and Takahashi, R., 1979, Chronopharmacological study of neuroleptics: III. Circadian rhythm of brain susceptibility to haloperidol, *Psychopharmacology* **63**:131–135.

Nagasaki, H., Kitahama, K., Valatz, J. L., and Jouvet, M., 1980, Sleep-promoting substance (SPS) and delta sleep-inducing peptide (DSIP) in the mouse, *Brain Res.* **192**:276–280.

Naiman, J., Poitras, R., and Engelsmann, F., 1972, Effect of chlorpromazine on REM rebound in normal volunteers, *Can. Psychiatr. Assoc. J.* **17**:463–469.

Nair, N. P. V., and Schwartz, G., 1978, Triazolam in insomnia: A standard controlled trial, *Curr. Ther. Res. Clin. Exp.* **23**:388–392.

Naitoh, P., Kales, A., Dollar, E. J., Smith, J. C., and Jacobson, A., 1969, Electroencephalographic activity after prolonged sleep loss, *Electroencephalogr. Clin. Neurophysiol.* **27**:2–11.

Nakamura, R. K., Kennedy, C., Gillin, J. C., Suda, S., Storch, F. I., Mendelson, W. B., and Sokoloff, L., 1983, Hypogenic center theory of sleep: No support from metabolic mapping in monkeys, *Brain Res.* **268**:372–376.

Nakazawa, Y., Tachibana, H., Kotorii, M., and Ogata, M., 1973, Effects of L-dopa on natural night sleep and on rebound of REM sleep, *Folia Psychiatr. Neurol. Jpn.* **27**:223–230.

Nakazawa, Y., Kotorii, T., Horikawa, S., Kororii, M., Ohshima, M., and Hasuzawa, H., 1979, Individual variations in the effects of flurazepam, clorazepate, L-dopa and thyrotropin-releasing hormone on REM sleep in man, *Psychopharmacology* **60**:203–206.

Nasrallah, H. A., Kuperman, S., and Coryell, W., 1980, Reversal of dexamethasone nonsuppression with sleep deprivation in primary depression, *Am. J. Psychiatry* **137**:1463–1464.

Nasrallah, H. B., and Coryell, W. H., 1982, Dexamethasone nonsuppression predicts the antidepressant effects of sleep deprivation, *Psychiatr. Res.* **68**:61–64.

Nathan, R. S., Sachar, E. J., Langer, G., Tabrizi, M. A., and Halpern, F. S., 1979, Diurnal variation in the response of plasma prolactin, cortisol, and growth hormone to insulin-induced hypoglycemia in normal man, *J. Clin. Endocrinol. Metab.* **49**:231–235.

Nathan, R. S., Sachar, E. J., Tabrizi, M. A., Asnis, G. M., Halbreich, U., and Halpern, F. S., 1982, Short communication: Diurnal hormonal responses thyrotropin-releasing hormone in normal men, *Psychoneuroendocrinology* **7**:235–238.

National Institute of Mental Health, 1984, Consensus conference report: Drugs and insomnia—the use of medication to promote sleep, *JAMA* **251**:2410–2414.

Naylor, G. J., and Le Poidevin, D., 1972, Sleep patterns in depressive states, *Br. J. Med. Psychol.* **45**:171–176.

Neff, N. H., and Yang, H. Y. T., 1974, Another look at the monoamine oxidase and the monoamine oxidase inhibitor drugs, *Life Sci.* **14**:2061–2074.

Neil, J. F., Merikanges, J. R., Foster, F. G., Merikanges, K. R., Spiker, D. G., and Kupfer, D. J., 1980, Waking and all-night sleep EEG's in anorexia nervosa, *Clin. Electroencephalogr.* **11**:9–15.

Neill, J. D., 1980, Neuroendocrine regulation of prolactin secretion, in: *Frontiers of Neuro-*

endocrinology (L. Martini and W. F. Ganong, eds.), Raven Press, New York, pp. 129–155.

Nelson, J. C., and Charney, D. S., 1980, Primary affective disorder criteria and the endogenous-reactive distinction, *Arch. Gen, Psychiatry* **37**:787–793.

Ness, R. C., 1978, The Old Hag phenomenon as sleep paralysis: A biocultural interpretation, *Cult. Med. Psychiatry* **2**:15–39.

Netick, A., Dugger, W. J., and Symmons, R. A., 1984, Ventilatory response to hypercapnia during sleep and wakefulness in cats, *J. Appl. Physiol.* **56**:1347–1345.

Nicassio, P., and Bootzin, R., 1974, A comparison of progressive relaxation and autogenic training as treatments for insomnia, *J. Abnorm. Psychol.* **83**:253–260.

Nicassio, P. M., Pate, J. K., Mendlowitz, D. R., and Woodward, N., 1985, Insomnia: nonpharmacologic management by private practice physicians, *So. Med. J.* **78**:556–560.

Nicholson, A. N., and Stone, B. M., 1979a, L-Tryptophan and sleep in healthy man *(Electroencephalogr. Clin. Neurophysiol.* **47**:539–545.

Nicholson, A. N., and Stone, B. M., 1979b, Diazepam and 3-hydroxydiazepam (temazepam) and sleep of middle age, *Br. J. Clin. Pharmacol.* **7**:463–468.

Nicholson, A. N., Spencer, M. B., Pascoe, P. A., and Stone, B. M., 1986, Sleep after transmeridian flights. *Lancet* **2**:1205–1208.

Nicoll, R. A., 1975a, Pentobarbital: Action on frog motoneurons, *Brain Res.* **94**:1–5.

Nicoll, R. A., 1975b, Presynaptic action of barbiturates in the frog spinal cord, *Proc. Natl. Acad. Sci. USA* **72**:1460–1463.

Nicoloff, J. T., 1970, A new method for the measurement of thyroidal iodine release in man, *J. Clin. Invest.* **47**:1912–1921.

Nicoloff, J. T., Fisher, D. A., and Appleman, M. D., 1970, The role of glucocorticords in the regulation of thyroid function in man, *J. Clin. Invest.* **49**:1922–1929.

Nielsen, M., Braestrup, C., and Squires, R. F., 1978, Evidence for a late evolutionary appearance of brain-specific benzodiazepine receptors: An investigation of 18 vertebrate and 5 invertebrate species, *Brain Res.* **141**:342–346.

Ninan, P., Insel, T. R., Cohen, R. M., Skolnick, P., and Paul, S. M., 1982, Benzodiazepine receptor mediated experimental 'anxiety' in primates, *Science* **218**:1332–1334.

Nokin, J., Vekemans, M., L'Hermite, M., and Robyn, C., 1972, Circadian periodicity of serum prolactin concentrations in man, *Br. Med. J.* **3**:561–572.

Nolen, W. A., van de Putte, J. J., Dijken, W. A., and Kamp, J. S., 1985, L-5HTP in depression resistant to re-uptake inhibitors. An open comparative study with tranylcypromine, *Br. J. Psychiatry* **147**:16–22.

Norman, S. E., Levin, B. E., and Cohn, M. A., 1986, Neuropsychological correlates of obstructive sleep apnea syndrome, *Sleep Res.* **15**:95.

Nurnberger, Jr., J., Sitaram, N., Gershon, E. S., and Gillin, J. C., 1983, A twin study of cholinergic REM induction, *Biol. Psychiatry* **18**:1161–1165.

Nutt, D., 1986, Benzodiazepine dependence in the clinic: Reason for anxiety? *Trends Pharmacol. Sci.* **7**:457–460.

Oakley, N., and Jones, B., 1980, The proconvulsant and diazepam-reversing effects of ethyl-B- carboline-3-carboxylate, *Eur. J. Pharmacol.* **68**:381–382.

Oately, K., and Goodwin, B. C., 1971, The explanation and investigation of biological rhythms, in: *Biological Rhythms and Human Performance* (W. P. Colauhoun, 1980, ed.), Academic Press, New York, pp. 1–38.

Ogunremi, O. O., Adamson, L., Barezinova, V., Hunter, W. M., Maclean, A. W., Oswald, I., and Percy-Robb, I. W., 1973, Two anti-anxiety drugs: A psychoendocrine study, *Br. Med. J.* **12**:202–205.

Ogura, C., Nakayawa, K., Majima, K., Nakamura, K., Ueda, H., Umezawa, Y., and Wardell, W. M., 1980, Residual effects of hypnotics: Triazolam, flurazepam, and nitrazepam, *Psychopharmacology* **68**:61–65.

Okawa, K. K., 1978, Comparison of triazolam .25 mg and flurazepam 15 mg in treating geriatric insomniacs, *Curr. Ther. Res. Clin. Exp.* **23**:381–387.

Okudaira, N., Fukuda, H., Nishihara, K., Ohtani, K., Endo, S., and Torii, S., 1983, Sleep apnea and nocturnal myoclonus in elderly persons in Vilcabamba, Ecuador, *J. Gerontol.* **38**:436–438.

Okuma, T., Hata, N., and Fujii, S., 1975, Differential effects of chlorpromazine, imipramine and amobarbital on REM sleep and REM density in man, *Folia Psychiatr. Neurol. Jpn.* **29**:25–37.

Onal, E., Lopata, M., and O'Connor, T., 1982, Pathogenesis of apneas in hypersomnia–sleep apnea syndrome, *Am. Rev. Respir. Dis.* **125**:167–174.

Orr, W. C., 1984, Sleep and breathing: An overview *Ear Nose Throat J.* **63**:11–21.

Orr, W. C., Imes, N. K., and Martin, R. J., 1979, Progesterone therapy in obese patients with sleep apnea, *Arch. Intern. Med.* **139**:109–111.

Orth, D. N., Island, D. P., and Liddle, G. W., 1967, Experimental alterations of the circadian rhythm in plasma cortisol (17-OHCS) concentration in man, *J. Clin. Endocrinol. Metab.* **27**:549–555.

Orzel, J. A., 1982, Acute myocardial infarction complicated by chronic amphetamine use, *Arch. Intern. Med.* **142**:644.

Oshtory, M. A., and Vijayan, N., 1980, Clonazepam treatment of insomnia due to sleep myoclonus, *Arch. Neurol.* **37**:119–120.

Oswald, I., 1959, Sudden bodily jerks on falling asleep, *Brain* **82**:92–103.

Oswald, I., 1962, Sleep mechanisms: Recent advances, *Proc. Roy. Soc. Med.* **55**:910–912.

Oswald, I., 1968, Insomnia: The abnormalities of sleep in man, in: *Proceedings of the XVth European Meeting on Electroencephalography* (H. Gastaut, L. Lugaresi, G. Berti, and G. Coccagna, eds.), Bologna, pp. 99–107.

Oswald, I., 1969, Sleep and dependence on amphetamine and other drugs, in: *Sleep: Physiology and Pathology* (A. Kales, ed.), Lippincott, London, pp. 317–330.

Oswald, I., 1970, Sleep, the great restorer, *New Scientist* **46**:170–172.

Oswald, I., and Priest, R. G., 1965, Five weeks to escape the sleeping pill habit, *Br. Med. J.* **2**:1093–1095.

Oswald, I., and Thacore, V. R., 1963, Amphetamine and phenmetrazine addiction, *Br. Med. J.* **2**:427–431.

Oswald, I., Berger, R. J., Jaramillo, B. A., Keddie, K. M. G., Olley, P. C., and Plunkett, G. B., 1963, Melancholia and barbiturates: A controlled EEG, body and eye movement study of sleep, *Br. J. Psychiatry* **109**:66–78.

Oswald, I., Berger, R. J., Evans, J. I., and Thacore, V. R., 1964, Effects of L-tryptophan upon human sleep, *Electroencephalogr. Clin. Neurophysiol.* **17**:603.

Oswald, I., Ashcroft, G. W., Berger, R. J., Eccleston, D., Evans, J. I., and Thacore V. R., 1966, Some experiments in the chemistry of normal sleep, *Br. J. Psychiatry* **112**:391–399.

Oswald, I., Adam, K., Allen, S., Burack, R., Spence, M., and Thacore, V., 1974, Alpha adrenergic blocker, thymoxamine, and mesoridazine both increase human REM sleep duration, *Sleep Res.* **3**:62.

Oswald, I., Thacore, V. R., Adam, K., Brezinova, V., and Burack, R., 1975, Alpha-adrenergic receptor blockade increases human REM sleep, *Br. J. Clin. Pharmacol.* **2**:107–110.

Oswald, I., Adam, K., Borrow, S., and Idzikowski, C., 1978, The effects of two hypnotics on sleep, subjective feelings and skilled performance, *Adv. Biosci.* **21**:51–63.

Othman, J., Rundell, O. H., and Orr, W. C., 1987, Not all narcoleptics are HLA DR2 positive, *Sleep Res.* **16**:403.

Othmer, E., Daughaday, W., and Guze, S., 1969, The effects of 24 hour REM deprivation on serum growth hormone levels in humans, *Electroencephalogr. Clin. Neurophysiol.* **27**:685.

Othmer, E., Goodwin, D., Levine, W., Malarky, W., Freeman, F., Halikas, J., and Daughaday, W., 1972, Sleep related growth hormone secretion in alcoholics, *Clin. Res.* **20**:726.

Othmer, E., Levine, W. R., Marlarkey, W. B., Corvalan, J. C., Hayden-Otto, M. P., Fishman, P. M., and Daughaday, W. H., 1974a, Body build and sleep-related growth hormone secretion, *Horm. Res.* **5**:156–166.

Othmer, E., Mendelson, W. B., Levine, W. R., Malarkey, W. B., and Daughaday, W. H., 1974b, Sleep-related growth hormone secretion and morning naps, *Steroids Lipids Res.* **5**:380–386.

Owen, M., and Bliss, E. L., 1970, Sleep loss and cortical excitability, *Am. J. Physiol.* **218**:171–173.

Owen, T. R., and Tyrer, P., 1983, Benzodiazepine dependence: A review of the evidence, *Drugs* **25**:385–398.

Pacold, S. T., Kirsteins, L., Hojvat, S., and Lawrence, A. M., 1978, Biologically active pituitary hormones in the rat brain amygdaloid nucleus, *Science* **199**:804–806.

Palaic, D. J., Desaty, J., Albert, J. M., and Panisset, J. C., 1971, Effect of ethanol on metabolism and subcellular distribution of serotonin in the rat brain, *Brain Res.* **25**:381–386.

Palfai, T., Wichlinski, L., Brown, H. A., and Brown, O. M., 1986, Effects of amnesic doses of reserpine or syrosingopine on mouse brain acetylcholine levels, *Pharmacol. Biochem. Behav.* **24**:1457–1459.

Papadimitriou, G. N., Christodoulou, G. N., Trikkas, G. M., Malliaras, D. E., Lykouras, E. P., and Stefanis, C. N., 1981, Sleep deprivation psychoprophylaxis in recurrent affective disorders, *Biol. Psychiatry* **160**:56–61.

Papousek, M., 1975, Chronobiologische aspekete der Zyklothymie, *Fortschr. Neurol. Psychiatr.* **43**:381–440.

Pappenheimer, J. R., Miller, T. B., and Goodrich, C. A., 1967, Sleep-promoting effects of cerebrospinal fluid from sleep-deprived goats, *Proc. Natl. Acad. Sci. USA* **58**:513–517.

Parker, D. C., and Rossman, L. G., 1971, Human growth hormone hyperglycemia, *J. Clin. Endocrinol. Metab.* **32**:65–69.

Parker, D. C., Rossman, L. G., and Vanderlaan, E. F., 1974a, Relation of sleep-entrained human prolactin release to REM-non-REM cycles, *J. Clin. Endocrinol. Metab.* **38**:646–651.

Parker, D. C., Rossman, L. G., Siler, T. M., Rivier, J., Yen, S. S. C., and Guillemin, R., 1974b, Inhibition of the sleep-related peak in physiologic human growth hormone release by somatostatin, *J. Clin. Endocrinol. Metab.* **38**:496–499.

Parker, D. C., Pekary, A. E., and Hershman, J. M., 1976, Effect of normal and reversed sleep–wake cycles upon nyctochemeral rhythmicity of plasma thyrotropin: Influence in sleep, *J. Clin. Endocrinol. Metab.* **43**:318.

Parker, D. C., Rossman, L. G., Pekary, A. E., Hershman, J. M., Kripke, D. F., and Gibson, W., 1981, Endocrine rhythms across reversal sleep–wake cycles, in: *The 24-Hour Workday: Proceedings of a Symposium on Variations in Work/Sleep Schedules*, Cincinnati, NIOSH, DHHS **95**981-127, pp. 151–180.

Parkes, J. D., and Fenton, G. W., 1973, Levo (−) amphetamine and dextro (+) amphetamine in the treatment of narcolepsy, *J. Neurol. Neurosurg. Psychiatry* **36**:1076–1081.

Parkes, J. D., Debono, A. G., Jenner, P., and Walters, J., 1977, Amphetamines, growth hormone and narcolepsy, *Br. J. Clin. Pharmacol.* **4**:343–349.

Parloff, M. B., Wolfe, B., Hadley, S., and Waskow, I. E., 1978, Assessment of psychoso-cial treatment of mental disorders: Current status and prospects, an invited paper of the Advisory Committee on Mental Health, Institute of Medicine, National Academy of Science, Feb. 1978.

Parmegiani, P. L., 1964, A study on the central representation of sleep behavior, in: *Progress in Brain Research, Topics in Basic Neurology* (W. Barsmann and J. L. Schade, eds.), Elsevier, Amsterdam, pp. 180–190.

Parmeggiani, P. L., 1980, Temperature regulation in sleep: A study in homeostastis, in: *Physiology and Sleep* (J. Orem and C. D. Barnes, eds.), Academic Press, New York, pp. 98–145.

Parmeggiani, P. L., and Rabini, C., 1970, Sleep and environmental temperature, *Arch. Ital. Biol.* **108**:369–387.

Pasnau, R. O., Naitoh, P., and Kollar, E. J., 1968, The psychological effects of 205 hours of sleep deprivation, *Arch. Gen. Psychiatry* **18**:496–505.

Passouant, P., Popoviciu, L., Velok, G., and Baldy-Moulinier, M., 1968, Etude poly-graphique des narcolepsies au cours du nychemere, *Rev. Neurol. (Paris)* **118**:431–441.

Pastel, R. H., and Fernstrom, J. D., 1984, The effects of clonidine on EEG wavebands associated with sleep in the rat, *Brain Res.* **300**:243–255.

Patel, Y. C., Alford, F. P., and Burger, H. G., 1972, The 24-hour plasma thyrotrophin profile, *Clin. Sci.* **43**:71–77.

Patel, Y. C., Baker, H. W. G., Burger, H. G., Johns, M. W., and Ledinek, J. E., 1974, Suppression of the thyrotrophin circadian rhythm by glucocorticoids, *J. Endocrinol.* **62**:421–422.

Paul, S. M., and Skolnick, P., 1982, Comparative neuropharmacology of antianxiety drugs, *Pharmacol. Biochem. Behav.* **17**:37–41.

Paul, S. M., Luu, M. D., and Skolnick, P., 1982, The effects of benzodiazepines on pre-synaptic calcium transport, in: *Pharmacology of Benzodiazepines* (E. Usdin, P. Skolnick, J. F. Tallman, J. R. Greenblatt, and S. M. Paul, eds.), MacMillan, London, pp. 87–92.

Pavel, S., and Eisner, C., 1984, A GABAergic habenulo-raphe pathway mediates both serotoninergic and hypnogenic effects of vasotocin in cats, *Brain Res. Bull.* **13**:623–627.

Pavel, S., Psatta, D., and Goldstein, R., 1977, Slow-wave sleep induced in cats by ex-tremely small amounts of synthetic and pineal vasotocin injected into the third ventri-cle of the brain, *Brain Res. Bull.* **2**:251–254.

Pavel, S., Goldstein, R., Popoviciu, L., Corfariu, O., and Foldes, A., 1979, Pineal vaso-tocin: REM sleep dependent release into cerebrospinal fluid of man, *Waking Sleeping* **3**:347–352.

Pavel, S., Goldstein, R., and Petrescu, M., 1980, Vasotocin, melatonin and narcolepsy: Possible involement of the pineal gland in its patho-physiological mechanism, *Pep-tides* **1**:281–284.

Pavel, S., Goldstein, R., Petresca, M., and Popa, M., 1981, REM sleep introduction in prepubertal boys by vasotocin: Evidence for the involvement of serotonin containing neurons, *Peptides* **2**:245–250.

Pawel, M. A., Sassin, J. F., and Weitzman, E. D., 1972, The temporal relation between HGH release and sleep stage changes at nocturnal sleep onset in man, *Life Sci.* **11**:587–593.

Pelham, R. W., Vaughn, G. M., Sandock, K. L., and Vaughn, M. H., 1973, Twenty-four hour cycle of a melanin-like substance in the plasma of human males, *J. Clin. Endo-crinol. Metab.* **37**:341–344.

Pellejero, T., Monti, J. M., Baglietto, J., Jantos, H., Pazos, S., Cichevski, V., and

Hawkins, M., 1984, Effects of methoxamine and alpha-adrenoceptor antagonists, prazosin and yohimbe on the sleep–wake cycle of the rat, *Sleep* **7**:365–372.

Penn, N. E., Kripke, D. F., and Scharff, J., 1981, Sleep paralysis among medical students, *J. Psychol.* **107**:247–252.

Perez-Cruet, J., Chase, T. N., and Murphy, D. L., 1974, Dietary regulation of brain tryptophan metabolism by plasma ratio of free tryptophan and neutral amino acids in humans, *Nature* **248**:693–695.

Perlow, M., McGregor, P., Fukushima, D., Hellman, L., and Weitzman, E., 1971, Seventy-two-hour polygraphic recording and 24-hour plasma cortisol measurement in the differential diagnosis of sleep disorders, presented at the 11th annual meeting of the Association for the Psychophysiological Study of Sleep.

Perlow, M., Sassin, J. F., Boyar, R., Hellman, L., MacGregor, P., and Weitzman, E. D., 1972, Reduction of twenty-four hour growth hormone secretion after clomiphene treatment, *Sleep Res.* **1**:188.

Peroutka, S. J., 1985, Selective labeling of 5-HT1a and 5-HT1b binding sites in bovine brain, *Brain Res.* **344**:167–171.

Peters, J., Santa-Cruz, F., Tower, B. B., and Rubin, R., 1981, Differential neuroendocrine responses to thyrotropin-releasing hormone during rapid eye movement and slow wave sleep in man, *J. Clin. Endocrinol. Metab.* **52**:975–981.

Petersen, E., Paschelke, G., Kehr, W., Nielson, M., and Braestrup C., 1982, Does the reversal of the anticonflict effect of phenobarbital by B-CCE and FG 7142 indicate benzodiazepine receptor-mediated anxiogenic properties? *Eur. J. Pharmacol.* **82**:217–221.

Petitjean, F., and Jouvet, M., 1970, Hypersomnie et augmentation de l'acide 5-hydroxyindolacetique cerebral par lesion isthmique chez le chat, *C. R. Acad. Sci. [D] (Paris)* **164**:2288–2293.

Petitjean, F., Buda, C., Janin, M., Sallanon, M., and Jouvet, M., 1985, Insomnia caused by administration of para-chlorophenylalanine: Reversibility by peripheral or central injection of 5-hydroxytryptophan and serotonin, *Sleep* **8**:56–67.

Pfaff, D., and Keiner, M., 1973, Atlas of estradiol-concentrating cells in the central nervous system of the female rat, *J. Comp. Neurol.* **151**:121–158.

Pflug, B., 1978, The influence of sleep deprivation on the duration of endogenous depressive epidosdes, *Arch. Psychiatr. Nervenkr.* **225**:173–177.

Pflug, B., and Tolle, R., 1971a, Therapy of endogenous depression by sleep deprivation: Practical and theoretical consequences, *Nervenarzt* **42**:117–124.

Pflug, B., and Tolle, R., 1971b, Disturbance of 24-hour rhythm, endogenous depression, and the treatment of endogenous depression by sleep deprivation, *Int. Pharmacopsychiat.* **6**:187–196.

Pflug, B., Johnsson, A., and Ekse, A. T., 1981, Manic-depressive states and daily temperature, *Acta Psychiatr. Scand.* **63**:277–289.

Philip, M., and Werner, C., 1979, Prediction of lofepramine-response in depression based on response to partial sleep deprivation, *Pharmakopsychiatr. Neuropsychopharmakol.* **12**:346–348.

Phillipson, E. A., 1977, Regulation of breathing during sleep, *Ann. Rev. Respir. Dis. Suppl.* **115**:217–244.

Phillipson, E. A., 1978, Respiratory adaptations in sleep, *Ann. Rev. Physiol.* **40**:133–156.

Phillipson, E. A., Sullivan, C. E., Read, D. J., Murphy, E., and Kozer, L. F., 1978, Ventilatory and waking responses to hypoxia in sleeping dogs, *J. Appl. Physiol.* **44**:512–520.

Phillipson, E. A., Bowes, G., Sullivan, C. E., and Woolf, G. M., 1980, The influence of sleep fragmentation on arousal and ventilatory responses to respiratory stimuli, *Sleep* **3**:281–288.

Phillis, J. W., and Wu, P. H., 1981, The role of adenosine and its nucleotides in central synaptic transmission, *Prog. Neurobiol.* **16**:187–239.

Pickel, V. M., Joh, T. H., and Reis, D. J., 1978, Immunocytochemical evidence for serotonergic innervation of noradrenergic neurons in nucleus locus ceruleus, in: *Interactions Between Putative Neurotransmitters in the Brain* (S. Grattini, J. F. Pujol, and R. Samanin, eds.), Raven Press, New York, pp. 369–399.

Piro, C., Fraioli, F., Sciarra, F., and Conti, C., 1973, Circadian rhythm of plasma testosterone, cortisol and gonadotropins in normal male subjects, *Steroid Biochem.* **4**:321–329.

Pishkin, V., Lovallo, W. R., Fishkin, S. M., and Shurley, J. T., 1980, Residual effects of temazepam and other hypnotic compounds on cognitive function, *J. Clin. Psychiatry* **41**:358–364.

Pohorecky, L. A., 1974, Effects of ethanol on central and peripheral noradrenergic neurons, *J. Pharmacol. Exp. Ther.* **189**:380–391.

Poirier, G., Montplasir, J., Decary, F., Momege, D., and Lebrun, A., 1986, HLA antigens in narcolepsy and idiopathic central nervous system hypersomnolence, *Sleep* **9**:153–161.

Poland, R. E., Rubin, R. T., Clank, R. B., and Gouin, P. R., 1972, Circadian patterns of urine 17-OHC and VMA excretion during sleep deprivation, *Dis. Nerv. Syst.* **33**:456–458.

Polc, P., Mohler, H., and Haefely, W., 1974, The effect of diazepam on spinal cord activities: Possible sites and mechanisms of action, *Naunyn Schmiedebergs Arch. Pharmacol.* **284**:319–337.

Pollack, C. P., McGregor, P., and Weitzman, E., 1975, The effects of flurazepam on daytime sleep after acute sleep–wake cycle reversal, *Sleep Res.* **4**:112.

Polzella, D. J., 1975, Effects of sleep deprivation on short-term recognition memory, *J. Exp. Psychol.* **104**:194–200.

Popoviciu, L., Corfarin, D. T., Tudosie, M., Foldes, A., and Pavel, S., 1982, Effects of arginine vasotocin on REM sleep in narcoleptics and in hypersomniacs, *Electroencephalogr. Clin. Neurophysiol.* **53**:325–328.

Porter, N. M., Clark, F. M., Green, R. D., and Radulovacki, M., 1986, Effects of chronic intracerebroventricular infusion of adenosine agonists and deoxycoformycin on brain adenosine receptors and sleep in the rat, abstract for Society for Neuroscience Meeting.

Post, R. M., Stoddard, F. G., Gillin, J. C., Buchsbaum, M., Runkle, D. C., Black, K., and Bunney, W. E., 1976, Slow and rapid alterations in motor activity, sleep and biochemistry in a cycling manic-depressive patient, *Arch. Gen. Psychiatry* **34**:470–477.

Post, R. M., Gerner, R. H., Carman, J. S., Gillin, J., Jimerson, D. S., Goodwin, F. K., and Bunney, W. E., 1978, Effects of a dopamine agonist piribedil in depressed patients, *Arch. Gen. Psychiatry* **35**:609–615.

Prange, A. J., Wilson, I. C., Lara, P. P., Alltop, L. B., and Breeses, G. R., 1972, Effect of thyrotropin releasing hormone in depression, *Lancet* **2**:999–1002.

Prange, A. J., Breese, G. R., Cott, J. M., Martin, B. R., Cooper, B. R., Wilson, I. C., and Plotnikoff, N. P., 1974, Thyrotropin releasing hormone: Antagonism of pentobarbital in rodents, *Life Sci.* **14**:447–455.

Pressman, M. R., Spielman, A. J., Korczyn, A. D., Rubenstein, A. E., Pollak, C. P., and Weitzman, E. D., 1984, Patterns of daytime sleepiness in narcoleptics and normals: A pupillometric study, *Electroencephalogr. Clin. Neurophysiol.* **57**:129–133.

Pressor, H. B., and Cain, U.S., 1983, Shift work among dual-earner couples with children, *Science* **219**:876–879.

Price, P. A., Schacter, M., Smith, S. J., Baxter, C. H., and Parkes, J. D., 1981, Gamma-hydroxybutyrate in narcolepsy, *Ann. Neurol.* **9:**198.

Price, W. J., and Holley, D. C., 1982, Sleep loss and the crash of flight 182, *J. Hum. Ergon.* **11:**291–301.

Prinz, P. N., Halter, J., Benedett, C., and Raskind, M., 1979, Circadian variation of plasma catecholamines in young and old men: Relation to rapid eye movement and slow wave sleep, *J. Clin. Endocrinol. Metab.* **49:**300–304.

Prinz, P. N., Vitiello, M. U., Smallwood, R. G., Schaene, R. B., and Halter, J. B., 1984, Plasma norepinephrine in normal young and aged men: Relationship with sleep, *J. Gerontol.* **39:**561–567.

Prinzmetal, M., and Bloomberg, W., 1935, The use of benzedrine for the treatment of narcolepsy, *JAMA* **105:**2051–2054.

Pscheidt, G. R., 1964, Monoamine oxidase inhibitors, *Int. Rev. Neurobiol.* **7:**191–229.

Pscheidt, G. R., Issekuty, B., and Himwich, H. E., 1961, Failure of ethanol to lower brain stem concentration of biogenic amines, *Q. J. Stud. Alcohol* **22:**550–553.

Pucilowski, O., and Valzelli, L., 1985, Evidence of norepinephrine-mediated suppression of para-chlorophenyl alanine-induced muricidal behavior, *Pharmacol. Res. Commun.* **17:**983–989.

Puder, R., Lacks, P., Bertelson, A. D., and Storandt, M., 1983, Short-term stimulus control treatment of insomnia in older adults, *Behav. Ther.* **14:**424–429.

Puig-Antich, J., Goetz, R., Hanlon, C., Davies, M., Thompson, J., Chambers, W. J., and Tabrizi, M. A., 1982, Sleep architecture and REM sleep measures in prepubertal children with major depression, *Arch. Gen. Psychiatry* **39:**932–939.

Puig-Antich, J., Novacenko, H., Davies, M., Chambers, W. J., Tabrizi, M. A., Krawiec, V., and Sachar, E. J., 1984a, Growth hormone secretion in prepubertal children with major depression. I. Final report on response to insulin-induced hypoglycemia during a depressive episode, *Arch. Gen. Psychiatry* **41:**455–460.

Puig-Antich, J., Goetz, R., Davies, M., Fein, M., Hanlon, C., Chambers, W. J., and Weitzman, E. D., 1984b, Growth hormone secretion in prepubertal children with major depression. II. Sleep-related plasma concentrations during a depressive episode, *Arch. Gen. Psychiatry* **41:**463–466.

Pujol, J. F., Buguet, A., Froment, J. L., Jones, B., and Jouvet, M., 1971, The central metabolism of serotonin in the cat during insomnia: A neurophysiological and biochemical study after *p*-chlorophenylalanine or destruction of the raphe system, *Brain Res.* **29:**195–212.

Pujol, J. F., Stein, D., Blondaux, F., Petitjean, J. L., Fremont, L., and Jouvet, M., 1973, Biochemical evidences for interaction phenomena between noradrenergic and serotoninergic systems in the cat brain, in: *Frontiers in Catecholamine Research* (E. Usdin, ed.), Pergamon Press, Oxford, pp. 771–772.

Quabbe, H. J., Schilling, E., and Helge, H., 1966, Pattern of growth hormone secretion during a 24-hour fast in normal adults, *J. Clin. Endocrinol. Metab.* **26:**1173–1177.

Quabbe, H. J., Vogt, C. B., Gregor, M., Stolz, B., and Witt, I., 1982, 24-Hour pattern of plasma prolactin in the male rhesus monkey and its relation to the sleep/wake cycle, *Endocrinology* **110:**969–975.

Radulovacki, M., Buckingham, R.L., Chen, E.H., and Kovacevic, R., 1977, Similar effects of tryptophan and sleep on cisternal cerebrospinal fluid 5-hydroxyir.doleacetic and homovanillic acids in cats, *Brain Res.* **129:**371–374.

Radulovacki, M., Wojcik, W.J., Walovitch, R., and Brodie, M., 1981a, Phenoxybenzamine and bromocriptine attenuate need for REM sleep in rats, *Pharmacol. Biochem. Behav.* **14:**371–375.

Radulovacki, M., Brodie, M., Walovitch, R., and Yanik, G., 1981b, Bromocriptine, dihy-droergotoxine and sleep in rats; Effects of repeated administration, *Gerontology* **27**:152–157.

Radulovacki, M., Virus, R.M., Djuricic-Nedelson, M., and Green, R.D., 1983, Hypnotic effects of deoxycorformycin in rats, *Brain Res.* **271**:392–395.

Radulovacki, M., Virus, R.M., Djuricic-Nedelson, M., and Green, R.D., 1984, Adenosine analogs and sleep in rats, *J. Pharmacol. Ther.* **228**:268–274.

Raffaele, R., Reggio, A., Tropea, R., Pennisi, G., Falsaperia, A., and Nicoletti F., 1983, Variations in the 5-hydroxyindoleacetic acid concentration in the cerebrospinal fluid during the sleep–wake cycle in man, *Ital. J. Neurol. Sci.* **1**:35–37.

Ragno, R.E., Dumont, C.H., and Sitar, D.S., 1982, Effect of ethanol ingestion on outcome of drug overdose, *Crit. Care Med.* **10**:180–185.

Rajagopal, K.R., Bennett, L.L., Dillard, T.A., Tellis, C.J., and Tenholder, M.F., 1986, Overnight nasal CPAP improves hypersomnolence in sleep apnea, *Chest* **90**:172–176.

Ralph, M.R., and Menaker, M., 1985, Bicuculline blocks circadian phase delays but not advances, *Brain Res.* **325**:362–365.

Randall, C.L., and Lester, D., 1974, Differential effects of ethanol and pentobarbital on sleep time in C57BL and BALB mice, *J. Pharmacol. Exp. Ther.* **188**:27–33.

Randall, C.L., Hughes, S.S., Williams, C.K., and Anton, R.F., 1983, Effect of prenatal alcohol exposure on consumption of alcohol and alcohol-induced sleep sleep time in mice, *Pharmacol. Biochem. Behav.* **18**:325–329.

Rangaraj, N., and Kalant, H., 1979, Interaction of ethanol and catecholamines on rat brain (Na + -K +) ATPase, *Can. J. Physiol. Pharmacol.* **57**:1098–1106.

Rangno, R.E., Dumont, D.C., and Sitar, D.C., 1982, Effect of ethanol ingestion on out-come of drug overdoses, *Critical Care Med.* **10**:180–185.

Rao, S., Sherbaniuk, R.W., Prosad, K., Lee, S.J.K., and Sproule, B.J., 1973, Cardio-pulmonary effects of diazepam, *Clin. Pharmacol. Ther.* **14**:182–189.

Rapoport, D.M., Sorkin, B., Garay, S.M., and Goldring, R.M., 1982, Reversal of the "Pickwickian syndrome" by long-term use of nocturnal nasal-airway pressure, *N. Engl. J. Med.* **307**:931–933.

Rapoport, D.M., Garay, S.M., and Goldring, R.M., 1983, Nasal CPAP in obstructive sleep apnea: Mechanisms of action, *Bull. Eur. Physiopath. Resp.* **19**:616–620.

Rapoport, D.M., Garay, S.M., Epstein, H., and Goldring, R.M., 1986, Hypercapnia in the obstructive sleep apnea syndrome, *Chest* **89**:627–635.

Read, D.J., Feest, T.G., and Nassim, M.A., 1981, Clonazepam: Effective treatment for restless legs syndrome in uraemia, *Br. Med. J.* **283**:885.

Rechtschaffen, A., 1968, Polygraphic aspects of insomnia: The abnormalities of sleep in man, in: *Proceedings of the XVth European Meeting on Electroencephalography* (H. Gestaut, L. Lugaresi, G. Berti, and G. Coccagna, eds.), Bologna, pp. 109–118.

Rechtschaffen, A., and Kales, A., 1968, A manual of standarized terminology, tech-niques, and scoring system for sleep stages of human subjects, Brain Information Service/Brain Research Institute, pp. 1-60.

Rechtschaffen, A., and Maron, L., 1964, The effect of amphetamines on the sleep cycle, *Electroencephalogr. Clin. Neurophysiol.* **16**:438–445.

Rechtschaffen, A., and Monroe, L. J., 1969, Laboratory studies of insomnia, in: *Sleep: Physiology and Pathology* (A. Kales, ed.), Lippincott, Philadelphia, pp. 158–169.

Rechtschaffen, A., Wolpert, E. A., Dement, W. C., Mitchell, S. A., and Fischer, C., 1963, Nocturnal sleep of narcoleptics, *Electroencephalogr. Clin. Neurophysiol.* **15**:599–609.

Rechtschaffen, A., Schulsinger, F., and Mednick, S. A., 1964, Schizophrenia and physi-ological indices of dreaming, *Arch. Gen. Psychiatry* **10**:89–93.

Rechtschaffen, A., Lovell, R. A., Freedman, D. W., Whitehead, P. K., and Aldrich, M., 1969, Effect of p-chlorophenylalanine on sleep in rats, *Psychophysiology* **6**:223.

Rechtscheffen, A., Molinari, S., Watson, R., and Wincor, M., 1970, Extraocular potentials: A possible indicator of PGO activity in the human, presented at Association for the Psychophysiogical Study of Sleep, Sante Fe, New Mexico.

Rechtschaffen, A., Gilliland, M. A., Bergmann, B. M., and Winter, J. B., 1983, Physiological correlates of prolonged sleep deprivation in rats, *Science* **221**:180–183.

Rees, A. J., Peters, D. K., Compston, D. A., and Batchelor, J. R., 1978, Strong asssociation between HLA-DRW2 and antibody-mediated Goodpasture's syndrome, *Lancet* **1**:966–968.

Reeves, R. L., 1977, Comparison of triazolam, flurazepam and placebo as hypnotics in geriatric practice, *J. Clin. Pharmacol.* **17**:319–323.

Reichlin, S., 1983, Somatostatin, *New Engl. J. Med.* **309**:1495–1501.

Reichlin, S., 1985, Neuroendocrinology, in: *Williams Textbook of Endocrinology* (J. D. Wilson and D. W. Foster, eds.), Saunders, Philadelphia, pp. 492–567.

Reimao, R., Lemmi, H., and Belluomini, J., 1984, Aspectos poligraficos dos movimentos periodicos do sono, *Arq. Neuropsiquiatr.* **42**:313–321.

Reimao, R., Lemmi, H., Akiskal, H., and Cocke, E., 1986, Obstructive sleep apnea treated with UPPP: A systematic follow-up study, *S. Med. J.* **79**:1064–1066.

Reindl, K., Falliers, C., Halberg, F., Chai, H., Hillman, D., and Nelson, W., 1969, Circadian acrophase in peak expiratory flow rate and urinary electrolyte excretion of asthmatic children: Phase shifting of rhythms by prednisone given at different circadian system phases, *Rass. Neurol. Veg.* **23**:5–26.

Reinhard, V., Kindel, K., Burmeister, P. L., Boehme, W., and Cramer, H., 1974, Melatonin: Influence on afternoon sleep pattern and plasma levels of HGH and cyclic AMP in healthy volunteers, *Proc. 2nd European Congress Sleep Res.* Rome, 1974.

Reivich, M., Isaacs, G., Evarts, E., and Kety, S., 1968, The effect of slow wave sleep and REM sleep on regional cerebral blood flow in cats, *J. Neurochem.* **15**:301–306.

Remmers, J. E., de Groot, W. J., and Sauaerland, E. K., 1976, Upper airway obstruction during sleep: Role of the genioglossus (Abst.), *Clin. Res.* **24**:33.

Rettie, A. E., Rettenmeier, A. W., Howald, W. N., and Baillie, T. A., 1987, Cytochrome P-450 catalyzed formation of delta-4 VPA, a toxic metabolite of valproic acid, *Science* **235**:890–894.

Reynolds, C. F., Coble, P., Black, R. S., Holzer, B., and Kupfer, D. J., 1980, Sleep disturbances in a series of elderly patients: Polysomnographic findings, *J. Am. Geriatr. Soc.* **28**:164–170.

Reynolds, C. F., Coble, P. A., Spiker, D. G., Neil, J. F., Holzer, B. C., and Kupfer, D. J., 1982, Prevalence of sleep apnea and nocturnal myoclonus in major affective disorders: Clinical and polysomnographic findings, *J. Nerv. Men. Dis.* **170**:565–567.

Reynolds, C. F., Taska, L. S., Sewitch, D. E., Restifo, K., Coble, P. A., and Kupfer, D. J., 1984a, Persistent psychophysiologic insomnia: Preliminary research diagnostic criteria and EEG sleep data, *Am. J. Psychiatry* **141**:804–805.

Reynolds, C. F., Kupfer, D. J., McEachran, A. B., Taska, L. S., Sewitch, D. E., and Coble, P. A., 1984b, Depressive psychopathology in male sleep apneics, *J. Clin. Psychiatry* **45**:287–290.

Reynolds, C. F., Kupfer, D. J., Taska, L. S., Hoch, C. C., Sewitch, D. E., Restifo, K., and Morycz R., 1985, Sleep apnea in Alzheimer's dementia: Correlation with mental deterioration, *J. Clin. Psychiatry* **46**:257–261.

Reyntjens, A., Gelders, Y. G., Hoppenbrouwers, M. J., and Bussche, G. V., 1986, Thymosthenic effects of ritanserin (R 55667), a centrally acting serotonin-S2 receptor blocker, *Drug Dev. Res.* **8**:205–211.

Richardson, G. S., Carskadon, M. A., Flagg, W., Van den Hoed, J., Dement, W. C., and Mitler, M. M., 1978, Excessive daytime sleepiness in man: Multiple sleep latency measurement in narcoleptic and control, *Electroencephalogr. Clin. Neurophysiol.* **45**:621–627.

Richter, C. P., 1957, Hormones and rhythms in man and animals, in: *Recent Progress in Hormone Research* (C. Pincus, ed.), Academic Press, New York, pp. 105–159.

Richter, C. P., 1965, *Biological Clocks in Medicine and Psychiatry*, C. Thomas, Springfield, IL, pp. 1–109.

Rickels, K., Gingrich, R., Morris, R. J., Rosenfeld, H., Perloff, M. M., Clark, E. L., and Schilling, A., 1975, Triazolam in insomniac family practice patients, *Clin. Pharmacol. Ther.* **18**:315–324.

Rietveld, W. J., 1985, Functional significance of the suprachiasmatic nucleus, in: *Circadian Rhythms in the Central Nervous System* (P. H. Redfern, I. C. Campbell, J. A. Davies, and K. F. Martin, eds.), VCH, Deerfield Beach, FL, pp. 45–55.

Risch, S. C., Cohen, R. M., Janowsky, D. S., Kalin, N. H., Sitaram, N., Gillin, J. C., and Murphy, D. L., 1981, Physotigmine induction of depressive symptomatology in normal human subjects, *Psychiatry Res.* **4**:89–94.

Ritvo, E. R., Ornitz, E. M., LaFranchi, S. C., and Walter, R. D., 1967, Effects of impramine on the sleep dream cycle: An EEG study in boys, *Electroencephalogr. Clin. Neurophysiol.* **22**:465–468.

Rockwell, D. A., Winget, C. M., Rosenblatt, L. S., Higgins, E. A., and Hetherington, N. W., 1978, Biological aspects of suicide: Circadian disorganization, *J. Nerv. Ment. Dis.* **166**:851–858.

Roehrs, T., Zorick, F., Kaffeman, M., Sicklesteel, J., and Roth, T., 1982, Flurazepam for short-term treatment of complaints of insomnia, *J. Clin. Pharmacol.* **22**:290–296.

Roehrs, T., Zorick, F., Sicklesteel, B. A., Wittig, R., and Roth, T., 1983, Age-related sleep-–wake disorders at a sleep disorder center, *J. Am. Geriatr. Soc.* **31**:364–370.

Roehrs, T., Zorick, F., Wittig, R., Paxton, C., Sicklesteel, J., and Roth, T., 1986a, Alerting effects of naps in patients with narcolepsy, *Sleep* **9**:194–199.

Roehrs, T., Kribbs, N., Zorick, F., and Roth, T., 1986b, Hypnotic residual effects of benzodiazepines with repeated administration, *Sleep* **9**:309–316.

Roehrs, T., Vogel, G., Vogel, F., Wittig, R., Zorick, F., and Paxton, C., 1986c, Dose effects of temazepam tablets on sleep, *Drugs Exp. Clin. Res.* **12**:693–699.

Roehrs, T., Jorick, N. J., Wittig, R. M., and Roth, T., 1986d, Dose determinants of rebound insomnia, *Br. J. Clin. Pharmacol.* **22**:143–147.

Roffwarg, H. P., Muzio, J. M., and Dement, W. C., 1966, Ontogenetic development of the human sleep–dream cycle, *Science* **152**:604–619.

Roffwarg, H. P., Sachar, E. D., Halpern, F., and Hellman, L, 1974, Plasma testosterone and sleep: Relationship to sleep stage variables, *Sleep Res.* **3**:172.

Roffwarg, H. P., Sachar, E. J., Halpern, F., and Hellman, L., 1982, Plasma testosterone and sleep: Relationship to sleep stage variables, *Psychosom. Med.* **44**:73–84.

Ronnekiev, O., Krulich, L., and McCann, S. M., 1973, An early morning surge of prolactin in the male rat and its pinealectomy, *Endocrinology* **92**:1339–1342.

Rosadini, P., Masturzo, P., Rodriguez, G., Murialdo, D., Montano, V., Bonura, M. L., and Polleri, A., 1983, Effects of a single oral dose of phenobarbital on prolactin, growth hormone and luteinizing hormone in normal women, *Acta Endocrinol.* **103**:309–314.

Rose, R. M., Kreuz, L. E., Holaday, J. W., Sulak, K. J., and Johnson, C., 1972, Diurnal variation of plasma testosterone and cortisol, *J. Endocrinol.* **54**:177–178.

Ross, D. H., Kibler, B. C., and Cardenas, H. L., 1977, Modification of glycoprotein residues as Ca^{2+} receptor sites after chronic ethanol exposure, *Drug Alcohol Depend.* **2**:305–315.

Ross, G. T., 1985, Disorders of the ovary and female reproductive tract, in: *Williams Textbook of Endocrinology* (J. D. Wilson and D. W. Foster, eds.), pp. 206–258.

Ross, R. T., 1982, Sudden infant death syndrome and progesterone, *Med. Hypotheses* **8**:461–463.

Roth, B., and Nevsimalova, S., 1975, Depression in narcolepsy and hypersomnia, *Arch Neurol. Neurochir. Psychiatry* **116**:291–300.

Roth, B., Bruhova, S., and Lehovsky, M., 1969, REM sleep and NREM sleep in narcolepsy and hypersomnia, *Electroencephalogr. Clin. Neurophysiol.* **26**:176–182.

Roth, B., Nevsimalova, S., and Rechtschaffen, A., 1972, Hypersomnia, with "sleep drunkenness," *Arch Gen. Psychiatry* **26**:456–462.

Roth, B., Nevsimalova, S., Sonka, K., and Docekal, P., 1986, An alternative to the multiple sleep latency test for determining sleepiness in narcolepsy and hypersomnia: Polygraphic score of sleepiness, *Sleep* **9**:243–245.

Roth, J., Glick, S. M., Yalow, R. S., and Berson, S. A., 1963, Hypoglocemia: Potent stimulus to secretion of growth hormone, *Science* **140**:987–988.

Roth, N., 1946, Problems in narcolepsy, *Bull. Menninger Clin.* **10**:160–170.

Roth, T., Kramer, M., Leston, W., and Lutz, T., 1974, The effects of sleep deprivation on mood, *Sleep Res.* **3**:154.

Roth, T., Kramer, M., and Lutz, T., 1976a, Intermediate use of triazolam: A sleep laboratory study, *J. Int. Med. Res.* **4**:59–63.

Roth, T., Kramer, M., and Lutz, T., 1976b, The nature of insomnia: A descriptive summary of a sleep clinic population, *Compr. Psychiatry* **17**:217.

Roth, T., Kramer, M., and Lutz, T., 1977, The effects of hypnotics on sleep, performance and subjective state, *Drugs Exp. Clin. Res.* **1**:279–287.

Rothman, M., 1984, Evaluation and management of alcohol-related psychiatric emergencies, in: *Psychiatric Emergencies—Clinical Emergency Medicine, Vol. 4* (W. R., Dubin, N., Hanke, and H. W., Ninckins, eds.), Churchill Livingston, New York, pp. 143–152.

Rowland, N. E., and Carlton, J., 1986, Neurobiology of an anorectic drug: Fenfluramine, *Prog. Neurobiol.* **27**:13–62.

Roy, A., 1977, Anorgasmia and cataplexy, *Arch. Sex. Behav.* **6**:437–441.

Roy-Byrne, P. P., Uhde, T. W., and Post, R. M., 1984, Antidepressant effects on one night's sleep deprivation: Clinical and theoretical implications, in: *Neurobiology of Mood Disorders* (R. M. Post and J. C. Ballinger, eds.), Williams & Williams, Baltimore, pp. 817–835.

Rubin, R. T., 1975, Sleep–endocrinology studies in man, *Prog. Brain Res.* **42**:73–80.

Rubin, R. T., Kales, A., and Clark, B. R., 1969, Decreased 17-hydroxycorticosteroid and VMA excretion during sleep following glutethimide administration in man, *Life Sci.* **8**:959–964.

Rubin, R. T., Kales, A., Adler, R., Fagan, T., and Odell, W., 1972, Gonadotropin secretion during sleep in normal adult men, *Science* **175**:196–198.

Rubin, R. T., Gouin, P. R., Kales, A., and Odell, W. D., 1973a, Luteinizing hormone, follicle stimulating hormone and growth hormone secretion in normal adult men during sleep and dreaming, *Psychosom. Med.* **35**:309–321.

Rubin, R. T., Gouin, P. R., Arenander, A. T., and Poland, R. E., 1973b, Human growth hormone release during sleep following prolonged flurazepam administration, *Res. Commun. Chem. Patholo. Pharmacol.* **6**:331–334.

Rubin, R. T., Poland, R. E., Rubin, L. E., and Gouin, P. R., 1974, The neuroendocrinology of human sleep, *Life Sci.* **14**:1041–1052.

Rubin, R. T., Gouin, P. R., Lubin, A., Poland, R. E., and Pirke, K. M., 1975a, Nocturnal increase of plasma testosterone in men: Relation to gonadotropins and prolactin, *J. Clin. Endocrinol. Metab.* **40:**1027–2033.

Rubin, R. T., Poland, R. E., Tower, B. B., and Gouin, P. R., 1975b, Nocturnal secretion of water and electrolyte-regulating hormones in normal adult men, presented at the Second International Sleep Research Congress, Edinburgh, June 20–July 4 1975.

Rudestam, K. E., 1980, *Methods of Self-Change,* Brooks/Cole Publishing, Co., Monterey, CA, pp. 1–255.

Rudolf, M., Geddes, D. M., Turner, J. A., and Saunders, K. B., 1978, Depression of central respiratory drive by nitrazepam, *Thorax* **33:**97–100.

Ruedy, J., 1973, Acute drug poisoning in the adult, *Can. Med. Assoc. J.* **109:**603–608.

Rundell, O. H., Lester, B. K., Griffiths, W. J., and Williams, H. L., 1972, Alcohol and sleep in young adults, *Psychopharmacologia* **26:**201–218.

Rush, A. J., Giles, D. E., Roffwarg, H. P., and Parker, C. R., 1982, Sleep EEG and dexamethasone suppression test findings in outpatients with unipolar major depressive disorders, *Biol. Psychiatry* **17:**327–341.

Rush, A. J., Schlesser, M. A., Roffwarg, H. P., Giles, D. E., Orsulak, P. J., and Fairchild, C., 1983, Relationships among the TRH, REM latency, and dexamethasone suppression tests: Preliminary findings, *J. Clin. Psychiatry* **44:**23–29.

Sachar, E. J., Hellman, L., Roffwarg, H. P., Halpern, F. S., Fukushima, D. K., and Gallagher, T. F., 1973a, Disrupted 24-hour patterns of cortisol secretion in psychotic depression, *Arch. Gen. Psychiatry* **28:**19–24.

Sachar, E. J., Frantz, A. G., Altman, N., and Sassin, J., 1973b, Growth hormone and prolactin in unipolar and bipolar depressed patients: Responses to hypoglycemia and L-dopa, *Am. J. Psychiatry* **130:**1362–1367.

Sack, D. A., Nurnberger, J., Rosenthal, N. E., Ashburn, E., and Wehr, T. A., 1985, Potentiation of antidepressant medications by phase advance of the sleep–wake cycle, *Am. J. Psychiatry* **142:**606–608.

Sagales, T., and Erill, S., 1975, Effects of central dopaminergic blockage with pimozide upon the EEG stages of sleep in man, *Psychopharmacology* **41:**53–56.

Sagales, T., Erill, S. T., and Domino, E. F., 1969, Differential effects of scopolamine and chlorpromazine on REM and NREM sleep in normal male subjects, *Clin. Pharmacol. Ther.* **10:**522–529.

Saito, H., and Saito, S., 1982, Plasma somatostatin in normal subjects and in various diseases: Increased levels in somatostatin-producing tumors, *Horm. Metab. Res.* **14:**71–76.

Saito, H., Saito, S., Kawano, N., and Tomita, S., 1983, Plasma somatostatin level during natural and interrupted nocturnal sleep in man, *Acta Endocrinol.* **104:**129–133.

Sakai, F., Meyer, J. S., Karacan, I., Yamaguchi, F., and Yamamoto, M., 1979, Narcolepsy: Regional cerebral blood flow during sleep and wakefulness, *Neurology* **29:**61–67.

Salin-Pascual, R., de la Fluente, J., and Fernandez-Guardiola, A., 1985, Effects of clonidine in narcolepsy, *J. Clin. Psychiatry* **46:**528–531.

Sallanon, M., Janin, M., Buda, C., and Jouvet, M., 1983, Serotoninergic mechanisms and sleep rebound, *Brain Res.* **268:**95–104.

Sallanon, M., Buda, C., Janin, M., and Jouvet, M., 1985, Implications of serotonin in sleep mechanisms: Induction, facilitation? in: *Sleep: Neurotransmitters and Neuromodulators* (A. Wauquier, J. M. Gaillard, J. M. Monti, and M. Radulovacki, eds.), Raven Press, New York, pp. 135–140.

Salvadorini, F., Galeone, F., Niucotera, M., Ombarato, M., and Saba, P., 1975, Clinical evaluation of CDP-choline (Nicholin): Efficacy as antidepressant treatment, *Curr. Ther. Res.* **18:**513–520.

Sampson, H., 1965, Deprivation of dreaming sleep by two methods: I. Compensatory REM time, *Arch. Gen. Psychiatry* **13**:79–86.

Samuels, S. I., and Rabinov, W., 1986, Difficulty reversing drug-induced coma in a patient with sleep apnea, *Anesth. Analg.* **65**:1222–1224.

Sanders, M. H., Moore, S. E., and Eveslage, J., 1983, CPAP via nasal mask: A treatment for occlusive sleep apnea, *Chest* **83**:144–145.

Sandyk, R., 1985, Efficacy of trazodone in narcolepsy, *Eur. Neurol.* **24**:335–337.

Sandyk, R., and Gillman, M., 1985a, Naloxone ameliorates narcolepsy, *Clin. Neuropharmacol.* **8**:96–97.

Sandyk, R., and Gillman, M., 1985b, Nomifensine exacerbates narcolepsy, *Neurology* **35**:138.

Sandyk, R., and Gillman, M., 1986, The opoid system in the restless legs and nocturnal myoclonus syndromes, *Sleep (Lett.)* **9**:370–371.

Sanford, J. R., 1975, Tolerance of debility in elderly dependents by supporters at home: Its significance for hospital practice., *Br. Med. J.* **3**:471–473.

Santiago, T. V., Scardella, A., and Edelman, N. H., 1984, Determinants of the ventilatory responses to hypoxia during sleep, *Am. Rev. Respir. Dis.* **130**:179–182.

Saskin, P., Spielman, A. J., Jelin, M. A., and Thorpy, M. J., 1984, Sleep restriction therapy for insomnia, *Sleep Res.* **13**:163.

Saskin, P., Moldofsky, H., and Lue, F. A., 1985, Periodic movements in sleep and sleep–wake complaint, *Sleep* **8**:319–324.

Sassin, J. F., 1970, Neurological findings following short-term sleep deprivation, *Arch. Neurol.* **22**:54–56.

Sassin, J. F., Parker, D. C., Mace, J. W., Gotlin, R. W., Johnson, L. C., and Rossman, L. G., 1969, Human growth hormone release: Relation to slow-wave sleep and sleep–waking cycles, *Science* **165**:513–515.

Sassin, J. F., Frantz, A. G., Weitzman, E. D., and Kapen, S., 1972a, Human prolactin: 24-Hour pattern with increased release during sleep, *Science* **177**:1205–1207.

Sassin, J., Hellman, L., and Weitzman, E., 1972b, A circadian pattern of growth hormone secretion in acromegalics, *Sleep Res.* **1**:189.

Sassin, J. F., Frantz, A. G., Kapen, S., and Weitzman, E. D., 1973, The nocturnal rise of human prolactin is dependent on sleep, *J. Clin. Endocrinol. Metab.* **37**:436–440.

Sastre, J. P., Sakai, K., and Jouvet, M., 1981, Are the gigantocelular tegmental field neurons responsible for paradoxical sleep? *Brain Res.* **229**:147–161.

Sauerland, E. K., and Harper, R. M., 1976, The human tongue during sleep: Electromyographic activity of the genioglossus muscle, *Esp. Neurol.* **51**:160–170.

Sauerland, E. K., Orr, W. C., and Hairston, L. E., 1981, EMG patterns of orogpharyngeal muscles during respiration in wakefulness and sleep, *Electromyogr. Clin. Neurophysiol.* **21**:307–316.

Sawyer, C. H., 1969, Some effects of hormones on sleep, *Exp. Med. Surg.* **27**:177–186.

Schachter, M., and Parkes, J. D., 1980, Fluvoxamine and clomipramine in the treatment of cataplexy, *J. Neurol. Neurosurg. Psychiatry* **43**:171–174.

Scharf, M. B., Brown, D., Woods, M., Brown, L., and Hirschowitz, J., 1985, The effects and effectiveness of gamma-hydroxbutyrate in patients with narcolepsy, *J. Clin. Psychiatry* **46**:222–225.

Schenck, J. M., 1969, Personality components in patients with sleep paralysis, *Psychiatr. Q.* **43**:343–348.

Schiavi, R. C., Davis, D. M., White, D., Edwards, A., Igel, G., and Fisher, C., 1974, Plasma testosterone during nocturnal sleep in normal men, *Steroids* **24**:191–202.

Schiavi, R. C., Fisher, C., White, D., Beers, P., Fogel, M., and Szechter, R., 1982, Hormonal variations during sleep in men with erectile dysfunction and normal controls, *Arch. Sex. Behav.* **11**:189–199.

Schiavi, R. C., Fisher, C., White, D., Beers, P., and Szechter, R., 1984, Pituitary–gonadal function during sleep in men with erectile impotence and normal controls, *Psychosom. Med.* **46**:239–254.

Schildkraut, J. J., 1974, Norepinephrine metabolism in subtypes of depressive disorders, *Psychopharmacol. Bull.* **10**:49–50.

Schilgen, B., and Tolle, R., 1980, Partial sleep deprivation as therapy for depression, *Arch. Gen. Psychiatry* **37**:267–271.

Schilgen, V. B., Bischofs, W., Blaszkiewicz, F., Bremer, W., Rudolf, G. A. E., and Tolle, R., 1976, Tolter und partieler Schlafentzug in der Behandlung von Depressionen, *Arneim-Forsch.(Drug Res.)* **26**:1171–1173.

Schilkrut, R., Chandra, O., Ossaald, M., Ruther, E., Baarfusser, B., and Matussek, N., 1975, Growth hormone release during sleep and with thermal stimulation in depressed patients, *Neuropsychobiology* **1**:70–79.

Schimizu, A., Hiyama, H., Yagasaki, A., Takahashi, H., Fujiki, A., and Yoshida, I., 1979, Sleep of depressed patients with hypersomnia: A 24 hour polygraphic study, *Waking Sleeping* **3**:335–339.

Schmidt, F. O., 1962, Macromolecular specificity and biological memory, in: *Macromolecular Specificity and Biological Memory* (F. O. Schmidt, ed.), MIT Press, Cambridge, MA, pp. 1–6.

Schmidt, H. S., 1982, Pupillometric assessment of disorders of arousal, *Sleep* **5**:s157–s164.

Schmidt, H. S., 1983, L-Tryptophan in the treatment of impaired respiration in sleep, *Bull. Eur. Physiolpathol. Respir.* **19**:625–629.

Schmidt, H. S., and Knopp, W., 1972, Sleep in Parkinson's disease: The effect of L-DOPA, *Psychophysiology* **9**:88–89.

Schmidt, H. S., and Wise, H. A., 1981, Significance of impaired penile tumescence and associated polysomnographic abnormalities in the impotent patient, *J. Urol.* **126**:348–352.

Schneider, E., Maxion, H., Zeigler, B., and Jacobi, P., 1974, Das schlafverhalten von Parkinsonkranken und seine Beeinflussung durch L-DOPA, *J. Neurol.* **207**:95–108.

Schneider-Helmert, D., 1981, Interval therapy with L-tryptophan in severe chronic insomniacs, *Int. Pharmacopsychiatry* **16**:162–173.

Schneider-Helmert, D., 1984, Effects of DSIP on narcolepsy, *Eur. Neurol.* **23**:353–357.

Schneider-Helmert, D., 1985, Clinical evaluation of DSIP, in: *Sleep: Neurotransmitters and Neuromodulators* (A. Wauquier, J. M. Gaillard, J. M. Mouti, and M. Radulovacki, eds.), Raven Press, New York, pp. 279–289.

Schoen, L., Kramer, M., Anand, V. K., and Weisenberger, S., 1984, Efficacy of UPPP in patients with obstructive sleep apnea, *Sleep Res.* **13**:164.

Schoenenberger, G. A., Maier, P. F., Tobler, H. J., Wilson, K., and Monnier, M., 1978, The delta EEG (sleep)-inducing peptide (DSIP), *Pflugers Archiv.* **376**:119–129.

Schoenhuber, R. Angiari, P., and Peserico, L., 1981, Narcolepsy symptomatic of a pontine glioma, *Ital. J. Neurol. Sci.* **4**:379–380.

Schramm, M., Thomas, G., Towart, R., and Franckowiak, G., 1983, Novel dihydropyridines with positive inotropic action through activation of Ca^{2++} channels, *Nature* **303**:535–537.

Schulte, F. J., and Parmelee, A., 1970, Thyroid hormone and brain development. An analysis of polygraphic data of hypothyroid babies before and during treatment, *Electroencephalogr. Clin. Neurophysiol.* **29**:212.

Schulte, F. J., Karsen, J. H., Engelbart, S., Bell, E. F., Castell, R., and Lenard, H. G.,

1973, Sleep patterns in hyperphenylalaminia: A lesson serotonin learned from phenylketonurea, *Pediatr. Res.* **7**:588–599.

Schulte, W., 1971, Zum Problem der Provocation und Kupierung von Melancholischen Phasen, *Schweizer Arch. Neurol. Neurochem. Psychiatr.* **109**:427–435.

Schultz, H., and Trojan, B., 1979, A comparison of eye movement density in normal subjects and in depressed patients before and after remission, *Sleep Res.* **8**:49.

Schultz, H., Lund, R., Cording, C., and Dirlich, G., 1979, Bimodal distribution of REM sleep latencies in depression, *Biol. Psychiatry* **14**:595–600.

Schultz, M. A., Schulte, F. J., Akiyama, Y., and Parmelee, A., 1968, Development of electroencephalographic sleep phenomena in hypothyroid infants, *Electroencephalogr. Clin. Neurophysiol.* **25**:351–358.

Schultz, W., 1966, Kombinierte Psycho und Pharmakotherapie bei Melancholikem, in: *Probleme der Pharmakopsychiatrischen Kombinations und Langzeibehand-lung* (H. Krantz and N. Petrilowitsch, eds.), Karger, Basel, pp. 150–169.

Schwartz, M. A., and Postma, E., 1970, Metabolism of flurazepam, a benzodiazepine, in man and dog, *J. Pharmacol. Sci.* **59**:1800–1806.

Schwartz, B. A., and Rockemaure, J., 1973, Syndrome pickwickien: Traitement par la chlorimipramine, *Nouv. Presse Med.* **2**:1520.

Schwartz, R. D., Skolnick, P., Hollingsworth, E. B., and Paul, S. M., 1984, Barbiturate and picrotoxin-sensitive chloride efflux in rat cerebral cortical synaptoneurosomes, *Fed. Eur. Biochem. Soc.* **175**:193–196.

Schwartz, R. D., Jackson, J. A., Weigert, D., Skolnick, P., and Paul, S. M., 1985, Characterization of barbiturate-stimulated chloride efflux from rat brain synaptoneurosomes, *J. Neurosci.* **5**:2963–2970.

Schwartz, W. J., Morton, M. T., Williams, R. S., Tamarkin, L., Baker, T. L., and Dement, W. C., 1986, Circadian timekeeping in narcoleptic dog, *Sleep* **9**:120–125.

Schweitzer, P. K., Sugerman, J. L., and Walsh, J. K., 1986, The use of triazolam in simulated shift work: I. Effects on daytime sleep, *Sleep Res.* **15**:44.

Schweitzer, P. K., Chambers, G. W., Birkenmeier, N., and Walsh, J. K., 1987, Nasal continuous positive airway pressure (CPAP) compliance at six, twelve and eighteen months, *Sleep Res.* **16**: 186.

Scollo-Lavizzari, G., Pralle, W., and de la Cruz, N., 1975, Activation effects of sleep deprivation and sleep in seizure patients, *Eur. Neurol.* **13**:1–5.

Scrima, L., 1981, An etiology of narcolepsy–cataplexy and a proposed cataplexy neuromechanism, *Int. J. Neurosci.* **15**:69–86.

Scrima, L., Broudy, M., Nay, K. N., and Cohn, M. A., 1982, Increased severity of obstructive sleep apnea after bedtime alcohol ingestion: Diagnostic potential and proposed mechanism, *Sleep* **5**:318–328.

Scrima, L., Stedman, D., Thomas, E., Johnson, F., and Hiller, F. C., 1986, Arousals after alcohol ingestion in asymptomatic nocturnal myoclonus subjects, *Sleep Res.* **15**:168.

Seidel, W. F., Roth, T., Roehrs, T., Zorick, F., and Dement, W. C., 1984, Treatment of a 12-hour shift of sleep schedule with benzodiazepines, *Science* **224**:1262–1264.

Seitzinger, S. P., Pilson, M. E., and Nixon, S. W., 1983, Ethanol modulation of opiate receptors in cultured neural cells, *Science* **222**:1246–1250.

Semba, J., 1983, Effects of REM deprivation on the monoamine metabolism in various regions of the rat brain, *Seishin Shinkeigaku Zasshi* **85**:349–360.

Shaar, C. J., and Clemens, J. A., 1974, The role of catecholamines in the release of anterior pituitary prolactin *in vitro*, *Endocrinology* **95**:1202–1212.

Shafor, R., Kripke, D., Timms, R., Ancoli-Israel, S., and Mitler, M. M., 1986, Insomnia and leg movements in sleep: Another look, *Sleep Res.* **15**:169.

Shapiro, W. R., 1975, Treatment of cataplexy with clomipramine, *Arch. Neurol.* **32**:653–656.

Shaywitz, B. A., Finkelstein, J., Hellman, L., and Weitzman, E.D., 1971, Growth hormone in newborn infants during sleep–wake periods, *Pediatrics* **48**:103–109.

Shepard, J. W., Schweitzer, P. K., Keller, C. A., Chun, D. S., and Dolan, G. F., 1984, Myocardial stress, *Chest* **86**:366–374.

Sherman, L., Kim, S., Benjamin, F., and Kolodny, H., 1971, Effect of chlorpromazine on serum growth-hormone concentration in man, *N. Engl. J. Med.* **284**:71–74.

Sherrey, J. H., and Megirian, D., 1975, Analysis of the respiratory role of pharyngeal constrictor motorneurons of cat, *Exp. Neurol.* **49**:839–851.

Shindler, J., Schachter, M., Brincat, S., and Parkes, J. D., 1985, Amphetamine, mazindol, and fencamfamin in narcolepsy, *Br. Med. J.* **290**:167–170.

Shipley, J. E., Kumar, A., Eiser, A., Feinberg, M., Flegel, P., and Greden, J. F., 1986, Clinical, EEG sleep, and DST correlates of sleep onset REM periods, *Sleep Res.* **15**:97.

Shute, C. C. D., and Lewis, P. R., 1967, The ascending cholinergic reticular system: Neocortical, olfactory and subcortical projections, *Brain* **90**:497–520.

Siegel, J. M., and McGinty, D. J., 1977, Pontine reticular formation neurons: Relationship of discharge to motor activity, *Science* **196**:678–680.

Siegel, J. M., Fahringer, H., Tomaszewski, K. S., Kaitin, K., Kilduff, T., and Dement, W. C., 1986, Heart rate and blood pressure changes associated with cataplexy in canine narcolepsy, *Sleep* **9**:216–221.

Sifakis, C., 1982, *The Encyclopedia of American Crime*, Facts on File, New York, p. 312.

Siffre, M., 1975, six months alone in a cave, *National Geographic* **147**:426–435.

Silver, J., and Billiar, R. B., 1976, An autoradiographic analysis of [^{3}H] alpha-bungarotoxin distribution in the rat brain after intraventricular injection, *J. Cell Biol.* **71**:956–963.

Simmons, F. B., Guilleminault, C., and Silvestri, R., 1973, Snoring and some obstructive sleep apnea can be cured by oropharyngeal surgery, *Arch. Otolaryngol.* **109**:503–507.

Simon, S., Schiffer, M., Glick, S. M., and Schwartz, E., 1967, Effect of medroxyprogesterone acetate upon stimulated release of growth hormone in men, *J. Clin. Endocrinol.* **27**:1633–1636.

Sitaram, N., Wyatt, R. J., Dawson, S., and Gillin, J. C., 1976, REM sleep induction by physostigmine infusion during sleep in normal volunteers, *Science* **191**:1281–1283.

Sitaram, N., Mendelson, W. B., Wyatt, R. J., and Gillin, J. C., 1977, Time-dependent induction of REM sleep and arousal by physostigimine infusion during human sleep, *Brain Res.* **122**:562–567.

Sitaram, N., Gillin, J. C., and Bunney, W. E., Jr., 1978a, Circadian effects on the time of switch, clinical ratings, and sleep in bipolar patients, *Acta Psychiatr. Scand.* **58**:267–278.

Sitaram, N., Moore, A. M., and Gillin, J. C., 1978b Induction and resetting of REM sleep rhythm in normal man by arecoline: Blockade by scopolamine, *Sleep* **1**:83–90.

Sitaram, N., Moore, A. J., and Gillin, J. C., 1979, Scopolamine induced muscarinic supersensitivity in man: Changes in sleep, *Psychiatry Res.* **1**:9–16.

Sitaram, N., Nurnberger, J. I., Gershon, E. S., and Gillin, J. C., 1980, Faster cholinergic REM sleep induction in euthymic patients with primary affective illness, *Science* **208**:200–202.

Sitaram, N., Moore, A. M., Vanskiver, C., Blendy, J., Nurnberger, J. I., Gershon, E. S., and Gillin, J. C., 1981, Hypersensitive cholinergic functioning in primary affective illness, in: Cholinergic Mechanisms (G. Pepeu and H. Ladinsky, eds.), Plenum Press, New York, pp. 947–962.

Sitaram, N., Nurnberger, J. I., Gershon, E. S., and Gillin, J. C., 1982, Cholinergic regulation of mood and REM sleep: A potential model and marker for vulnerability to depression, *Am. J. Psychiatry* **139:**571–576.

Skatrud, J. B., Dempsey, J. A., and Kaiser, D. G., 1978, Ventilatory response to medroxyprogesterone acetate in normal subjects: Time course and mechanism, *J. Appl. Physiol.* **44:**939–944.

Skatrud, J. B., Dempsey, J. A., Iber, C., and Berssenbrugge, A., 1981, Correction of CO1² retention during sleep in patients with chronic obstructive pulmonary disease, *Am. Rev. Respir. Dis.* **124:**260–268.

Skolnick, P., Paul, S. M., and Marangos, P. J., 1979, Brain benzodiazepine levels following intravenous administration of 34-diazepam: Relationship to the potentiation of purinergic depression of central nervous system neurons, *Can. J. Physiol. Pharmacol.* **57:**1040–1042.

Skolnick, P., Paul, S. M., and Barker, J. L., 1980, Pentobarbital potentiates GABA-enhanced (³H)-diazepam binding to benzodiazepine receptors, *Eur. J. Pharmacol.* **65:**125–127.

Skolnick, P., Mendelson, W. B., and Paul, S. B., 1981a, Benzodiazepine receptors in the central nervous system, in: *Psychopharmacology of Sleep* (D. Wheatley, ed.), Raven Press, New York, pp. 117–134.

Skolnick, P., Paul, S., Crawley, J., Rice, K., Barber, S., Webber, R., and Cain M., 1981b, 3-Hydroxymethyl-B-carboline antagonizes some pharmacologic properties of diazepam, *Eur. J. Pharmacol.* **69:**525–527.

Skolnick, P., Moncada, V., Barber, J., and Paul, S., 1981c, Pentobarbital: Dual actions to increase brain benzodiazepine receptor affinity, *Science* **211:**1448–1450.

Skolnick, P., Schweri, M., Williams, E., Moncada, V., and Paul, S. M., 1982, An *in vitro* test which differentiates benzodiazepine agonists and antagonists, *Eur. J. Pharmacol.* **78:**133–136.

Slater, I. H., Jones, G. T., and Moore, R. A., 1978, Inhibition of REM sleep by fluoretine, a specific inhibitor of serotonin uptake, *Neuropharmacology* **17:**383–389.

Smallwood, R. G., Vitiello, M. V., Giblin, E. C., and Prinz, P. N., 1983, Sleep apnea: Relationship to age, sex, and Alzheimer's dementia, *Sleep* **6:**16–22.

Smith, J. W., Johnson, L. C., and Burdick, J. A., 1971, Sleep, psychological and clinical changes during alcohol withdrawal in NAD-treated alcoholics, *Q. J. Stud. Alcohol* **32:**982–994.

Smith, P. L., Hapouik, E. F., Allen, R. P., and Bleecker, E. R., 1983, The effects of protriptyline in sleep disordered breathing, *Am. Rev. Respir. Dis.* **127:**8–13.

Smith, R. C., 1985, Relationship of periodic movements in sleep (nocturnal myoclonus) and the Babinski sign, *Sleep* **8:**239–243.

Smythe, G. A., and Lazarus, L., 1974, Suppression of human growth hormone secretion by melatonin, and cyproheptadine, *J. Clin. Invest.* **54:**116–121.

Snyder, F., 1963, The new biology of dreaming, *Arch. Gen. Psychiatry* **8:**381–391.

Snyder, F., Hobson, J. A., Moneson, D. F., and Goldfrank, F., 1964, Changes in respiration, heart rate, and systolic blood pressure in human sleep, *J. Appl. Physiol.* **19:**417–422.

Snyder, F., 1968, Electroencephalographic studies of sleep in depression, in: *Computers and Electronic Devices in Psychiatry* (N. S. Kline and E. Lasha, eds.), Grune & Stratton, New York, pp. 272–301.

Snyder, F., 1969a, Dynamic aspects of sleep disturbance in relation to mental illness, *Biol. Psychiatry* **1:**119–130.

Snyder, F., 1969b, Disturbance of EEG sleep patterns in relation to acute psychosis, in: *Schizophrenia: Current Concepts and Research* (S. D. Sanker, ed.), PJD Publication, Hicksville, NY, pp. 751–724.

Snyder, F., 1972a, NIH studies of EEG sleep in affective illness, in: *Recent Advances in the Psychobiology of the Depressive Illnesses* (T. Williams, M. Katz, and J. Shields, eds.), DHEW, Washington, D.C., pp. 171–192.

Snyder, F., 1972b, Electroencephalographic studies of sleep in psychiatric disorders, in: *The Sleeping Brain* (M. H. Chase, ed.), Brain Information Research Institute, Los Angeles, pp. 376–393.

Snyder, S., 1972, Catecholamines and serotonin, in: *Basic Neurochemistry* (R. W. Albers, G. J. Siegel, R. Katzman, and B. W. Agranoff, eds.), Little, Brown, Boston, pp. 89–104.

Snyder, S., and Hams, G., 1982, Serotoninergic agents in the treatment of isolated sleep paralysis, *Am. J. Psychiatry* **139:**1202–1205.

Snyder, S., Karacan, I., and Salis, P. J., 1981, Effects of disulfiram on the sleep of chronic alcoholics, *Curr. Alcohol.* **8:**159–166.

Snyder, S., Karacan, I., Thornby, J., and Moore, C., 1984, Sleep patterns of sober chronic alcoholics, *Sleep Res.* **13:**182.

Snythe, G. A., and Lazarus, L., 1973, Growth hormone regulation by melatonin and serotonin, *Nature* **244:**230–231.

Souetre, E., Salvati, E., Pringuey, D., and Darcourt, G., 1985, Sleep and mood of depressed patients are improved by a phase advance process, presentation to Fourth World Congress of Biological Psychiatry, Sept. 8–13, Philadelphia, PA.

Soulairac, A., Schaub, C., Franchimont, P., Aymard, N., and Cauwienberge, H., 1968, Etude de l'activation pharmacologique du pole central de l'axe hypothalamohypophysaire, *Ann. Endocrinol.* **29:**45–54.

Sours, J. A., 1963, Narcolepsy and other disturbances in the sleep–waking rhythm: A study of 115 cases with review of the literature, *J. Nerv. Ment. Dis.* **137:**525–542.

Spielman, A. J., Saskin, P., and Thorpy, M. J., 1974, Sleep restriction therapy for chronic insomnia: Outcome as a function of pre-treatment total sleep time, *Sleep Res.* **13:**167.

Spielman, A. J., Saskin, P., and Thorpy, M. J., 1983, Sleep restriction treatment of insomnia, *Sleep Res.* **12:**286.

Spielman, A. J., Adler, J. M., Glovinsky, M. R., Pressmawn, M. R., Thorpy, M. J., Ellman, S. J., and Ackerman, K. D., 1986, Dynamics of REM sleep in narcolepsy, *Sleep* **9:**175–182.

Spielman, A. J., Saskin, P., and Thorpy, M. J., 1987, Treatment of chronic insomnia by restriction of time in bed. *Sleep* **10:**45–56.

Spiker, D. G., Foster, F. G., Coble, P., Love, D., and Kupfer, D. J., 1977, The sleep disorder in depressed alcoholics, *Sleep Res.* **6:**161.

Spiker, D. G., Coble, P., Cofsky, J., Foster, F. G., and Kupfer, D. J., 1978, EEG sleep and severity of depression, *Biol. Psychiatry* **13:**485–488.

Spilotis, B. E., August, G. P., Hung, W., Sonis, W., Mendelson, W. B., and Bercu, B. B., 1984, Growth hormone neurosecretory dysfunction, *JAMA* **251:**2223–2251.

Spinweber, C. L., and Johnson, L. C., 1982, Effects of triazolam (0.5 mg) on sleep, performance, memory and arousal threshold, *Psychopharmacology* **76:**5–12.

Spinweber, C. L., Ursin, R., Hilbert, R. P., and Hildebrand, R. L., 1983, L-Tryptophan: Effects on daytime sleep latency and the waking EEG, *Electroencephalogr. Clin. Neurophysiol.* **55:**652–661.

Spitz, I. M., Calderon, C., Gordon, C. R., Oksenberg, M., Ron, N., Laufer, N., and Livshin, Y., 1981, Dissociation between sleep-related and TRH-induced prolactin secretion in seminiferous tubule failure, *Metabolism* **31:**10–13.

Spooner, C. E., and Winters, W. D., 1965, Evidence for a direct action of monoamines on the chick central nervous system, *Experientia* **21:**256–258.

Squires, R., 1981, GABA receptors regulate the affinities of anions required for brain specific benzodiazepine binding, in: *GABA and Benzodiazepine Receptors* (E. Costa, G., Di-
Chara, G. Gessa, eds.), Raven Press, New York, pp. 129–138.

Squires, R. F., and Braestrup, C., 1977, Benzodiazepine receptors in rat brain, *Nature*
266:732–734.

Squires, R. F., Casoda, J. E., Richardson, M., and Saederup, E., 1982, (35s) *t*-Butylbicyclo-
phosphorothionate bind with high affinity to brain specific sites, *Mol. Pharmacol.*
23:326–336.

Stahl, S. M., Layzer, R. B., Aminoff, M. J., Townsend, J. J., and Feldon, S., 1980, Continuous cataplexy in a patient with a midbrain tumor: The limp man syndrome, *Neurology* **30**:1115–1119.

Starobinski, A., 1921, Un Cas de psychose maniaque-depressive à un jour d'alternance,
Ann. Med. Psychol. **11**:344–347.

Stein, D., Jouvet, M., and Pujol, J. F., 1974, Effects of alpha-methyl-para-tyrosine upon
cerebral amine metabolism and sleep states in the cat, *Brain Res.* **72**:360–365.

Steiner, E., Villen, T., Hallberg, M., and Rane, A., 1984, Amphetamine secretion in breast
milk, *Eur. J. Clin. Pharmacol.* **27**:123–124.

Steinmark, S. W., and Borkovec, T. D., 1974, Active and placebo treatment effects on
moderate insomnia under counterdemand and positive demand instructions, *J. Abnorm. Psychol.* **83**:157–163.

Stepanski, E., Lamphere, J., Badia, P., Zorick, F., and Roth, T., 1984, Sleep fragmentation
and daytime sleep, *Sleep* **7**:18–26.

Stern, E., Parmelee, A. H., Akiyama, Y., Schultz, M. A., and Wenner, W. H., 1969, Sleep
cycle characteristics in infants, *Pediatrics* **43**:65–70.

Stern, W. C., and Morgane, P. J., 1972, Effects of catecholamine and modulating drugs on
sleep in the cat, *Psychophysiology* **2**:86.

Stern, W. C., Forbes, W. B., Jalowiec, J. E., and Morgane, P. J., 1975a, Growth hormone
administration and sleep in the rat, presented at the Second International Sleep Research Congress, June 30–July 4, Edinburgh.

Stern, W. C., Miller, M., Resnick, O., and Morgane, P. J., 1975b, Distribution of [125]I-
labeled rat growth hormone in regional brain areas and peripheral tissue of the rat,
Am. J. Anat. **144**:503–507.

Stern, W. C., Miller, M., Jalowiec, J. E., Forbes, W. B., and Morgane, P. J., 1975c, Effects
of growth hormone on brain biogenic amine levels, *Pharmacol. Biochem. Behav.* **3**:1115–
1118.

Stern, W. C., Jalowiec, J. E., Shabskelowitz, H., and Morgane, P. J., 1975d, Effects of
growth hormone on sleep–waking patterns in cats, *Horm. Behav.* **6**:189–196.

Stewart, J. K., Clifton, D. K., Koerker, D. J., Rogol, A. D., Jaffe, T., and Goodner, C. J.,
1985, Pulsatile release of growth hormone and prolactin from the primate *in vitro*,
Endocrinology **116**:1–5.

Stiel, J. N., Island, D. P., and Liddle, G. W., 1970, Effect of glucorticoids on plasma
growth hormone in man, *Metabolism* **19**:158–164.

Stokes, J. A., and Harris, R. A., Alcohol and synaptosomal calcium transport, *Mol. Pharmacol.* **22**:99–104.

Stone, C. A., Wenger, H. C., Ludden, C. T., Stavorski, J. M., and Ross, C. A., 1981,
Antiserotonin–antihistaminic properties of cyproheptadine, *J. Pharmacol. Exp. Ther.*
131:73–84.

Stopa, E. G., King, J. C., Lydic, R., and Schoene, W. C., 1984, Human brain contains
vasopressin and vasoactive intestinal polypeptide neuronal subpopulations in the
SCN region, *Brain Res.* **297**:159–163.

Stotsky, B. A., Cole, J. O., Tang, Y. T., and Gahm, I. G., 1971, Sodium butabarbital (Butisol sodium) as an hypnotic agent for aged psychiatric patients with sleep disorders, *Am. Geriatr. Soc.* **19**:860–870.

Stoyva, J., and Metcalf, D., 1968, Sleep patterns following chronic exposure to cholinesterase-inhibiting organophosphate compounds, *Psychophysiology* **5**:206.

Strain, G. M., Olcott, B. M., Archer, R. M., and McClintock, B. K., 1984, Narcolepsy in a bull, *J. Am. Vet. Med. Assoc.* **185**:538–541.

Strohl, K. P., Hensley, M. J., Hallett, M., Saunders, N. A., and Ingram, R. H., 1980, Activation of upper airway muscles before onset of inspiration in normals, *J. Appl. Physiol.* **49**:638–642.

Strohl, K. P., Hensley, M. J., Saunders, N. A., Brown, R., and Ingram, R. H., 1981, Progesterone administration and progressive sleep apnea, *JAMA* **245**:1230–1232.

Strong, R., and Wood, G. W., 1984, Membrane properties and aging: *In vivo* and *in vitro* effects of ethanol on synaptosomal γ-aminobutyric acid (GABA) release, *J. Pharmacol. Exp. Ther.* **229**:726–730.

Sugerman, J. L., Stern, J., and Walsh, J., 1984, Waking function in psychophysiological and subjective insomnia, *Sleep Res.* **13**:169.

Sullivan, C. E., 1980, Breathing in sleep, in: *Physiology and Sleep* (J. Orem and C. D. Barnes, eds.), Academic Press, New York, pp. 214–272.

Sullivan, C. E., Murphy, E., Kozar, L. F., and Phillipson, E. A., 1979, Ventilatory responses to CO_2 and lung inflation in tonic versus phasic REM sleep, *J. Appl. Physiol.* **47**:1304–1310.

Sullivan, C. E., Issa, F. G., Berthon-Jones, M., and Eues, L., 1981, Reversal of obstructive sleep apnea by continous positive airway pressure applied through the nose, *Lancet* **1**:862–865.

Sullivan, C. E., Berthon-Jones, M., and Issa, F. G., 1983, Remission of severe obesity–hypoventilation syndrome after short-term treatment during sleep with nasal continous positive airway pressure, *Am. Rev. Respir. Dis.* **128**:177–181.

Sullivan, C. E., Issa, F. G., Bethon-Jones, M., McCauley, V. B., and Costal, L.J.V., 1984, Home treatment of obstructive sleep apnea with continuous positive airway pressure applied through a nose mask, *Bull. Eur. Physiopathol. Respir.* **20**:49–54.

Sultan, C., Amilhau, D., Descomps, B., Bonardet, A., Passouant, P., and Jean, R., 1980, La Secretion de prolactine pendant le sommeil en periode peripubertaire. Resultats preliminaires, *Ann. Biol. Clin.* **38**:157–160.

Sunshine, A., 1975, Comparison of the hypnotic activity of triazolam, flurazepam hydrochloride and placebo, *J. Clin. Pharmacol. Ther.* **5**:573–577.

Sutoo, D., and Sano, K., 1984, Modulating effects of biogenic amines on calcium and ethanol-induced sleeping time, *Alcohol* **1**:141–144.

Sutton, F. D., Zwillich, C. W., Creagh, C. E., Pierson, D. J., and Weil, J. V., 1975, Progesterone for outpatient treatment of Pickwickian syndrome, *Ann. Intern. Med.* **83**:476–479.

Suzdak, P. D., Schwartz, R. D., Skolnick, P., and Paul, S. M., 1986, Ethanol stimulates gamma-aminobutyric acid receptor-mediated chloride transport in rat brain synaptoneurosomes, *Proc. Natl. Acad. Sci. USA* **83**:4071–4075.

Svendsen, K., and Christensen, P. G., 1981, Duration of REM sleep latency as predictor of effect of anti-depressant therapy, *Acta Psychiatr. Scand.* **64**:238–243.

Sweeney, C. R., Hendricks, J. C., Beech, J., and Morrison, A. R., 1983, Narcolepsy in a horse, *J. Am. Vet. Med. Assoc.* **183**:126–128.

Symonds, C. P., 1953, Nocturnal myoclonus, *J. Neurol. Neurosurg. Psychiatry* **16**:166–171.

Taasan, U. C., Block, A. J., Boysen, P. G., and Wynne, J. W., 1981, Alcohol increases sleep apnea and oxygen desaturation in asymptomatic men, *Am. J. Med.* **71**:240–245.

Tabakoff, B., Ritzmann, R. F., and Boggan, W. O., 1975, Inhibition of the transport of 5-hydroxyindoleacetic acid from brain by ethanol, *J. Neurochem.* **24**:1043–1051.

Tabakoff, B., and Hoffman, P. L., 1983, Neurochemical aspects of tolerance to and physical dependence on alcohol, in: *The Biology of Alcoholism* (B. Kissin and H. Begleiter, eds.), Plenum Press, New York, p. 199.

Tabushi, K., and Himwich, H. E., 1971, Electroencephalographic study of the effects of methysergide on sleep in the rabbit, *Electroencephalogr. Clin. Neurophysiol.* **31**:491–497.

Takahashi, S., Kondo, H., Yoshimura, M., Ochi, Y., and Yoshimi, T., 1973, Growth hormone responses to administration of 1-5-hydroxytryptophan (1-5-HTP) in manic-depressive psychoses, *Folia Psychiatr. Neurol. Jpn.* **27**:197–205.

Takahashi, S., Kondo, S., Yoshimura, M., and Ochi, K., 1974, Growth hormone responses to administration of *l*-5-hydroxytryptophan (*l*-5-HTP) in manic-depressive psychosis, in: *Psychoneuroendocrinology* (Workshop Conf. Int. Soc. Psychoneuroendocrinology) (N. Hatotan and T. Mieken, eds.), Karger, Basel, pp. 32–38.

Takahashi, Y., 1974, Growth hormone secretion during sleep: A review, in: *Biological Rhythms in Neuroendocrine Activity* (M. Kawakami, ed.), Igaku-Shoin, Tokyo, pp. 316–325.

Takahashi, Y., Kipnis, D. M., and Daughaday, W. H., 1968, Growth hormone secretion during sleep, *J. Clin. Invest.* **47**:2079–2090.

Takebe, K., Kunita, H., Sawano, S., Horiuchi, Y., and Mashimo, K., 1969, Preliminary communications: Circadian rhythms of plasma growth hormone and cortisol after insulin, *J. Clin. Endocrinol. Metab.* **29**:1630–1633.

Talwalker, P. K., Ratner, A., and Meites, J., 1963, *In vitro* inhibition of pituitary prolactin synthesis and release of hypothalamic extract, *Am. J. Physiol.* **205**:213–218.

Tamarkin, L., Craig, C. J., Garrick, N. A., and Wehr, T. A., 1983, Effect of clorgyline (MAO type A inhibitor) on locomotor activity in the Syrian hamster, *Am. J. Physiol.* **245**:R215–R221.

Tan, T. L., Kales, J. D., Kales, A., Soldatos, C. R., and Bixler, E. O., 1984, Biopsychobehavioral correlates of insomnia, IV: Diagnosis based on DSM-III, *Am. J. Psychiatry* **141**:357–363.

Tanner, J. M., 1972, Human growth hormone, *Nature* **237**:433–439.

Tanner, J. M., Whitehouse, R. H., Hughes, P.C.R., and Vince, F. P., 1971, Effect of human growth hormone treatment for 1 to 7 years on growth of 100 children, with growth hormone deficiency, low birthweight, inherited smallness, Turner's syndrome and other complaints, *Arch. Dis. Child.* **46**:745–782.

Tansella, M., Zimmermann-Tansella, A., and Lader, M., 1974, The residual effects of N-desmethyldiazepam in patients, *Psychopharmacologia* **38**:81–90.

Tarter, R. E., and Edwards, K. L., 1985, Neuropsychology of alcoholism, in: *Alcohol and the Brain: Chronic Effects* (R. E. Tarter and D. H. Van Thiel, eds.), Plenum, NY, pp. 217–244.

Taub, J. M., and Berger, R. J., 1973, Sleep stage patterns associated with acute shifts in the sleep–wake cycle, *Electroencephalogr. Clin. Neurophysiol.* **35**:613–619.

Taub, J. M., Hawkins, D. R., and Van de Castle, R. L., 1978, Electrographic analysis of the sleep cycle in young depressed patients, *Biol. Psychol.* **7**:203–214.

Taub, J. M., 1982, Sleep pattern variation as a function of age in affective disorders, *Int. J. Neurosci.* **17**:219–232.

Telsted, W., Sorensen, O., Larsen, S., Lillevold, P. E., Stensrud, P., and Nyberg-Hansen, R., 1984, Treatment of the restless legs syndrome with carbamazepine: A double blind study, *Br. Med. J.* **288**:444–446.

Tenen, S. S., and Hirsch, J. D., 1980, Beta-carboline-3-carboxylate antagonizes diazepam activity, *Nature* **288**:609–610.

Tepas, D. I., 1982, Adaptation, to shiftwork: Fact or fallacy? *J. Human Ergon.* **11**:1–12.

Tepas, D. I., Walsh, J. K., and Armstrong, D. R., 1981a, Comprehensive study of the sleep of shift workers, in: *Biological Rhythms, Sleep and Shift Work: Advances in Sleep Research* (L. C. Johnson et al. eds.), Spectrum, New York, pp. 347–356.

Tepas, D.I., Walsh, J.K., Moss, P.O., and Armstrong, D., 1981b, Polysomnographic correlates of shift worker performance in the laboratory, *Adv. Biosciences* **301**:179–186.

Thase, M. E., Himmelhoch, J. M., Mallinger, A. G., Jarrett, D. B., and Kupfer, D. J., 1986, EEG sleep and DST findings in anergic bipolar depression, presentation at Society of Biological Psychiatry, 41st annual convention, May 7–11, Washington, D.C.

Thomson, G., 1985, The mode of inheritance of the HLA-linked gene predisposing to narcolepsy, *Tissue Antigens* **26**:201–203.

Thoresen, C. E., Coates, T. J., Kirmil-Gray, K., and Rosekind, M. R., 1978, Treating insomnia: A self-management approach, *Sleep Res.* **7**:252.

Thoresen, C. E., Rosekind, M. R., Burnett, K. F., Stavosky, J., Jacobsen, S., Dexter, G., and Miles, L., 1981a, Ambulatory physiological monitoring in the natural environment of normal and sleep disturbed subjects with latency, maintenance, and combined complaints, *Sleep Res.* **10**:237.

Thoresen, C. E., Coates, T. J., Kirmil-Gray, K., and Rosekind, M. R., 1981b, Behavioral self-management in treating sleep-maintenance insomnia, *J. Behav. Med.* **4**:41–52.

Thorpy, M. J., Sher, A., and Spielman, A. J., 1984a, Uvulo-palato-pharyngoplasty (UPPP) for obstructive sleep apnea: II. Early results, *Sleep Res.* **13**:171.

Thorpy, M. J., Sher, A., and Spielman, A. J., 1984b, Uvulo-palato-pharyngoplasty for obstructive sleep apnea: III. Follow-up response, *Sleep Res.* **13**:172.

Ticku, M. K., and Olsen, R. W., 1978, Interaction of barbiturates with dihydropicortonin-binding sites related to the GABA receptor-ionophore system, *Life Sci.* **22**:1643–1652.

Tietz, E. I., Chiu, T. H., and Rosenberg, H. C., 1985, Pre- versus postsynaptic localization of benzodiazepine and B-carboline binding sites, *J. Neurochem.* **44**:1524–1534.

Tilley, A. J., Wilkenson, R. T., Warren, P.S.G., Watson, W. B., and Drud, M., 1982, The sleep and performance of shift workers, *Hum. Factors* **24**:629–641.

Timms, R. M., 1982, Sexual dysfunction and chronic obstructive pulmonary disease, *Chest* **81**:398–399.

Tissot, R., 1965, The effects of certain drugs on the sleep cycles in man, in: *Progress in Brain Research* (K. Akert, C. Bally, and J. P. Schade, eds.), Elsevier, New York, pp. 175–177.

Tobler, I., and Borbely, A. A., 1980, Effect of delta sleep inducing peptide (DSIP) arginine vasotocin (AUT) on sleep and motor activity in the rat, *Waking Sleeping* **4**:139–153.

Tobler, I., and Borbely, A., 1982, Sleep regulation after reduction of brain serotonin: Effect of *p*-chlorophenylalanine combined with sleep deprivation in the rat, *Sleep* **5**:145–153.

Torda, C., 1967, Effect of serotonin depletion on sleep in rats, *Brain Res.* **6**:375–377.

Torda, C., 1968, Contribution to serotonin theory of dreaming (LSD infusion) *NY State J. Med.* **68**:1135–1138.

Torsvall, L., Akerstedt, T., and Gillberg, M., 1981, Age, sleep, and irregular work hours: A field study with EEG recording, catecholamine excretion, and self-ratings, *Scand. J. Work Envir. Health* **7**:196–203.

Touchon, J., Besset, A., Baldy-Moulinier, M., Billiard, M., Uziel, A., and Passouant, P., 1981, Aspects electrophysiologiques de l'epilepsie ethylique, *Rev. Electroenceph. Neurophysiol. Clin.* **11**:514–519.

Touchon, J., Billiard, M., Besset, A., De Lustrac, C., and Moulinier, M., 1984, Sleep organization in alcoholic epilepsy, *Sleep Res.* **13**:183.

Toyoda, J., 1964, The effects of chlorpromazine and imipramine on the human nocturnal sleep electroencephalogram, *Folia Psychiatr. Neurol. Jpn.* **18**:198–221.

Toyoda, J., Saraki, K., and Kurihara, M., 1966, A polygraphic study on the effect of atropine on human nocturnal sleep, *Folia Psychiatr. Neurol. Jpn.* **20**:275–289.

Trenchard, D., and Meanock, C., 1982, Obstructive apnea and paradoxical rib cage movements induced by diaphragm pacing: A probable mechanism and suggestions for treatment, *Am. Rev. Respir. Dis.* **125**:784–785.

Trulson, M. E., 1985, Dietary tryptophan does not alter the function of brain serotonin neurons, *Life Sci.* **37**:1067–1072.

Trulson, M. E., and Sampson, H. U., 1986, Ultrastructural changes of the liver following L-tryptophan ingestion in rats, *J. Nutr.* **116**:1109–1115.

Trzepacz, P. T., Violette, E. J., and Sateia, M. J., 1984, Response to opiods in three patients with restless legs syndrome, *Am. J. Psychiatry* **141**:993–995.

Tsuda, K., Sakurai, H., Seino, Y., Seino, S., Tanigawa, Tanigawa, K., Kuzuya, H., and Imura, H., 1981, Somatostatin-like immunoreactivity in human peripheral plasma following affinity chromatography, *Diabetes* **30**:471–474.

Tufik, S., 1981, Changes in response to dopaminergic drugs in rats submitted to REM-sleep deprivation, *Psychopharmacology* **72**:257–260.

Tune, G. S., 1969, Sleep and wakefulness in a group of shift workers, *Br. J. Ind. Med.* **26**:54–58.

Turek, F. W., and Losee-Olson, S., 1986, A benzodiazepine used in the treatment of insomnia phase-shifts the mammalian circadian clock, *Nature* **321**:167–168.

Turkington, R. W., 1972, Prolactin secretion in patients, treated with various drugs, *Arch. Intern. Med.* **130**:349–354.

Tusiewicz, K., Moldofsky, H., Bryan, A. C., and Bryan, M. H., 1977, Mechanics of the rib cage and diaphragm during sleep, *J. Appl. Physiol.* **43**:600–602.

Tyler, D. B., 1955, Psychological changes during experimental sleep deprivation, *Dis. Nerv. Syst.* **16**:293–299.

Uchizono, K., Inoni, S., Iriki, M., Ishikawa, M., Komoda, Y., and Nagasaki, H., 1975, Purification of the sleep-promoting substances from sleep-deprived rat brain, in: *Peptides: Chemistry, Structure and Biology* (R. Walker and J. Memhofer, eds.), Ann Arbor Publishers, Ann Arbor, pp. 667–671.

Uchizono, K., Higashi, A., Iriki, M., Nagasaki, H., Ishikawa, M., Komoda, Y., Inone, S., and Honda, K., 1978, Sleep-promoting fractions obtained from brain stem of sleep-deprived rats, in *Integrative Control Functions of the Brain*, Vol. 1 (M. Ito, ed.), Elsevier, Amsterdam, pp. 392–396.

Underwood, L. E., 1984, Report of the conference on uses and possible abuses of biosynthetic human growth hormone, *N. Engl. J. Med.* **311**:606–608.

Underwood, L. E., Azumi, K., Voina, S. J., and Van, Wyk J. J., 1971, Growth hormone levels during sleep in normal and growth-hormone deficient children, *Pediatrics* **48**:946–954.

Ungerstedt, U., 1971, Stereotaxic mapping of the monoamine pathways in the rat brain, *Acta Physiol. Scand. (Suppl.)* **367**:1–48.

Ursin, R., 1972, Differential effect of para-chlorophenylalanine on the two slow wave stages in the cat, *Acta Physiol. Scand.* **86**:278–285.

Valley, V., and Broughton, R., 1981, Daytime performance deficits and physiological vigilance in patients with narcolepsy–cataplexy compared to controls, *Rev. EEG Neurophysiol.* **11**:133–139.

Valley, V., and Broughton, R., 1983, The physiological (EEG) nature of drowsiness and its relation to performance deficits in narcoleptics, *Electroencephalogr. Clin. Neurophysiol.* **55**:243–251.

Valzelli, L., Bernasconi, S., and Dalessandro, M., 1983, Time courses of p-CPA-induced depletion of brain serotonin and muricidal aggression in the rat, *Pharmacol. Res. Commun.* **15**:387–395.

Van Bemmel, A. L., and Van den Hoofdakker, R. H., 1981, Maintenance of therapeutic effects of total sleep deprivation by limitation of subsequent sleep, *Acta Psychiatr. Scand.* **63**:453–462.

Van Cauter, E., L'Hermite, M., Copinschi, G., Refetoff, S., Desir, D., and Robyn, C., 1981, Quantitative analysis of spontaneous variations of plasma prolactin in normals, *Am. J. Physiol.* **241**:355–363.

Van Cauter, E., Desir, D., Refetoff, S., Spire, J. P., Noel, P., L'Hermite, M., and Robyn, C., 1982, The relationship between episodic variations of plasma prolactin and REM–non-REM cyclicity is an artifact, *J. Clin. Endocrinol. Metab.* **54**:70–75.

Van den Burg, W., and Van den Hoofdakker, R., 1975a, Total sleep deprivation on endogenous depression, *Arch. Gen. Psychiatry* **32**:1121–1125.

Van den Burg, W., and Van den Hoofdakker, R.H., 1975b, Two nights of total sleep deprivation as an antidepressive treatment, in: *Sleep 1974* (P. Levin and W.P. Koella, eds.), Karger, New York, pp. 478–481.

Van den Hoed, J., Lucas, E. A., and Dement, W. C., 1973, Hallucinatory experiences during cataplexy in patients with narcolepsy, *Am. J. Psychiatry* **136**:1210–1212.

Van den Hoofdakker, R. H., Beersma, D. G. M., Bouhuys, A. L., and Dols, L. C. W., 1985, Effects of total sleep deprivation on mood and chronophysiology in depression (Abstr. 206.4), *Fourth World Congress of Biological Psychiatry*, Society for Biological Psychiatry, Philadelphia, 124.

Van Loon, G. R., 1973, Brain catecholamines and ACTH secretion, in: *Frontiers in Neuroendocrinology* (W. F. Ganong and L. Martini, eds.), Oxford University Press, New York, pp. 209–247.

Van Praag, H. M., 1984, In search of the mode of action of antidepressants: 5-HTP/tyrosine mixtures in depression, in: *Frontiers in Biochemical and Pharmacological Research in Depression* (E. Usdin, ed.), Raven Press, New York, pp. 301–314.

Van Riezen, H., 1972, Different central effects of 5-HT antagonists mianserine and cyproheptadine, *Arch. Int. Pharmacodyn. Ther.* **198**:256–269.

Vanhaelst, L., Van Cauter, E., Degaute, J. P., and Golstein, J., 1972, Circadian variations of serum thyrotropin levels in man, *J. Clin. Endocrinol. Metab.* **35**:479–482.

Vanhaelst, L., Golstein, J., Van Cauter, E., L'Hermite, M., and Robyn, C., 1973, Etude simultanee des varitations circadiennes des taux sanguins de la thyreotriping (THS) et de la prolactine hypophysaires chez l'homme, *Compt. Rend. Acad. Sci. (Paris)* **276**:1875–1877.

Vanhoutte, P. M., and Paoletti, R., 1987, The WHO classification of calcium antagonists, *Trends in Pharmacol. Sci.* **8**:4–5.

Vaughan, T., Wyatt, R. J., and Green, R., 1972, Changes in REM sleep of chronically anxious depressed patients given alpha-methyl-paratyrosine (AMPT) *Psychophysiology* **9**:96.

Velluci, S. V., 1984, Chlordiazepoxide-induced potentiation of hexobarbitone sleeping time is reduced by ACTH, *Pharmacol. Biochem. Behav.* **21**:39–41.

Vernikos-Danellis, J, and Winget, C. M., 1979, The importance of light, postural and social cues in the regulation of the plasma cortisol rhythms in man, in: *Chronopharmacology* (A. Reinberg and F. Halbert, eds.), Pergamon Press, New York, pp. 101–106.

Vespignani, H., Barroche, G., Escaillas, J. P., and Weber, M., 1984, Importance of mazindol in the treatment of narcolepsy, *Sleep* **7**:274–275.

Vigneri, R., and D'Agata, R., 1971, Growth hormone release during the first year of life in relation to sleep–wake periods, *J. Clin. Endocrinol. Metab.* **33**:561–563.

Vincent, J. D., Favarel-Garriogues, J.,Bourgeois, M., and Dugy, B., 1968, Night sleep of the schizophrenic at the start of evolution (trans.), *Ann. Med. Psychol. (Paris)* **2**:227–235.

Vitiello, M. V., Prinz, P. N., and Halter, J. B., 1983, Sodium-restricted diet increases nighttime plasma norepinephrine and impairs nighttime sleep patterns in man, *J. Clin. Endocrinol. Metab.* **56**:553–556.

Vogel, G. W., 1968, REM deprivation. III. Dreaming and psychosis, *Arch. Gen. Psychiatry* **18**:312–329.

Vogel, G. W., 1975, A review of REM sleep deprivation, *Arch. Gen. Psychiatry* **32**:749–761.

Vogel, G. W., 1979, REM sleep and the prevention of endogenous depression, *Waking Sleeping* **3**:313–318.

Vogel, G. W., 1983, Evidence for REM sleep deprivation as the mechanism of action of antidepressant drugs, *Prog. Neuropsychopharmacol. Biol. Psychol.* **7**:343–349.

Vogel, G. W., 1986, REM and depression, presented at International Symposium on the Neurobiology of Sleep/Wakefulness Cycle, May 28–31, 1986, Tbilisi, Georgia, USSR.

Vogel, G. W., and Traub, A. C., 1968a, REM deprivation. I. The effect on schizophrenic patients, *Arch. Gen. Psychiatry* **18**:287–300.

Vogel, G. W., and Traub, A. C., 1968b, Further studies on REM deprivation of depressed patients, *Psychophysiology* **5**:239.

Vogel, G. W., Traub, A. C., and Ben-Horin, P., 1968, REM deprivation, II: The effects on depressed patients, *Arch. Gen. Psychiatry* **18**:301–311.

Vogel, G. W., Hickman, S., Thurmond, J., and Barrowclough, A., 1971, The effect of Dalmane (flurazepam) on the sleep cycle of good and poor sleepers, paper presented at Annual Meeting of the Psychophysiological Study of Sleep, June 3–5.

Vogel, G. W., Rudman, A., Thurmond, A., Barrowclough, B., Seisler, D., and Hickman, J., 1972, Human growth hormone and slow-wave sleep, *Psychophysiology* **9**:102.

Vogel, G. W., Thompson, F. C., Jr., Thurmond, A., and Rivers, B., 1973, The effect of REM deprivation on depression, *Psychosomatics* **14**:104–107.

Vogel, G. W., Thurmond, S., Gibbons, P., Sloan, K., and Walker, M., 1975a, REM sleep reduction effects on depression syndromes, *Arch. Gen. Psychiatry* **32**:765–777.

Vogel, G. W., Thurmond, A., Gibbons, P., Edwards, K., Sloan, K. B., and Sexton, K., 1975b, The effects of triazolam on the sleep of insomniacs, *J. Psychopharmacol.* **41**:65–69.

Vogel, G. W., Barker, K., Gibbons, P., and Thurmond, A., 1976, A comparison of the effects of flurazepam 30 mg and triazolam 0.5 mg on the sleep of insomniacs, *J. Psychopharmacol.* **47**:81–86.

Vogel, G. W., Vogel, F., McAbee, R. S., and Thurmond, A. J., 1980, Improvement of depression by REM sleep deprivation, *Arch. Gen. Psychiatry* **37**:247–253.

Vogel, J., Beer, B., and Clody, D., 1971, A simple and reliable conflict procedure for testing anti-anxiety agents, *Psychopharmacology* **21**:1–7.

Volk, S., Simon, O., Schultz, H., Hansert, E., and Wilde-frenz, J., 1984, The structure of wakefulness and its relationship to daytime sleep in narcoleptic patients, *Electroencephalogr. Clin. Neurophysiol.* **57**:119–128.

Voloschin, L. M., and Tramezzani, J. H., 1984, Relationship of prolactin release in lactating rats to mild ejection, sleep state, and ultrasonic vocalization, *Endocrinology* **114**:618–623.

Von Economo, C., 1929, Schlaftheorie, *Ergeb. Physiol.* **28**:312–339.

Wagman, A. M. I., and Allen, R. P., 1974, Effects of alcohol ingestion and abstinence on slow wave sleep of alcoholics, *Adv. Exp. Med. Biol.* **59**:453–466.

Wagner, D. R., Pollak, C. P., and Weitzman, E. D., 1983, Nocturnal nasal-airway pressure for sleep apnea, *N. Engl. J. Med.* **308**:461–462.

Waldhorn, R. E., 1985, Sleep apnea syndrome, *Am. Family Physician* **32**:149–166.

Walsh, J. K., Tepas, D. I., and Moss, P. D., 1981, The EEG sleep of night and rotating shift workers, in: *Biological Rhythms, Sleep, and Shift Work: Advances in Sleep Research* (L. C. Johnson *et al.*, eds.), Spectrum, New York, pp. 371–381.

Walsh, J. K., Smitson, S. A., and Kramer, M., 1982, Sleep-onset REM sleep: Comparison of narcoleptic and obstructive sleep apnea patients, *Clin. Electroencephalogr.* **13**:57–60.

Walsh, J. K., Muehlbach, M. J., and Schweitzer, P. K., 1984, Acute administration of triazolam for the daytime sleep of rotating shift workers, *Sleep* **7**:223–229.

Walsh, J. K., Sugerman, J. L., Schweitzer, P. K., and Duntley, S., 1986, The use of triazolam in simulated shift work: II. Physiological sleep tendency and performance, *Sleep Res.* **15**:46.

Wambebe, C., 1983, Influence of some GABAergic agents on nitrazepam-induced sleep in the domestic fowl (*Gallus domesticus*), *Nippon Yakurigaku Zasshi* **33**:1111–1118.

Ware, J., 1841, Treatment of delirium tremens, *Med. Commun. Mass. Med. Sci.* **6**:175–182.

Ware, J. C., 1983, Tricyclic antidepressants in the treatment of insomnia, *J. Clin. Psychiatry* **44**:25–28.

Wasserman, M. D., Pollak, C. P., Spielman, A. J., and Weitzman, E. D., 1980, Theoretical and technical problems in the measurement of nocturnal penile tumescence for the differential diagnosis of impotence, *Psychosom. Med.* **42**:575–585.

Watson, R., Hartmann, E., and Schildkraut, J. J., 1972, Amphetamine withdrawal: Affective state, sleep patterns, and MHPG excretion, *Am. J. Psychiatry* **129**:263–269.

Wauquier, A., 1983, Drug effects on sleep–wakefulness patterns in dogs, *Neuropsychobiology* **10**:60–64.

Webb, W. B., 1983, Are there permanent effects of night shift work on sleep? *Biol. Psychol.* **16**:273–283.

Webb, W. B., and Agnew, H. W., 1970, Sleep stage characteristics of long and short sleepers, *Science* **168**:146–147.

Webb, W. B., and Agnew, H. W., 1971, Stage 4 sleep: Influence of time course variables, *Science* **174**:1354–1356.

Webb, W. B., and Agnew, H. W., 1972, Sleep and waking in an environment free of time cues, *Psychophysiology* **9**:133.

Webb, W. B., and Agnew, H. W., 1973, Effects on performance of high and low energy expenditure during sleep deprivation, *Percept. Mot. Skills* **37**:511–514.

Webb, W. B., and Agnew, H. W., 1974, The effects of chronic limitation of sleep length, *Psychophysiology* **11**:265–274.

Webb, W. B., and Agnew, H. W., 1975, Sleep efficiency for sleep–wake cycles of varied length, *Psychophysiology* **12**:637–641.

Webb, W. B., and Friel, J., 1971, Sleep stage and personality characteristics of "natural" long and short term sleepers, *Science* **171**:587–588.

Webster, B. R., Guansing, A. R., and Paice, J. C., 1972, Absence of diurnal variation of serum TSH, *J. Clin. Endocrinol. Metab.* **34**:899–901.

Weeke, J., 1973, Circadian variation of the serum thyrotropin level in normal subjects, *Scand. J. Clin. Lab. Invest.* **31**:337–342.

Weeke, J., and Gundersen, H. J. G., 1978, Circadian and 30 minute variations in serum TSH and thyroid hormones in normal subjects, *Acta Endocrinol.* **89**:659–672.

Weeke, J., Hansen, A. P., and Lundek, K., 1975, Inhibition by somatostatin of basal levels of serum thyrotropin (TSH) in normal men, *J. Clin. Endocrinol. Metab.* **41**:168.

Wehr, T. A., and Goodwin, F. K., 1983, Introduction, in: *Circadian Rhythms in Psychiatry* (T. A. Wehr and F. K. Goodwin, eds.), Boxwood Press, Pacific Grove, CA, pp. 1–15.

Wehr, T. A., and Wirz-Justice, A., 1982, Circadian rhythm mechanisms in affective illness and in anti-depressant drug action, *Pharmacopsychiatry* **15**:31–39.

Wehr, T. A., Wirz-Justice, A., Goodwin, F. K., Duncan, W., and Gillin, J. C., 1979, Phase-advance of the circadian sleep–wake cycle as an antidepressant, *Science* **206**:710–713.

Wehr, T. A., Muscattola, G., and Goodwin, F. K., 1980, Urinary MHPG circadian rhythm: Early timing (phase advance) in manic-depressives compared with normal subjects, *Arch. Gen. Psychiatry* **37**:257–266.

Wehr, T. A., Goodwin, F. K., Wirz-Justice, A., Breitmaier, J., and Craig, C., 1982, 48-hour sleep–wake cycles in manic-depressive illness, *Arch. Gen. Psychiatry* **39**:559–565.

Wehr, T. A., Gillin, J. C., and Goodwin, F. K., 1983, Sleep and circadian rhythms in depression, in: *New Perspectives in Sleep Research* (M. Chase, ed.), Spectrum, Jamaica, New York, pp. 195–225.

Weiner, N., 1980, Drugs that inhibit adrenergic nerves and block adrenergic receptors, in: *The Pharmacological Basis of Therapeutics* (A. G. Gilman, L. S. Goodman and A. Gilman, eds.), Macmillan, New York, pp. 176–210.

Weiss, M. F., 1973, The treatment of insomnia through the use of electrosleep: An EEG study, *Sleep Res.* **2**:174.

Weitzman, E. D., Goldmacher, D., Kripke, D., MacGregor, P., Kream, J., and Hellman, L., 1968a, Reversal of sleep–waking cycle: Effect on sleep stage pattern and certain neuroendocrine rhythms, *Trans. Am. Neurol. Assoc.* **93**:153–157.

Weitzman, E. D., Rapport, M. M., McGregor, P., and Jacobs, J., 1968b, Sleep patterns of the monkey and brain serotonin concentration: Effect of p-chlorophenylalanine, *Science* **160**:1361–1363.

Weitzman, E. D., McGregor, P., Moore, C., and Jacobs, J., 1969, The effects of alpha-methylparatyrosine on sleep patterns of the monkey, *Life Sci.* **8**:751–757.

Weitzman, E. D., Kripke, D. F., Goldmacher, D., McGregor, P., and Nogeire, C., 1970, Acute reversal of the sleep-waking cycle in man, *Arch. Neurol.* **22**:483–489.

Weitzman, E. D., Fukushima, D., Nogeire, C., Roffwarg, H., Gallagher, T. F., and Hellman, L., 1971, Twenty-four hour pattern of the episodic secretion of cortisol in normal subjects, *J. Clin. Endocrinol.* **33**:14–22.

Weitzman, E. D., Perlow, M., Sassin, F. J., Fukushima, D., Burack, B., and Hellman, L., 1972, Persistence of the twenty-four hour pattern of episodic cortisol secretion and growth hormone release in blind subjects, *Trans. Am. Neurol. Assoc.* **97**:197–199.

Weitzman, E. D., Nogeire, C., Perlow, M., Fukushima, D., Sassin, J., McGregor, P., and Gallagher, T. F., 1974, *J. Clin. Endocrinol.* **38**:1018–1030.

Weitzman, E. D., deGraaf, A. S., Sassin, J. F., Hansen, T., Gotligsen, O.B., Perlow, M., and Hellman L., 1975, Seasonal patterns of sleep stages and secretion of cortisol and growth hormone during 24 hour periods in northern Norway, *Acta Endocrinol.* **78**:65–76.

Weitzman, E. D., Czeisler, C. A., and Moore-Ede, M. C., 1979, Sleep–wake, neuroendocrine and body temperature circadian rhythms under entrained and non-entrained (free-running) conditions in man, in: *Biological Rhythms and Their Central Mechanisms* (M. Suda, O. Hayaishi, and H. Nakagawa, eds.), Biomedical Press, Elsevier/North-Holland, pp. 199–227.

Weitzman, E. D., Czeisler, C. A., Zimmerman, J. C., and Ronda, J. M., 1980, Timing of REM and stages 3 and 4 sleep during temporal isolation in man, *Sleep* **2**:391–407.

Weitzman, E. D., Czeisler, C. A., Coleman, R. M., Spielman, A. J., Zimmerman, J. C., and Dement, W., 1981, Delayed sleep phase syndrome: A chronobiological disorder with sleep-onset insomnia, *Arch. Gen. Psychiatry* **38**:737–746.

Weldon, V. W., Gupta, S. K., Hamond, M. W., Paliara, A. S., Jacobs, L. S., and Daughaday, W. H., 1973, The use of L-DOPA in the diagnosis of hyposomatotropism in children, *J. Clin. Endocrinol. Metab.* **36**:42–46.

Wells, W., 1898, Some nervous and mental manifestations occurring in connection with nasal disease, *Am. J. Med. Sci.* **116**:677–682.

Westlund, K. N., Denney, R. M., Kochersperger, L. M., Rose, R. M., and Abell, C. W., 1985, Distinct monoamine oxidase A and B populations in primate brain, *Science* **234**:181–183.

Westphal, C., 1877, Eigenthumliche mit Einschlafen verbundene Anflle, *Arch. Psychiatry* **7**:631–625.

Wetterberg, L., Arendt, J., Paunier, L., Sionenko, P. C., van Donselar, W., and Heyden, T., 1976, Human serum melatonin changes during the menstrual cycle, *J. Clin. Endocrinol. Metab.* **42**:185–188.

Wever, R., 1964, Ein Mathematisches modell fur biologische Schwingungen, *Z. Tierpsychol.* **21**:359–372.

Wever, R., 1975,The circadian multi-oscillatory system of man, *Int. J. Chronobiol.* **3**:19–55.

Wever, R. A., 1979, *The Circadian System of Man: Results of Experiments under Temporal Isolation*, Springer-Verlag, New York, pp. 1–276.

White, D. P., Zwillich, C. W., Pickett, C. K., Douglas, N. J., Findley, L. J., and Weil, J. V., 1982, Central sleep apnea: Improvement with acetazoamide therapy, *Arch. Int. Med.* **142**:1816–1819.

Whybrow, P. C., and Prange, A. J., 1981, A hypothesis of thyroid–catecholamine–receptor interaction, *Arch. Gen. Psychiatry* **38**:106–113.

Williams, D. L., MacLean, A. W., and Cairns, J., 1983, Dose-response effects of ethanol on the sleep of young women, *J. Stud. Alcohol* **44**:515–523.

Williams, H. L., and Salamy, A., 1972, Alcohol and sleep, in: *The Biology of Alcoholism*, vol. 2 (B. Kissin and H. Begleiter, eds.), Plenum Press, New York/London, pp. 435–4830.

Williams, H. L., Lubin, A., and Goodnow, J. J., 1959, Impaired performance with acute sleep loss, *Psychol. Monogr.* **73**:1–26.

Williams, H. L., Lester, B. K., and Coulter, J. D., 1969, Monoamines and the EEG stages of sleep, *Acta Nerv. Super.* **11**:188–192.

Williams, R. L., Karacan, I., and Hursch, C. J., 1974, *EEG of Human Sleep: Clinical Applications*, Wiley, New York.

Williamson, M. J., Paul, S. M., and Skolnick, P., 1978, Demonstration of [³H]diazepam binding to benzodiazepine receptors *in vivo*, *Life Sci.* **28**:1935–1940.

Willumeit, H. P., Ott, H., and Neubert, W., 1984, Simulated car driving as a useful technique for the determination of residual effects and alcohol interaction after short- and long-acting benzodiazepines, in: *Sleep, Benzodiazepines, and Performance* (I. Hindmarch, H. Ott, and T. Roth, eds.), Springer-Verlag, Berlin, pp. 182–192.

Wilson, R., Raynal, S., Guilleminault, C., Zarcone, V., and Dement, W., 1973, REM sleep latencies in daytime sleep recordings of narcoleptics, *Sleep Res.* **2**:166.

Wirz-Justice, A., Puringer, W., and Hole, G., 1976, Sleep deprivation and clomipramine in endogenous depression, *Lancet* **2**:912.

Wirz-Justice, A., Kafka, M. S., Naber, D., and Wehr, T. A., 1980a, Circadian rhythms in rat brain alpha and beta-adrenergic receptors are modified by chronic imipramine, *Life Sci.* **27**:341–347.

Wirz-Justice, A., Wehr, T. A., Goodwin, F. K., Kafka, M. S., Naber, D., Marangos, P. J., and Campbell, I. C., 1980b, Antidepressant drugs slow circadian rhythms in behavior and brain neurotransmitter receptors, *Psychopharmacol. Bull.* **16**:45–47.

Wirz-Justice, A., Tobler, I., Kafka, M. S., Naber, D., Marango, P. J., Borbely, A. A., and Wehr, T. A., 1981, Sleep deprivation: Effects on circadian rhythms of rat brain neurotransmitter receptors, *Psychiatry Res.* **5**:67–76.

Wise, C. D., Berger, B. D., and Stein, L., 1972, Benzodiazepines: Anxiety-reducing activity by reduction of serotonin turnover in the brain, *Science* **177**:180–183.

Wixon, H. N., and Hunt, W. A., 1980, Effect of acute and chronic ethanol treatment on gamma-aminobutyric acid levels and on aminoxyacetic acid-induced GABA accumulation, *Subst. Alcohol Actions Misuse* **1**:481–491.

Wolf, H., 1901, Trionalkur, *Centralblatt Nervenheilkune*, **2**:286–283.

Wolff, G., and Money, J., 1973, Relationship between sleep and growth in patients with reversible somatotropin deficiency (psychosocial dwarfism), *Psychol. Med.* **3**:18–27.

Wolin, S. J., and Mello, N. K., 1973, The effects of alcohol on dreams and hallucinations in alcohol addicts, *Ann. NY Acad. Sci.* **215**:266–302.

Woolf, P. D., Lantiqua, R., and Lee, L. A., 1979, Dopamine inhibition of stimulated growth hormone secretion: Evidence for dopaminergic modulation in insulin and L-dopa induced growth hormone secretion in man, *J. Clin. Endocrinol. Metab.* **49**:326–330.

Wurtman, R. J., and Cardinali, D. P., 1974, The pineal organs, in: *Textbook of Endocrinology* (R. H. Williams, ed.), W. B. Saunders, Philadelphia, pp. 832–840.

Wyatt, R. J., 1972, The serotonin–catecholamine dream bicycle: A clinical study, *Biol. Psychol.* **5**:33–63.

Wyatt, R. J., and Gillin, J. C., 1975, Development of tolerance to and dependence on endogenous neurotransmitters, in: *Neurobiological Mechanisms of Adaption and Behavior* (A. J. Mandell, ed.), pp. 47–59.

Wyatt, R. J., and Murphy, D. L., 1976, Low platelet monoamine oxidase activity and schizophrenia, *Schizophr. Bull.* **2**:77–89.

Wyatt, R. J., Chase, T. N., Scott, J., Snyder, F., and Engelman, K., 1970a, Effect of L-dopa on the sleep of man, *Nature* **228**:999–1001.

Wyatt, R. J., Engelman, K., Kupfer, D. J., Fram, D. H., Sjoerdsma,A., and Snyder, F., 1970b, Effects of L-tryptophan (a natural sedative) on human sleep, *Lancet* **2**:842–846.

Wyatt, R. J., Chase, T. N., Kupfer, D. J., Scott, J., Snyder, F., Sjoerdsma, A., and Engelman, K., 1971a, Brain catecholamine and human sleep, *Nature* **233**:63–65.

Wyatt, R. J., Fram, D. H., Buchbinder, R., and Snyder F., 1971b, Treatment of intractable narcolepsy with a monoamine oxidase inhibitor, *N. Engl. J. Med.* **285**:987–991.

Wyatt, R. J., Fram, D., Kupfer, D. J., and Snyder, F., 1971c, Total prolonged drug-induced REM sleep suppression in anxious-depressed patients, *Arch. Gen. Psychiatry* **24**:145–155.

Wyatt, R. J., Zarcone, V., Engelman, K., Dement, W. C., Snyder, F., and Sjoerdsma, A., 1971d, Effects of 5-hydroxytryptophan on the sleep of normal human subjects, *Electroencephalogr. Clin. Neurophysiol.* **30**:505–509.

Wyatt, R. J., Gillin, J. C., and Vaughan, T., 1972a, Adrenal corticol and neuro-transmitter activity during human sleep, *Proc. Fifth Int. Congr. Pharmacol.* **4**:134–144.

Wyatt, R. J., Vaughan, T., Galanter, M., Kaplan, J., and Green, R., 1972b, Behavioral changes of chronic schizophrenic patients given L-5-hydroxytryptophan, *Science* **177**;1124–1126.

Wyatt, R. J., Kaplan, J., and Vaughan, T., 1973, Tolerance and dependence to serotonin, *Arch. Gen. Psychiatry* **29**:597–599.

Wyatt, R. J., Neff, N. H., Vaughan, T., Franz, J., and Ommaya, A., 1974, Ventricular fluid 5-hydroxyindoleacetic acid concentrations during human sleep, *Adv. Biochem. Psychopharmacol.* **11**:193–197.

Wyler, A. R., Wilkus, R. J., and Troupin, A. S., 1975, Methysergide in the treatment of narcolepsy, *Arch. Neurol.* **32:**265–268.

Wynne, J. W., Block, A. J., Hemenway, J., Hunt, L. A., Shaw, D., and Flick, M. B., 1978a, Disordered breathing and oxygen desaturation during sleep in patients with chronic obstructive pulmonary disease, *Chest* **73:**301–303.

Wynne, J. W., Block, A. J., Hunt, L. A., and Flick, M. R., 1978b, Disordered breathing and oxygen desaturation during daytime naps, *John Hopkins Med. J.* **143:**3–7.

Yamaoka, S., 1980, Modification of circadian sleep rhythms by gonadal steroids and the neural mechanisms involved, *Brain Res.* **185:**385–398.

Yamashita, I., Moroji, T., Yamajaki, K., Kato, H., Sakahita, A., Onodera, I., and Ito, K., 1969, Neuroendocrinological studies in mental disorders and psychotropic drugs. Part I. On the circadian rhythm of the plasma adrenocortical hormone in mental patients and methamphetamine, *Folia Psychiatr. Neurol. Jpn.* **23:**143–158.

Yen, S. S. C., Tsai, C. S., Naftolin, F., Vandenberg, G., and Ajabor, L., 1972, Pulsatile patterns of gonadotropin release in subjects with and without ovarian function, *J. Clin. Endocrinol. Metab.* **34:**671–675.

Yoshimura, M., Ochi, Y., Miyazaki, T., Shiomi, K., and Hachiya, T., 1973, Effect of L-5-HTP on the release of growth hormone, TSH and insulin, *Endocrinol. Jpn.* **20:**135–141.

Yoss, E. R., and Daly, D. D., 1957, Criteria for the diagnosis of the narcoleptic syndrome, *Proc. Staff Meeting Mayo Clinic* **32:**320–328.

Yoss, R. E., and Daly, D. D., 1960a, Narcolepsy, *Med. Clin. North Am.* **44:**953–968.

Yoss, R. E., and Daly, D. D., 1960b, Narcolepsy, *Arch. Intern. Med.* **106:**168–171.

Yules, R. B., Freedman, D. X., and Chandler, K. A., 1966, The effect of ethyl alcohol on man's electroencephalographic sleep cycle, *Electroencephalogr. Clin. Neurophysiol.* **20:**109–111.

Yules, R. B., Lippman, M. E., and Freedman, D. X., 1967, Alcohol administration prior to sleep: The effect on EEG stages, *Arch. Gen. Psychiatry* **16:**94–97.

Zaccaria, M., Giordano, G., Ragazzo, E., Sicolo, N., Foresta, C., and Scandellari, C., 1985, Lack of effect of diazepam administration on hGH and hPRL secretion in normal and acromegalic subjects, *J. Endocrinol. Invest.* **8:**161–170.

Zammit, G., Rosenbaum, A., Stokes, P., Davis, J., Zorick, F., and Roth, T., 1986, The DST and sleep EEG in two types of depressed patients: Placebo responders and persistent depressives, *Sleep Res.* **15:**98.

Zarcone, V., 1973, Narcolepsy, *N. Engl. J. Med.* **288:**1156–1166.

Zarcone, V., and Hoddes, E., 1975, Effects of 5-hydroxytryptophan on fragmentation of REM sleep in alcoholics, *Am. J. Psychiatry* **132:**74–76.

Zarcone, V., Hollister, L., and Dement, W. C., 1970, The effect of L-dihydroxyphenylalanine (L-Dopa) on the sleep of two depressed patients, *Psychophysiology* **7:**314–315.

Zarcone, V., Kales, A., Scharf, M., Tan, T. L., Simmons, J. Q., and Dement, W. C., 1973, Repeated oral ingestion of 5-hydroxytryptophan: The effect on behavior and sleep processes in two schizophrenic children, *Arch. Gen. Psychiatry* **28:**843–846.

Zarcone, V., Hoddes, E., and Smythe, H., 1973, Oral 5-hydroxytryptophan effects on sleep, in: *Serotonin and Behavior* (J. Barchas and E. Usdin, eds.), Academic Press, New York, pp. 499–509.

Zarcone, V., Schrier, L., and Barchas, J., 1977, Alcohol, sleep and cerebrospinal fluid changes in alcoholics, *Adv. Exp. Med. Biol.* **85a:**593–500.

Zetler, G., 1980, Effects of cholecystokinin-like peptides on rearing activity and hexobarbital-induced sleep, *Eur. J. Pharmacol.* **66:**137–139.

Zorick, F., Roth, T., Kramer, M., and Flessa, H., 1977, Intensification of excessive daytime sleepiness by lymphoma, *Sleep Res.* **6:**199.

Zorick, F. J., Salis, P. J., Roth, T., and Kramer, M., 1979, Narcolepsy and automatic behavior: A case report, *J. Clin. Psychiatry* **40**:194–197.

Zorick, F., Roehrs, T., Koshorek, G., Sicklesteel, J., and Hartse, K., 1982, Patterns of sleepiness in various disorders of excessive daytime somnolence, *Sleep* **5S**:S165–174.

Zorick, F., Fujita, S., Conway, W., Sicklesteel, J., Roehrs, T., and Roth, T., 1984a, Uvulo-palato-pharyngoplasty: One year follow-up, *Sleep Res.* **13**:176.

Zorick, F., Kribbs, N., Roehrs, T., Roth, T., and 1984b, Polysomnographic and MMPI characteristics of patients with insomnia, *Psycopharmacology* **1**:2–10.

Zorick, F., Roehrs, T., Wittig, R., Lamphere, J., Sicklesteel, J., and Roth, T., 1986, Sleep–wake abnormalities in narcolepsy, *Sleep* **9**:189–193.

Zung, W. W. K., 1969, Antidepressant drugs and sleep, *Exp. Med. Surg.* **27**:124–137.

Index